UICC PROJECT ON EVALUATION OF SCREENING FOR CANCER

CANCER SCREENING

Edited by

A. B. MILLER
Professor, Department of Preventive Medicine
and Biostatistics, University of Toronto

J. CHAMBERLAIN
Director, DHSS Cancer Screening Evaluation Unit,
The Institute of Cancer Research, University of London

N. E. DAY
Professor, Department of Community Medicine,
University of Cambridge

M. HAKAMA
Professor, Department of Public Health,
University of Tampere, Finland

P. C. PROROK
Chief, Screening Section, Division of Cancer Prevention and Control,
National Cancer Institute, Bethesda, USA

A report of the workshop to update conclusions on screening for cancer of sites previously considered, and to evaluate some new sites, held at Selwyn College, Cambridge, UK, April 2–5 1990

Published on behalf of

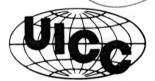

International Union Against Cancer

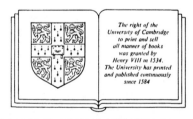

The right of the
University of Cambridge
to print and sell
all manner of books
was granted by
Henry VIII in 1534.
The University has printed
and published continuously
since 1584

CAMBRIDGE UNIVERSITY PRESS

Cambridge
New York • Port Chester • Melbourne • Sydney

CAMBRIDGE UNIVERSITY PRESS
Cambridge, New York, Melbourne, Madrid, Cape Town,
Singapore, São Paulo, Delhi, Tokyo, Mexico City

Cambridge University Press
The Edinburgh Building, Cambridge CB2 8RU, UK

Published in the United States of America by Cambridge University Press, New York

www.cambridge.org
Information on this title: www.cambridge.org/9780521116947

Published for the International Union Against Cancer
by Cambridge University Press 1991

First published 1991
First paperback edition 2011

A catalogue record for this publication is available from the British Library

ISBN 978-0-521-41041-0 Hardback
ISBN 978-0-521-11694-7 Paperback

Contents

Contents

SECTION 6   SCREENING FOR PROSTATE CANCER

State of the Art on Screening for Prostate Cancer

SECTION 7   SCREENING FOR NEUROBLASTOMA

State of the Art on Screening for Neuroblastoma

SECTION 8   SCREENING FOR STOMACH CANCER

State of the Art on Screening for Stomach Cancer

SECTION 9   SCREENING FOR NASOPHARYNGEAL CANCER

State of the Art on Screening for Nasopharyngeal Cancer

Contributors

C. Åhrén, M.D., Ph.D.
Department of Pathology, Sahlgrenska Hospital, Göteborg, Sweden

I. Andersson, M.D.
Department of Diagnostic Radiology, Lund University, Malmö General Hospital, Malmö, Sweden.

M. Asztély, M.D. Ph.D.
Department of Radiology, Sahlgrenska Hospital, Göteborg, Sweden.

C.J. Baines, M.D. M.Sc.
Department of Preventive Medicine and Biostatistics, University of Toronto, Toronto, Ontario, Canada.

S.G. Baker, Sc.D.
Screening Section, Biometry Branch, Division of Cancer Prevention and Control, National Cancer Institute, Bethesda Md, U.S.A.

R.C. Bast Jr, M.D.
Duke University Medical Center, Durham, Nc, U.S.A.

J.H.M. Blom, *M.D.*
Department of Urology, Erasmus University, Rotterdam, Dr Molewaterplein 40,
3015 GD Rotterdam, The Netherlands

J.H. Bond, M.D.
Department of Medicine, School of Medicine, University of Minnesota, Minneapolis Mn, U.S.A.

G. M. Bradley, M.D.
Department of Laboratory Medicine and Pathology, School of Medicine,
University of Minnesota, Minneapolis Mn, U.S.A.

D.P. Byar, M.D.
Division of Cancer Prevention and Control, National Cancer Institute, Bethesda Md, U.S.A.

J. Chamberlain, M.B., F.R.C.P., F.F.P.H.M.
Cancer Screening Evaluation Unit, Section of Epidemiology, Institute of Cancer Research: Royal Cancer Hospital, Belmont, Sutton, Surrey, U.K.

T.R. Church, Ph.D.
Division of Environmental and Occupational Health, School of Public Health, University of Minnesota, Minneapolis Mn, U.S.A.

R.J. Connor, Dr. Eng.
Screening Section, Biometry Branch, Division of Cancer Prevention and Control, National Cancer Institute, Bethesda Md., U.S.A.

A.W. Craft, M.D., F.R.C.P.
Children's Cancer Unit, Department of Child Health, University of Newcastle upon Tyne, Newcastle upon Tyne, U.K.

H. Cuckle, B.A., M.Sc., D.Phil.
Department of Environmental and Preventive Medicine, The Medical College of St Bartholomew's Hospital, University of London, Charterhouse Square, London, U.K.

J. Cuzick, Ph.D.
Department of Mathematics, Statistics and Epidemiology, Imperial Cancer Research Fund, Lincoln's Inn Fields, London, U.K.

G. Dale, B.Sc., M.D.
Departments of Child Health and Clinical Biochemistry, University of Newcastle upon Tyne, Newcastle upon Tyne, U.K.

A.P. Davies, M.R.C.O.G.
Gynaecological Oncology Unit, Department of Obstetrics and Gynaecology, The Royal London Hospital, Whitechapel, London, U.K.

N.E. Day, B.A., Ph.D.
Department of Community Medicine, University of Cambridge Medical School, Cambridge, U.K.

V.R. Doherty, M.B.
Department of Dermatology, Western Infirmary, Glasgow, Scotland

S.W. Duffy, B.Sc., MSc.
MRC Biostatistics Unit, Cambridge, U.K.

F. Ederer, F.A.C.E.
The Emmes Corporation, Washington D.C., U.S.A.

G. Eklund, Ph.D.
Epidemiological Unit, Karolinska Institute and Hospital, Stockholm, Sweden.

N. Einhorn, M.D., Ph.D.
Gynecological Oncology Department, Radiumhemmet, Karolinska Hospital, Stockholm, Sweden.

R. Ellman,
Cancer Screening Evaluation Unit, Section of Epidemiology, Institute of Cancer Research: Royal Cancer Hospital, Belmont, Sutton, Surrey, U.K.

J.M. Elwood, M.D.
Cancer Epidemiology Unit, Department of Preventive and Social Medicine, University of Otago, Dunedin, New Zealand.

B. Engarås, M.D.
Department of Surgery, Sahlgrenska Hospital, Göteborg, Sweden.

G.C.J. Fagerberg, M.D.
Department of Radiology, Medical University of Linköping, Linköping, Sweden.

C. Fenger
Department of Surgical Gastroenterology and Pathology, Odense University Hospital
and Institute of Social Medicine, Aarhus University, Odense C., Denmark.

A. Fukao
Department of Public Health, Tohoku University School of Medicine, Seiryomachi,
Sendai, Japan.

A.C. Geller, M.P.H.
Department of Dermatology, Boston University School of Medicine, Boston, Ma, U.S.A.

J.D.F. Habbema, Ph.D.
Department of Public Health and Social Medicine, Erasmus University, Rotterdam, The
Netherlands.

E. Haglind, M.D., Ph.D.
Department of Surgery, Sahlgrenska Hospital, Göteborg, Sweden.

M. Hakama, Sc.D.
Department of Public Health, University of Tampere, Tampere, Finland.

P. Hall, M.D., Ph.D.
WellCare MediHall AB, Stockholm, Sweden

J.D. Hardcastle, M.A., M.Chir., F.R.C.P., F.R.C.S.
Department of Surgery, University of Nottingham, Nottingham, U.K.

S. Hisamichi, M.D.
Department of Public Health, Tohoku University School of Medicine, Seiryomachi,
Sendai, Japan

B.M. van Ineveld, M.Sc.
Department of Public Health and Social Medicine, Erasmus University, Rotterdam, The
Netherlands.

I. Jacobs, M.B., B.S.
Gynaecological Oncology Unit, Department of Obstetrics and Gynaecology, The Royal
London Hospital, Whitechapel, London, U.K.

L. Janzon, M.D.
Department of Community Health Sciences, Lund University, Malmö General Hospital,
Malmö, Sweden

H. Kawakatsu, M.D.
Department of Pediatrics, Kyoto Prefectural University of Medicine, Kawaramachi,
Kamikyoku, Kyoto, Japan.

J. Kewinter, M.D., Ph.D.
Department of Surgery, Sahlgrenska Hospital, Gothenburg, Sweden

R.C. Knapp, M.D.
Harvard Medical School, Boston, Ma, U.S.A.

J. Knight, M.Sc.
Department of Preventive Medicine and Biostatistics, University of Toronto, Toronto, Ontario, Canada.

H.K. Koh, M.D.
Boston University Schools of Medicine and Public Health, Boston, Ma, U.S.A.

S. Komatsu
Department of Public Health, Tohoku University School of Medicine, Seiryomachi, Sendai, Japan

H.J. de Koning, M.D.
Department of Public Health and Social Medicine, Erasmus University, Rotterdam, The Netherlands.

V. Koroltchouk, M.D.
Cancer and Palliative Care Unit, World Health Organization, Geneva.

O. Kronborg, M.D.
Department of Surgical Gastroenterology, Odense University Hospital, Odense C., Denmark.

R.A. Lew, Ph.D.
University of Massachusetts Medical Center, Worcester, Ma, U.S.A.

K. Magnus, Ph.D.
The Cancer Registry of Norway, Montebello, Oslo, Norway.

J.S. Mandel, Ph.D., M.P.H.
Division of Environmental and Occupational Health, School of Public Health, University of Minnesota, Minneapolis Mn., U.S.A.

Y. Matsuda, M.D.
Department of Pediatrics, Kyoto Prefectural University of Medicine, Kawaramachi, Kamikyoku, Kyoto, Japan.

T. Matsumura, M.D.
Department of Pediatrics, Kyoto Prefectural University of Medicine, Kawaramachi, Kamikyoku, Kyoto, Japan.

A.B. Miller, M.B., F.R.C.P.
Department of Preventive Medicine and Biostatistics, University of Toronto, Toronto, Ontario, Canada.

D.R. Miller, Sc.D.
University of Massachusetts Medical Center, Worcester, Ma, U.S.A.

S. Moss, Ph.D.
Cancer Screening Evaluation Unit, Section of Epidemiology, Institute of Cancer Research: Royal Cancer Hospital, Belmont, Sutton, Surrey, U.K.

S. Narod, M.D.
Department of Preventive Medicine and Biostatistics, University of Toronto, Toronto, Ontario, Canada.

M. Nishikouri
Department of Health and Environment, Miyagi Prefectural Office, Sendai, Japan.

J. Olsen
Department of Surgical Gastroenterology and Pathology, Odense University Hospital
and Institute of Social Medicine, Aarhus University, Odense C., Denmark.

D. Oram, F.R.C.O.G.
Gynaecological Oncology Unit, Department of Obstetrics and Gynaecology, The Royal
London Hospital, Whitechapel, London, U.K.

L. Parker, Ph.D.
Lecturer in Epidemiology, Children's Cancer Unit, Department of Child Health,
University of Newcastle upon Tyne, Newcastle upon Tyne, U.K.

D.M. Parkin, M.D.
Unit of Descriptive Epidemiology, International Agency for Research on Cancer, Lyon
Cédex, France.

F. Pettersson, M.D.
Department of Gynecology, Karolinska Hospital, Stockholm, Sweden.

P.C. Prorok, Ph.D.
Biometry Branch, Division of Cancer Prevention and Control, National Cancer Institute,
Bethesda Md., U.S.A.

A.J. Sasco, M.D., Dr P.H.
Unit of Analytical Epidemiology, International Agency for Research on Cancer, Lyon
Cédex, France.

T. Sawada, M.D.
Department of Pediatrics, Kyoto Prefectural University of Medicine, Kawaramachi,
Kamikyoku, Kyoto, Japan.

D.A. Schoenfeld, Ph.D.
Biostatistics Department, Harvard Medical School, Boston, Ma, U.S.A.

L.M. Schuman, M.D.
Division of Epidemiology, School of Public Health, University of Minnesota,
Minneapolis Mn, U.S.A.

K. Sjövall, M.D., Ph.D.
Department of Gynecology, Karolinska Hospital, Stockholm, Sweden.

C.R. Smart, M.D.
Early Detection Branch, Division of Cancer Prevention and Control, National Cancer
Institute, Bethesda Md., U.S.A.

D.C. Snover, M.D.
Department of Laboratory Medicine and Pathology, School of Medicine, University of
Minnesota, Minneapolis Mn, U.S.A.

M.C. South, B.A., MSc.
Department of Chemical and Process Engineering, University of Newcastle upon Tyne,
Newcastle upon Tyne, U.K.

H.H. Storm, M.D.
Section of Cancer Registration, The Danish Cancer Registry, Danish Cancer Society,
Copenhagen, Denmark.

N. Sugawara
Cancer Detection Centre, Miyagi Cancer Society, Kamisugi, Sendai, Japan

J. Svanvik, M.D., Ph.D.
Department of Surgery, Sahlgrenska Hospital, Göteborg, Sweden

L. Tabár, M.D.
Department of Mammography, Central Hospital, Falun, Sweden.

A. Takano
Miyagi Prefectural Cancer Registry, Miyagi Cancer Society, Kamisugi 6-chome, Sendai,
Japan.

W.M. Thomas, M.B., B.Ch., F.R.C.S.
Department of Surgery, University of Nottingham, Nottingham, U.K.

T. To, Ph.D.
Department of Preventive Medicine and Biostatistics, University of Toronto, Toronto,
Ontario, Canada.

Y. Tsubono
Department of Public Health, Tohoku University School of Medicine, Seiryomachi,
Sendai, Japan.

I. Tsuji
Department of Public Health, Tohoku University School of Medicine, Seiryomachi,
Sendai, Japan.

H. Tulinius, M.D.
Director Icelandic Cancer Registry, Reykjavik, Iceland.

J. Wahrendorf, Ph.D.
Institute of Epidemiology and Biometry, German Cancer Research Center, Heidelberg,
Federal Republic of Germany.

N. Wald, M.B., B.S., D.Sc., F.R.C.P., F.F.C.M.
Department of Environmental and Preventive Medicine, The Medical College of
St Bartholomew's Hospital, University of London, Charterhouse Square, London, U.K.

C. Wall, M.Sc.
Department of Preventive Medicine and Biostatistics, University of Toronto, Toronto,
Ontario, Canada.

S.E. Williams, M.S.
Department of Surgery, School of Medicine, University of Minnesota, Minneapolis Mn,
U.S.A.

V.R. Zurawski Jr, Ph.D.
Centecor, Malvern Pa, U.S.A.

Preface

This is the fifth monograph arising from the meetings of the UICC Project on Evaluation of Screening for Cancer since the Project was initiated in its present form in 1982. The Project has been organized by the same core committee (the editors of the present monograph) throughout, and operates as part of the Programme on Detection and Diagnosis of the International Union Against Cancer (UICC). The first monograph arose from a workshop held in Venice, Italy, and considered General Principles on the Evaluation of Screening for Cancer and Screening for Lung, Bladder and Oral Cancer and was published as UICC Technical Report number 78 in 1984. The second monograph arose from a workshop held in Lyon, France, and considered Screening for Cancer of the Cervix, Endometrium and Ovary and was published as part of the IARC Scientific Publications number 76 on Screening for Cancer of the Cervix in 1986. The third monograph arose from a workshop held in Göteborg, Sweden, on Screening for Gastrointestinal Cancer and the fourth from a workshop held in Helsinki, Finland, on Screening for Breast Cancer, both being published by Hans Huber, Toronto, in 1988.

The present monograph is based on a workshop held at Selwyn College, Cambridge, U.K., with the support of the Cancer Research Campaign, the Imperial Cancer Research Fund and the UICC on 2–5 April, 1990. The workshop was held to update our conclusions on screening for most of the cancer sites that we had previously considered, and to evaluate screening for a number of new sites, as well as to consider again various methodological issues in this field. We elected not to reconsider screening for lung, bladder, oral, endometrial and liver cancer in light of the lack of new knowledge since we previously considered these sites. Instead we included in our deliberations for the first time screening for malignant melanoma, prostate cancer, neuroblastoma and nasopharyngeal cancer. A summary report on the meeting and its main conclusions has been published (Miller et al., *Int J Cancer* 46:761-769, 1990).

As in the previous monographs arising from this Project, the present monograph consists of a 'State of the Art' message for each site, including recommendations for research and our conclusion on the applicability of screening for the relevant site in public health terms, the papers presented at the workshop and a summary of the discussions on screening for the site. We believe the monograph will be useful to those interested in screening for cancer, including government and non-government organizations concerned with cancer control, cancer researchers, and members of National Cancer Societies and of international organisations concerned with cancer.

The monograph was produced in camera-ready form on a MacIntosh system at the University of Toronto. We wish to express our grateful thanks to Gail Bryant for her expertise and the many hours she put into the work.

The Editors

State of the Art on Breast Cancer Screening

Screening for breast cancer by mammography every 1 to 3 years can reduce breast cancer mortality substantially in women age 50-70. In women under age 50 there is little evidence for a benefit, at least in the first 10 years after screening is initiated. The cost-effectiveness of screening every 2-3 years by mammography for women age 50-70 compares well with many other medical procedures.

The time taken for a reduction in breast cancer mortality to appear will depend on the initial quality of the screening modalities used. The level of effect in the target population will be strongly dependent on the degree of compliance and on the quality of the mammography. The effect on mortality will be reduced if the screening sensitivity is inadequate.

Physical examination, for women over 50, has lower sensitivity than mammography, and in some studies was inferior to mammography in specificity and predictive value. In programmes with high quality mammography physical examination may not be a cost-effective adjunct to mammography as a screening procedure.

The introduction of mass screening into a population should be planned in a way such that the initial and long-term outcome measures can be evaluated.

Non-randomised studies of the effectiveness of breast screening in which screened women are compared with women who refused screening will give an incorrect estimate of the effect of screening in the population if the non-compliers are at substantially different underlying risk from the rest of the population. The results of studies in which this source of bias is not specifically examined need to be treated with extra caution. Study designs which specify women who attended, who refused and who had no opportunity to be screened may reduce this problem.

Recommendations for Research
The relative benefit of different screening intervals, and their cost-effectiveness.
Measures to guarantee high compliance with invitations to screening.
The effectiveness of physical examination alone, when mammography is inappropriate or unavailable for all.
The effectiveness of breast self-examination both alone and as an adjunct to other screening tests for breast cancer.

1 Sensitivity and specifity of screening in the UK Trial of Early Detection of Breast Cancer

UK TRIAL OF EARLY DETECTION OF BREAST CANCER GROUP *

* J Chamberlain, D Coleman, R Ellman, S Moss, +
B Thomas, J Price, PS Boulter, N Gibbs (Guildford)
APM Forrest, FE Alexander, TJ Anderson, AE Kirkpatrick, A Hill (Edinburgh)
M Vessey (Oxford), M Summerly (Stoke), P Bradfield (Southmead), P Preece (Dundee)

+ Cancer Screening Evaluation Unit, Institute of Cancer Research Section of Epidemiology, Sutton, Surrey , U.K.

1 INTRODUCTION

The UK Trial of Early Detection of Breast Cancer (TEDBC) is a comparison between geographically separate District Health Authorities offering different services to their female population between the ages of 45 and 64. Two districts, Edinburgh and Guildford, invited every woman in this age range to be screened every year for seven years. Two further districts, Huddersfield and Nottingham, invited every woman in the age range to a class teaching breast self-examination (BSE) and provided them with a self-referral breast clinic. The remaining four districts (Dundee, Oxford, Southmead and Stoke) served as a control group for comparison. The entire study population (240,000 women) is being followed up so that breast cancer incidence and mortality comparisons can be made over several years. Details of the method (UK TEDBC, 1981) and first analysis of breast cancer mortality (UK TEDBC, 1988) have been published. The latter found an apparent 20% reduction in mortality in the screened populations compared with the controls after 6-7 years but this was not statistically significant; there was no difference in mortality between the BSE districts and the controls.

This paper concentrates on the sensitivity and specificity of screening in the two screening districts. Except where otherwise indicated the results presented here are limited to "well women" who came to be screened in response to invitation. A small number of symptomatic women who were referred to the screening clinic either by their general practitioners or by themselves are excluded. Biopsy rates in the whole population of screening districts and control districts are also compared.

The screening procedure employed was a combination of physical examination and mammography. Physical examination was used every year and mammography in the first, third, fifth and seventh rounds; the mammographic technique was a single mediolateral oblique view of each breast, although in Edinburgh in the first round a cephalo-caudal view was also taken.

2 SENSITIVITY
Three different measures of sensitivity are presented.

2.1 Relative Sensitivity of Mammography and Physical Examination
The simplest shows the relative sensitivities of mammography and physical examination when used in combination, taking all screen-detected cancers as the denominator. Results are presented separately for the first (prevalence) screen, and for the subsequent (incidence) screens when mammography and physical examination were used, in rounds 3, 5 and 7.

Table 1   Relative sensitivities of mammography & physical examination at the prevalence screen (Edinburgh & Guildford combined)

Mammography Opinion	Physical Opinion			
	Normal/ diffuse	Localised Benign	Suspicious	Total
Normal/dyplasia	2	5	3	10
Localized benign	10	6	2	18
Suspicious	39	24	90	153
Total	51	35	95	181

$$\text{Relative sensitivity of mammography} = \frac{18 + 153}{181} = 94.5\%$$

$$\text{Relative sensitivity of physical} = \frac{35 + 95}{181} = 71.8\%$$

One hundred and eighty-one cancers were detected at the prevalence screen, 91 in Edinburgh and 90 in Guildford. Table 1 shows that, taking the cut-off point between normal and abnormal as a verdict of localized benign or suspicious, 171 of the 181 cancers (94.5%) were detected by mammography and 130 (71.8%) by physical examination. Taking each centre separately the sensitivities were very similar; 95.6% for mammography in Edinburgh (which used two views for this screen) and 93.3% in Guildford. The sensitivity of physical examination was 71.4% in Edinburgh and 72.2% in Guildford.

Table 2 Relative sensitivities of mammography & physical examination
at the incidence screens (Edinburgh & Guildford combined)

Mammography Opinion	Physical Opinion			
	Normal/ diffuse	Localised Benign	Suspicious	Total
Normal/dyplasia	9	14	3	26
Localized benign	35	11	6	52
Suspicious	101	25	59	185
Total	145	50	68	263

Relative sensitivity of mammography $= \dfrac{52 + 185}{263} = 90.1\%$

Relative sensitivity of physical $= \dfrac{50 + 68}{263} = 44.9\%$

Table 2 shows comparable findings for the 263 cancers which were detected in screening rounds 3, 5 and 7. Two hundred and thirty-seven (90.1%) were positive on mammography, but only 118 (44.9%) on physical examination. Within Edinburgh, 100 out of 110 cancers were detected by mammography (90.9%), and in Guildford 137 out of 153 cancers (89.5%). For physical examination 52 out of 110 (47.3%) were positive in Edinburgh and 66 out of 153 (43.1%) in Guildford.

2.2 Sensitivity Classing Interval Cancers in 12 Months after Screening as False Negatives

The second, traditional, method takes account of interval cancers presenting with symptoms during the one year period before the next screen was due, and assumes that these were false negatives to the previous screen. Sensitivity is defined as the proportion of screen-detected cancers out of the sum of screen-detected and interval cancers. Results are presented separately for the first screen, for subsequent screens when mammography was used (rounds 3, 5 and 7), and for physical only screens (rounds 2, 4 and 6). This method credits screening with the detection of cancers which might not otherwise have surfaced for many years, (if at all).

Taking Edinburgh and Guildford together, 14 interval cancers presented in the 12 months following the prevalence screen, at which 181 cancers had been detected. The sensitivity of the first screen is therefore 181/181 + 14, i.e. 92.8%. For the subsequent screens in rounds 3, 5 and 7 when mammography was used with physical examination, 25 interval cancers presented within 12 months, and 263 were detected at screening, giving a sensitivity of 91.3%.

In rounds 2, 4 and 6 when physical examination was used on its own (after a combined mammographic and physical screen the previous year) 41 interval cancers presented in the 12 months following screening at which 76 cancers had been detected, giving a sensitivity of 65%. Table 3 shows all these results separately for Edinburgh and Guildford.

Table 3   Interval cancers presenting within 12 months of different screening rounds

	Edinburgh	Guildford	Total
Cancers detected at first screen	91	90	181
Interval cancers within 12 months	8	6	14
Sensitivity	91.9%	93.8%	92.8%
Cancers detected in Rounds 3,5 and 7	110	153	236
Interval cancers within 12 months	8	17	25
Sensitivity	93.2%	90.0%	91.3%
Cancers detected by physical examination in Rounds 2,4 and 6	37	39	76
Interval cancers within 12 months	21	20	41
Sensitivity	64.0%	66.0%	65.0%

2.3 Sensitivity for Detecting Cancers Expected in 1-year & 2-year Intervals after Screening

The third method (Tabar et al, 1987) is based on knowledge of the expected annual incidence of cancer in the absence of screening. Subtraction of observed interval cancers from the expected number gives the number of cancers in each year following the screen whose diagnosis was advanced by screening. This can then be expressed as a proportion of the expected incidence. Within the context of a randomized controlled trial the expected

Table 4   Proportion of cancers expected at intervals after screening whose diagnosis was advanced by screening

Interval after screen	Type of Screen		
	First mammography + clinical	Subsequent mammography + clinical	Clinical
0-11 months			
Woman-years	31690	68057	68628
Expected cancers (E)	56.1	120.8	121.9
Observed interval cancers (O)	15	26	41
% detected at screen (E-O)/E	73.3	78.5	66.4
12-23 months			
Woman-years	6654	6948	-
Expected cancers (E)	11.7	12.4	-
Observed interval cancers (O)	7	7	-
% detected at screen (E-O)/E	40.2	43.5	-

incidence can be taken as the incidence in the control group who have not been offered screening, after adjusting for any differences in incidence between acceptors and non-acceptors of screening in the study group. In this non-randomized trial the incidence of breast cancer in the combined comparison districts has been used as the expected incidence, after making appropriate adjustments for differences between acceptors and non-acceptors, and where relevant for differences in incidence in different age-groups. In calculating sensitivity by this method, symptomatic women from the screening population who were referred to the screening clinic before invitation are included; two interval cancers occurred among those women within 12 months of a negative screen.

From the incidence of breast cancer in the combined comparison districts (1.77 per 1000 woman-years), 56.1 cases would be expected in the year following the 1st screen, had these women not been screened. Fifteen interval cancers presented during this year. The sensitivity of the first screen is therefore 56.1 minus 15 divided by 56.4, i.e. 73.3% (Table 4). One fifth of these women did not attend for the physical only screen due after one year, and among them seven interval cancers arose 12 to 23 months after the first screen. The expected incidence (from the comparison centres) in these 6654 women is 11.7. Therefore in the second year after first screening sensitivity fell to 11.7 - 7/11.7, i.e. 43.5%. Table 4 also shows that following subsequent mammographic and physical screens in rounds 3, 5 and 7, the sensitivity for detecting cancers expected in the ensuing year was 78.5% and in the second year 43.5%. Data are only available for one year following a physical only screen in rounds 2,4 and 6, because the number of women who failed to attend one year later for a subsequent mammographic screen was too small to calculate sensitivity in this way. Physical examination advanced the date of diagnosis of 66.4% of cases expected in the ensuing 12 months.

An analysis has also been done of sensitivity among women of different ages. The women included in this trial were aged 45 to 64 at entry. When examined in five year age-groups there was no difference between sensitivity in those aged 45 to 49 and those aged 50 to 54 at entry. The data are therefore presented in two 10-year groups, 45 to 54 and 55 to 64. Table 5 shows the proportion of cancers whose diagnosis was advanced by screening in different age-groups. This table combines all screens in which mammography and physical examination were used (rounds 1, 3, 5 and 7), and also shows the sensitivity in different age-groups for physical examination alone in rounds 2, 4 and 6. In women aged 55 and over screening was 84% sensitive in the first year after mammographic screening, falling to 59% in the second year. Comparable sensitivities for younger women were 70% in the first year falling to only 24% in the second year following screening.

Table 5   Proportion of cancers expected whose diagnosis was advanced by screening according to age at entry and type of screen

	Type of Screen					
Interval after screen	Rounds 1,3,5 & 7 Age at entry			Rounds 2,4,6 Age at entry		
	45-54	55-64	All ages	45-64	55-64	All ages
0-11 months						
Woman-years	55112	44635	99747	37762	30886	68628
Expected cancers (E)	91.2	85.7	176.9	62.7	59.2	121.9
Observed interval cancers (O)	27	14	41	23	18	41
% detected at screen (E-O)/E	70.4	83.7	76.8	63.3	69.6	66.4
12-23 months						
Woman-years	7216	6386	13602	-	-	-
Expected cancers (E)	11.8	12.3	24.1			
Observed interval cancers (O)	9	5	14			
% detected at screen (E-O)/E	23.7	59.3	41.9			

Table 6 compares the findings following any mammographic screen for Edinburgh and Guildford.

Table 6 Proportion of cancers whose diagnosis was advanced by screening in rounds 1,3,5 &7 in Edinburgh and Guildford

Interval after screen	Screening Centre		Total
	Edinburgh	Guildford	
0-11 months			
Woman-years	46363	54091	10454
Expected cancers (E)	82.5	96.2	178.8
Observed interval cancers (O)	17	24	41
% detected at screen (E-O)/E	79	75	77
12-23 months			
Woman-years	5237	8448	13685
Expected cancers (E)	9.3	15.0	24.4
Observed interval cancers (O)	8	6	14
% detected at screen (E-O)/E	14	60	43

3 SPECIFICITY

Specificity is defined as the ability of screening correctly to classify women without cancer as negative. At each screen, including the subsquent interval before the next screen, women can be classified as cancer detected (true positives), interval cancer (false negatives), positive but cancer not diagnosed (false positives) or negative and cancer not diagnosed (true negatives). Specificity is measured as the proportion of true negative results out of all those in whom cancer is not diagnosed.

The procedure adopted in both Edinburgh and Guildford for investigating women with positive findings (i.e. suspicious of cancer or localised benign) was to recall the women for further mammographic views and clinical assessment, including cyst aspiration, ultrasound, and fine needle aspiration as appropriate. Following this assessment (which could continue for several visits to the clinic) the women were either referred for biopsy or returned to routine screening (a few being kept under continuing surveillance or refusing investigation).

Figures 1, 2 and 3 illustrate these outcomes of screening for the first mammographic and physical screen, for subsequent mammographic and physical screens, and for physical only screens.

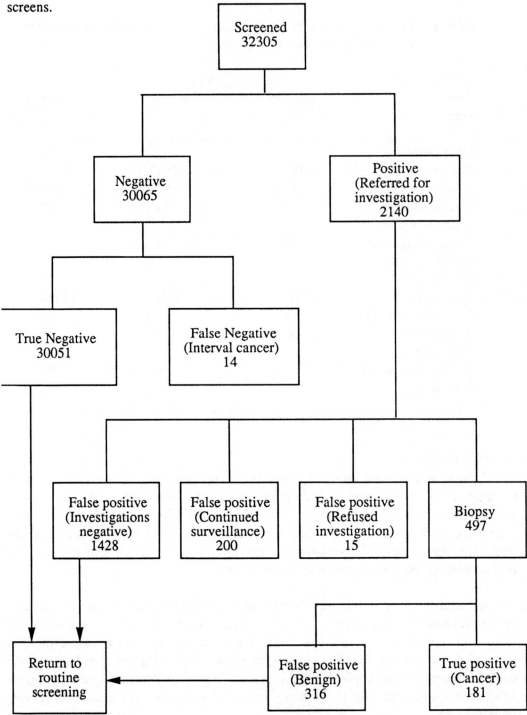

Figure 1. Outcome of routine screening in rounds 1 in Edinburgh and Guildford

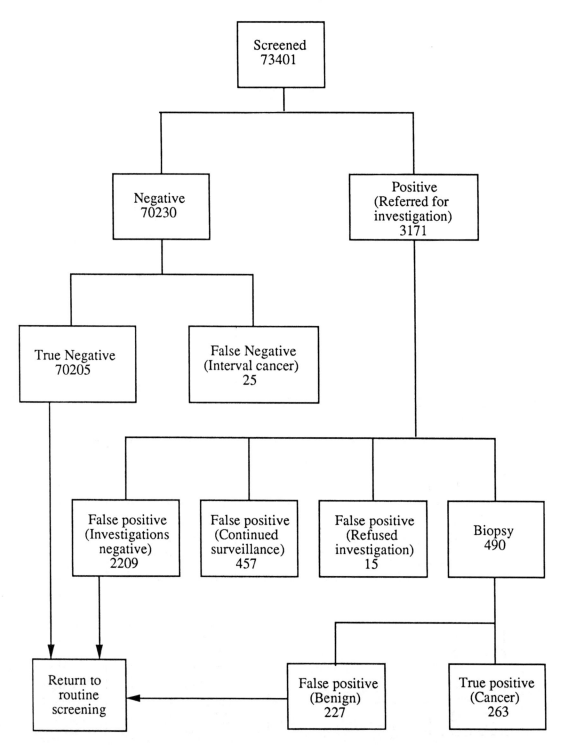

Figure 2. Outcome of routine screening in rounds 3,5 & 7 in Edinburgh and Guildford

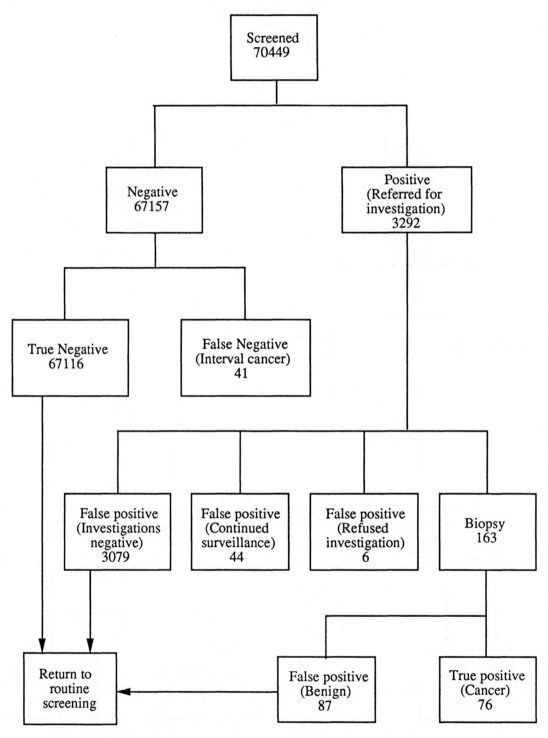

Figure 3. Outcome of routine screening by physical examination alone in rounds 2,4 & 6 in Edinburgh and Guildford

Table 7 Specificity and predictive value of routine screening in round 1

		Cancer Present	Cancer Absent	Total
		True +ve	False +ve	
Test Result	+ve	181	1,959	2,140
	-ve	False -ve	True -ve	
		14	30,051	30,065
Total		195	32,010	32,205

$$\text{Specificity} = \frac{30,051}{32,010} = 0.94$$

Predictive value of a
$$\text{referral for investigation} = \frac{181}{2,140} = 0.08$$

Table 8 Specificity and predictive value of routine screening in rounds 3, 5 and 7

		Cancer Present	Cancer Absent	Total
		True +ve	False +ve	
Test Result	+ve	263	2,908	3,171
	-ve	False -ve	True -ve	
		25	70,205	70,230
Total		288	73,113	73,401

$$\text{Specificity} = \frac{70,205}{73,113} = 0.96$$

Predictive value of a
$$\text{referral for investigation} = \frac{263}{3,171} = 0.08$$

From the figures it is possible to illustrate the division of screening findings into true and false positives, and true and false negatives. Tables 7, 8 and 9 show these, giving the specificity and predictive value of a positive screening result.

Table 9   Specificity and predictive value of routine screening by physical examination alone in rounds 2,4 & 6

		Cancer Present	Cancer Absent	Total
		True +ve	False +ve	
Test Result	+ve	76	3,216	3,292
	-ve	False -ve	True -ve	
		41	67,116	67,157
Total		117	70,332	70,449

$$\text{Specificity} = \frac{67,116}{70,332} = 0.95$$

$$\text{Predictive value of a referral for investigation} = \frac{76}{3,292} = 0.02$$

Specificity at the prevalence screen was 94% (i.e. 6% of women without cancer were recalled for further investigation). In subsequent rounds it improved slightly increasing to 95% at physical only rounds, and 96% at subsequent mammographic rounds. In each round, Edinburgh had higher specificity than Guildford as shown in Table 10.

Table 10   Specificity and predictive value of screening in different rounds in Edinburgh and Guildford

	Specificity		Positive Predictive Value	
	Edinburgh	Guildford	Edinburgh	Guildford
Round 1	96%	92%	14.8%	5.9%
Rounds 2, 4, 6	97%	94%	4.1%	1.6%
Rounds 3, 5, 7	97%	95%	10.2%	7.3%

The predictive value of a positive screening result - i.e. the probability that a woman referred for further investigation will have cancer was 8% for mammographic screening rounds but only 2% for physical only rounds, with Edinburgh again having higher values than Guildford.

Some workers regard the initial investigations of women with positive screening results as part of the screening process itself ("2nd stage screening") in which case only referrals for biopsy would be regarded as positives. If this definition is used, specificity of the first screen increases to 0.987, of further mammographic and physical rounds to 0.996 and of physical only rounds to 0.999. The predictive value of a biopsy referral is 36% in the first round, 54% in subsequent mammographic and physical rounds, and 47% in physical only rounds. There was less difference between Edinburgh and Guildford in biopsy referrals than in all referrals for investigation, with Guildford having higher predictive values than Edinburgh except for Round 1.

4 BIOPSY RATES

Concern is frequently expressed about the extra workload of surgery and histopathology which is generated by screening. In this trial, data about all breast biopsies were collected from histopathology laboratories in the four comparison districts where no screening was provided, as well as from the screening districts themselves. Details of cytopathology were not collected because it was very seldom used in 1979/80 when this study was started. It is possible to compare the breast biopsy rate, subdivided into benign and malignant, between

Table 11 Biopsy rates per 1,000 women in successive years of the trial

	Years	1	2	3	4	5	6	7
Comparison	Total	2.60	2.64	2.72	2.84	2.71	2.67	2.31
Centres	Benign	1.03	1.13	1.00	0.94	0.84	0.79	0.78
	Malignant	1.57	1.51	1.72	1.90	1.87	1.88	1.53
Edinburgh	Total	12.47	5.43	5.87	2.99	4.02	2.55	2.57
	Benign	7.99	2.78	3.29	1.16	1.58	1.14	0.92
	Malignant	4.48	2.65	2.58	1.83	2.44	1.41	1.65
Guildford	Total	11.18	3.64	5.53	2.59	3.55	2.49	4.24
	Benign	7.04	2.13	2.05	0.80	1.21	0.59	1.23
	Malignant	4.14	1.51	3.48	1.79	2.34	1.90	3.01

screening and comparison districts during the course of the trial. To ensure comparability with the comparison districts, data from the screening districts include biopsies performed in non-attenders, and in women with previous negative screening results, as well as those in women referred from screening. Table 11 shows the biopsy rates per 1000 women in successive years of the trial. It can be seen that there is a 4 to 5-fold increase in biopsies in screening districts in the first year after entry, when two thirds of the population had a first mammographic and physical screen. In subsequent years when women were offered mammographic and physical screens, the biopsy rate was still raised, at about twice the rate in the comparison districts (except for the final year in Edinburgh). In the second year, when physical screening alone was offered, the biopsy rate was above that in the comparison districts but in subsequent physical only years it was marginally lower than that in the comparison districts.

5   DISCUSSION

The sensitivity of screening in the UK TEDBC gives comparable figures to many previous series regarding the relative sensitivities of mammography and physical examination, and the overall sensitivity using the traditional method of including all screen-detected cancers in the numerator. Using the proportional incidence method, which gives a more realistic indicator of the impact of screening, at least in the short term, the sensitivity in this trial is similar to that in the Swedish Two- Counties trial (Tabar et al, 1987) for the first 12 months after screening, but falls off more markedly in the second 12 month period. Moreover, whereas in the Swedish trial the age cut-off point between higher and lower sensitivity was age 50, in this trial women aged 50 to 54 had an almost identical experience to those aged 45 to 49 and it was only after age 55 that sensitivity improved. Whatever method of calculating sensitivity is used, screening by physical examination performs less well than screening which includes mammography, suggesting that the potential for reducing mortality by physical screening alone is less.

The probability of an unaffected woman being referred for further investigation of a screen-detected abnormality is one of the unwanted side-effects of screening. In this trial, the specificity calculations show that 3 to 8% of women fell into this category, with the proportion being higher at the prevalence screen than at subsequent screens and higher in Guildford than in Edinburgh. The main concern about these false positive referrals is that they cause the women great anxiety, although one study in Guildford (Ellman et al, 1989) found that the level of psychological morbidity among women referred for investigation from screening was less than that in symptomatic women and was transient. The system of multidisciplinary assessment of referred women in this trial has almost certainly contributed to the low benign biopsy rate, with only 1% of unaffected women referred for biopsy following the prevalent screening and 0.5% or less at subsequent screens. However the effect which the screening programme has on the total number of biopsies in the population (including those in which cancer is diagnosed) is very considerable in the years during which screening is first introduced, and remains about double the expected rate in rounds when mammographic screening is repeated.

REFERENCES

Ellman R, Angeli N, Christians A et al. Psychiatric morbidity associated with screening for breast cancer. Br J Cancer 1989; 60:781-84.

Tabar L, Fagerberg G, Day NE et al. What is the optimum interval between mammographic screening examinations? Br J Cancer 1987; 55:547-51.

UK Trial of Early Detection of Breast Cancer Group. Trial of early detection of breast cancer: a description of method. Br J Cancer 1981; 44:618-27.

UK Trial of Early Detection of Breast Cancer Group. First results on mortality reduction in the UK Trial of Early Detection of Breast Cancer. Lancet 1988; ii:411-16.

2 Screening for Breast Cancer in Finland

M. HAKAMA

University of Tampere, Tampere, and Finnish Cancer Registry, Helsinki, Finland

1 INTRODUCTION

A screening programme can be spontaneously implemented or implemented through active planning resulting in an organized programme. Spontaneous programmes have so far shown smaller effects than organized ones. Opportunistic screening has no means to prevent unnecessary frequent screening causing high marginal cost.

Spontaneous screening for breast cancer is likely to pay most attention to high sensitivity without accepting the responsibility to avoid low specificity which is a consequence of the high sensitivity. For a high technology screening programme, such as mammography for breast cancer, low specificity results in high cost and prevalent adverse effects. Furthermore, in countries with limited resources for work-up of the screen positive cases, there is the danger of saturating the surgical services and preventing other competing activities. Therefore, screening for breast cancer must have high specificity.

The other reason which makes active planning important relates to the needs for evaluation. There are a number of examples of spontaneously adopted health service activities. Many problems were faced, when the evaluation of the effect of such activities was attempted. It was often practically and sometimes ethically impossible to estimate the magnitude of the effect. When such an attempt was made, many biases prevented reliable conclusions. Breast self examination is an example of a rather spontaneously adopted activity, reliable evaluation of which continues to pose considerable problems (WHO, 1984).

The need to evaluate any health service activity and the necessity to use the resources to maximize the effect and prevent saturation of services have led in Finland to an organized programme of mammographic screening (Hakama, 1988). The organized programme, a public health policy, was implemented as an experiment. Therefore evaluation of its effect can be undertaken rapidly, reliably, and without high expenditures. The objective of the evaluation is to contrast the effectiveness of the organized programme to normal clinical practice supplemented by spontaneous screening.

2   DESIGN OF THE PROGRAMME

In Finland the health services are organized by local municipalities or conglomerations of them comprising a central hospital district. The National Board of Health is responsible for general quidelines and expert advice. After acceptance by the National Board of Health any activity is subsidized by the central government. In 1986 the National Board of Health gave final advice on organizing screening for breast cancer. Because this guaranteed the state subsidizing the municipalities for the expenses, the screening activities organized by the municipal health services rapidly expanded.

The Finnish population is 5 million. There are about 450 municipalities ranging from 0.5 million inhabitants (Helsinki) to a few hundred in remote areas. The central hospital districts number 21.

The bases of most of the present organized mass screening programmes are formal agreements between individual municipalities and the Cancer Society of Finland. Women to be screened are identified from the national population registry. The Cancer Society of Finland provides letters of invitation to those asked to attend as well as notification forms. The cancer organizations provide expertise to interpret the mammograms. Traditionally there is a close contact between the local Cancer Society detection clinic and the central hospital ensuring immediate referrals of positive cases. The notification cards are centrally filed at the Finnish Cancer Society financed Cancer Registry. The Finnish Cancer Registry is also responsible for automatic data processing for feedback of the mass screening information to the mass screening registry on magnetic tapes. The mass screening registry also contains information derived from the national population registry and nationwide cancer registry thus ensuing inferences on nonattendance, interval cancer and mortality from breast cancer and other causes.

The National Board of Health recommendation for the birth cohorts to be screened involves a random element. Women at the age of 50 and above will be screened every second year. The municipalities were recommended to start in 1987 by screening three birth cohorts which can be increased according to a systematic schedule. The cohorts with even years of birth were randomized to be screened first and only with the expansion of the programme also the odd year born cohorts will be included.

In 1987 254 out of the total of 460 municipalities joined the programme and about 57,000 women were invited to be screened. This implies that on average three cohorts were screened even if there were differences between the municipalities. Some of them did not screen at all, some had started before 1987 i.e. before the official recommendation, which modified the cohorts subjected to screening, and some did not strictly follow the recommendation for the number or age of the cohorts to be screened. About half of the women invited for screening belonged to the recommended cohorts (Table 1).

Table 1. Percentage distribution of women invited to attend the organized screening and relative risk to be invited (woman born 1928 have unit risk) in Finland in 1987 by birth cohort.

Year of birth	Per cent of invitations	Relative risk to be invited
1913-1927	8	0.03
1928	20	1.00
1929-1931	8	0.13
1932	13	0.65
1933-1935	10	0.16
1936	18	0.90
1937-1948	23	0.10
Total	100	

Large municipalities followed the recommendation to a lesser extent than small ones, therefore most of the municipalities agreed to screen the recommended cohorts born in 1928, 1932 and 1936. For example, Helsinki, the capital of Finland with 10 per cent of the total population, screened only those at 50 years of age i.e. the cohort born 1937. In 1988 the number of municipalities increased to 286 and cohorts born in 1930, 1934 and 1938 were recommended to be screened. Some municipalities preferred not to join the programme organized by the Cancer Society of Finland, and some form of organized screening covered practically the total country in 1989.

In the details there is and will be variation in implementing the design and all the municipalities will not follow the recommendations. However, the basic design will remain: The effectiveness of the screening programme will be monitored and evaluated with a comparable control population the size of which will decrease as the programmes expand by time.

The time span from start to full coverage is only 5 years. The power of the design depends on the extent it is followed by the municipalities and can not be accurately estimated. Postponement of the inclusion of new cohorts by some of the municipalities will improve the chances for adequate comparisons. Even if there were deviations from the basic design serious enough to prevent experimental evaluation, nonexperimental cohort or case-control designs are stil available. The women in the cohorts actually invited to be screened are identified, their screening history is known and they are monitored for deaths. The extra expenses in the organized programme devoted to evaluation only are marginal and probably much less than those required by any a posteriori attempts to arrive at reliable estimates of effectiveness.

3   IMPLEMENTING THE PROGRAMME

During the two first years of the organized programme, 1987 and 1988, the Cancer Society of Finland invited 126,000 women to be screened. Altogether 88.5 per cent attended and there were 5,000 screen positivies, 418 (0.37%) cancers were diagnosed (Table 2).

Table 2 Extent of the organized screening programme for breast cancer in Finland in 1987 and 1988

	Number	per cent
Number of invitations	126 255	100
Attenders	111 682	88.5
Screen positives	5 080	4.55
Positive cytology	998	0.89
Malignant	418	0.37

Breast cancer incidence at age 50 to 59 years was 156 per 100,000 in 1985—1986. Hence, the screen detected cancers equalled the numbers of clinically detected cases expected to surface during the average of a 2.4 year period.

4   DISCUSSION

The detection rate of 0.37% is less than that in the most of other screening programmes (Day and Miller, 1988). Part of the difference can be accounted for by the low risk of breast cancer in Finland (Hakulenin et al, 1986). However, even when related to the background risk the detection rate is rather low. The ratio of screening prevalence to annual incidence is about 3 years in other studies (Day and Miller,1988) which may indicate lack of sensitivity of the Finnish programme.

On the other hand it is possible that not all the cancers detected at screening would have surfaced clinically even if left untreated. An analysis by flow cytometry indicated that the malignant potential of the screen detected cases was low (Kallioniemi et al, 1988) and even less than the malignancy of clinically diagnosed five year survivors (Kallioniemi et al, 1989).

Because of high cost high specificity was emphasised when the screening programme was implemented. The proportion of screen positives (4.6%) is low for a public health policy. The results were analysed by central hospital district and the range of screen positives was from 2.3 to 6.0 per cent in the 14 areas with sufficient number of mammography (Hakama et al, 1990). This implies that there are means to improve the specificity. The sensitivity varied as well (ratio of prevalence to incidence from 1.6 to 5.0) without correlation to specificity. Therefore, it seems that specificity can be improved without loss in the yield.

Specificity is related also to experience and, in fact, the per cent of screen positives decreased from 5.1 to 4.0 in 1987—1988.

The Finnish experience from the two first years of organized screening for breast cancer as a public health policy shows that the programme was technically feasible, attendance rate was high, the experimental design was satisfactorily followed and the health authorities were rapidly informed of the results in terms of process indicators (Elovainio et al, 1987). Results on effectiveness cannot be provided but it is possible that such a public health policy is less sensitive than a specificly designed randomized preventive trial. There may also be some overdiagnosis, i.e. not all the histologically malignant cancer cases would have surfaced clinically even if left untreated. These aspects emphasize the importance of experience of both the radiologists and the pathologists involved.

It is also important to design any public health policy in such a way that its effectiveness, benefits and harms can be evaluated. The optimal method of evaluation is the randomised experiment. Finally, the Finnish experience shows that the experimental design can and should be applied not only in clinical and preventive medicine but also in health services for a public health policy.

REFERENCES
Day N, Miller AB (eds). Screening for Breast Cancer. Hans Huber, Toronto, 1988.
Elovainio L, Kajantie R, Louhivuori K,Hakama M. Syöpäjärjestöjen rintasyöpäseulonnat 1987. Duodecim 1989:105:1184-1190.
Hakama M. Design of the Finnish Breast Cancer Screening Study. In: Screening for Breast Cancer. Day NE, Miller AB, (eds). Toronto,Hans Huber, 1988; pp. 59-62.
Hakama M, Elovainio L, Kajantie R, Louhivuori K. Breast cancer screening as public health policy in Finland. Submitted 1990.
Hakulinen T, Andersen A, Malker B, Pukkala E, Schou G,Tulinius H. Trends in Cancer Incidence in the Nordic Countires. Acta Path. Microbiol. Immunol. Scand. Sect. A 1986:94:Suppl. 288:1-151.
Kallioniemi O-P, Kärkkäinen A, Auvinen O, Mattila J, Koivula T, Hakama M. DNA flow cytometric analysis indicates that many breast cancers detected in the first round of mammographic screening have a low malignant potential. Int. J. Cancer 1988:42:697-702.
Kallioniemi O-P, Kärkkäinen A, Mattila J, Auvinen O, Koivula T, Hakama M. Mammografiaseulonnassa todettavien rintasyöpien biologiset ominaisuudet — virtaussytometrinen tutkimus. Duodecim 1989:105:1532-1538.
WHO. Self-examination in the detection of breast cancer: Memorandum from a WHO meeting. Bull. Wld Hlth Org., 1984; 62:861-869.

3 The Swedish Two-County Trial of Mammographic Screening for Breast Cancer: Recent Results on Mortality and Tumour Characteristics

L. TABÁR [1], C. J. G. FAGERBERG [2], M. C. SOUTH [3], N. E. DAY [3] and S. W. DUFFY [3]

[1] Mammography Department, Central Hospital, Falun, Sweden.
[2] Department of Radiology, Medical University of Linköping, Linköping, Sweden.
[3] MRC Biostatistics Unit, Cambridge, U.K.

1 INTRODUCTION

The desire to control breast cancer has a long history. Despite continuing efforts to control the disease through a variety of therapeutic methods in different combinations, no substantial change in mortality has been demonstrated. This, together with a lack of knowledge about the etiology of breast cancer, has naturally intensified interest in detecting and treating it at an earlier stage; the hope is that by advancing the time of diagnosis, treatment will result in a more favourable outcome.

Breast cancer is a common malignancy, therefore the stimulus for continued investigations comes not only from within the medical profession, but from increased public awareness and demand. What happened in Sweden in the mid 1970s illustrates this well; the response of women to the spread of information about the results of both a study in the US (HIP) (Shapiro et al, 1971), and a Swedish pilot project in which modern screen film mammography was successfully tested (Lundgren and Jakobsson, 1976), led to pressure for the introduction of mass screening for breast cancer with mammography. However, there was a need for further trials to be conducted, with different designs and under different circumstances, in order to try to answer the many questions sorrounding this issue (Tabar and Dean, 1987). Therefore the Swedish National Board of Health and Welfare designed a randomised controlled trial which was accepted by two counties, Kopparberg (W) and Ostergotland (E). The major question to be answered was whether population based screening with single-view mammography could significantly reduce mortality from breast cancer.

The purpose of this article is to describe the results of the Swedish two-county (W-E) trial after an average of 10 years follow-up and to provide insights into the mechanism of early detection.

2 MATERIAL AND METHODS

Of the 134,867 women aged 40-74 living in the two counties at the time of randomization, 77,080 were randomized to the study group and 55,985 to the control group. Women with breast cancer diagnosed prior to randomization were not included in the study, giving a total trial population of 133,065. The number and age distribution of women invited to screening (active study population, ASP) and women not invited (control group or passive study population, PSP) are given in Table 1.

Table 1   Age Distribution of Women in the W-E Trial. Data are percentages of women in each age group.

Age at randomization	ASP			PSP		
	W	E	Total	W	E	Total
40-49	24.8	26.7	25.7	27.1	28.3	27.9
50-59	30.4	30.5	30.5	29.9	30.1	30.0
60-69	31.0	29.7	30.4	29.9	28.6	29.1
70-74	13.8	13.1	13.4	13.1	13.0	13.0
Total	100.0	100.0	100.0	100.0	100.0	100.0
Number of Women in trial	38589	38491	77080	18582	37403	55985

The slight differences in the age distribution are a result of cluster rather than individual randomization and necessitate adjustment for age when analysing the results. Subsequent references to age in the text imply age at randomization.

The explanation for the differing sizes of the ASP and PSP is that the small administrative units, municipalities and parishes, on which randomization was based, were allocated to the two groups in the ratio 1 : 1 in E-county and 2 : 1 in W-county. The procedure has been described in detail elsewhere (Tabar et al, 1988). It could be argued that some allowance for the cluster randomization procedure should be made during the mortality analysis, since it could lead to extra-Poisson variation. However, the result obtained by negative binomial analysis, which allows for the possibility of some variation between clusters, matches almost exactly that found using a standard Poisson regression analysis. This indicates that cluster randomization has not produced population imbalances affecting the result. However, a supplementary analysis which adjusts for pre-trial breast cancer mortality within clusters is planned. The required data is already available for Kopparberg and work is currently underway to collect similar data for Ostergotland, so that such an analysis can be carried out.

The identification of the women aged 40-74 and still resident in the counties was made through the Swedish population registry. Individual letters of invitation were sent out to women in the active study population. Those aged 70-74 at the time of randomization received invitations to two screening rounds only. The average interval between screens was about 24 months for women aged 40-49 and 33 months for those aged 50 and over.

The only screening modality used was single view screen-film mammography (the medio-lateral oblique projection) without physical examination (Fagerberg and Tabar, 1988; Tabar and Gad, 1981; Fagerberg et al, 1985).

Screening started in Kopparberg county in October 1977 and in Ostergotland in May 1978. Table 2 shows the women years of observation and years of follow-up in the two counties since the date of randomization and up to the end of 1989. The average length of follow-up since date of randomization in the W-E trial, both groups combined, is 9.9 years. In 1986, the year after the first publication of positive findings, screening started in the control group.

Table 2 Women years of observation and average years of follow-up in the two counties from date of randomization to December 31st 1989.

| | ASP | | PSP | |
County	Woman yrs observed	Average yrs follow-up	Woman yrs observed	Average yrs follow-up
Kopparberg	392,924	10.2	190,193	10.2
Ostergotland	373,551	9.7	365,048	9.8
Both Counties	766,475	9.9	555,241	9.9

The stage of carcinomas diagnosed in the W-E trial was determined according to the UICC p-TNM histopathologic classification (1978). Treatment of an individual case was based on this determination, and was independent of the woman's allocation to study or control group. The cause of death was defined according to written guide-lines strictly applied in all cases by a committee of surgeons, pathologists and radiologists. The guide-lines for classification of death have been published (Tabar et al, 1989).

Crude mortality analysis was carried out using Poisson log-linear regression using population size as the denominator. Further analysis, using person years at risk as the denominator, has also been carried out and the significance of factors potentially affecting mortality were assessed using the chi-squared (change in scaled deviance) statistic. Cox's proportional hazards regression has been used in the survival analysis among breast cancer cases (Cox, 1972).

3 RESULTS
The attendance rates for successive screening rounds in the W-E trial are shown in Table 3.

Table 3   Attendance rates for the W-E Trial.

Age at Entry	1st screen	2nd screen	3rd screen
40-49	93.2%	89.2%	88. 4%
50-59	91.8%	87.7%	86.2%
60-69	87.9%	80.9%	77.8%
70-74	78.7%	66.8%	–

Details of further assessment procedures required by those who attended screening appear elsewhere (Tabar et al, 1988). Out of cases referred to surgical biopsy, 50% at the first screening round and 75% at the second round proved to be cancers at histopathological examination.

Table 4 shows the number of women with breast cancer detected during the trial, according to age and study group. Those women who had bilateral breast cancer have only been included once, the more advanced tumour being considered.

After the prevalence round of screening in the control arm, no excess of cases is seen in either group. The overall rate of detection is 18.4 breast cancers per 1,000 women in the study group and 18.6 per 1,000 in the control group.

Figures 1 and 2 show the rates of breast cancers per 1,000 women according to size at detection and node status, within ASP and PSP, age 40-74, again after the prevalence round of screening in the control arm. The rate of detection of tumours smaller than 20mm is significantly higher in the ASP than in the PSP (p< 0.001). Significantly fewer cases with nodal or distant metastases were detected in the ASP relative to the PSP (p<0.001).

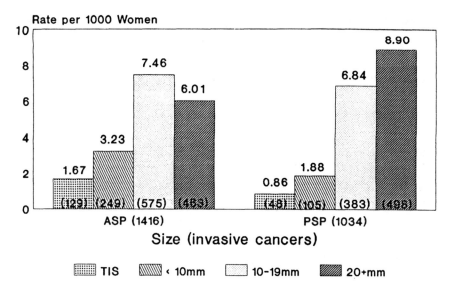

Figure 1   Rates of Breast Cancer per 1,000 women (and number of cases) in the W-E Trial in ASP and PSP by tumour size. Women age 40-74 on entry.

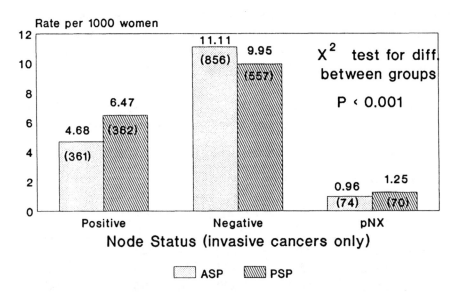

Figure 2 Rates of Breast Cancer per 1,000 women (and number of cases) in W-E Trial in the ASP and PSP by Node Status. Women age 40-74 on entry.

Table 4   Breast cancers detected by age and group, before and after
commencement of screening the control group.

(a) Before screening controls

Age	ASP	PSP	Total
40-49	237	113	350
50-59	368	221	589
60-69	518	278	796
70-74	255	140	395

(b) During screening of controls

Age	ASP	PSP	Total
40-49	18	47	65
50-59	13	94	107
60-69	5	141	146
70-74	4	6	10

The numbers of cases detected with different size and nodal status characteristics are given
in Tables 5 and 6, tabulated by detection mode. In Table 5 there were eight cases for
which the size was not recorded. Omitted are cases detected between randomization and
screening, or after screening ceased (ages 70 - 74).

Table 5   Size distribution of breast cancers diagnosed according to
screening status of the case at detection.   Ages 40 - 74.

SIZE

(a) Before screening controls

	TIS	<20 MM	> 20 mm	Total
Controls	22	299	427	748
First screen	45	284	96	425
Later screen	56	330	94	480
Interval	18	129	148	295
Refusers	7	32	93	132
Total	148	1074	858	2080

Table 5 contd.

(b) During screening of controls

Controls (first screen)	26	189	71	286
Later screen (ASP)	1	18	3	22
Interval (ASP)	0	9	4	13
Refusers (ASP)	0	2	2	4
Total	27	218	80	325

Table 6 Node status of breast cancers diagnosed according to screening status of the case at detection.   Age 40 - 74.

NODE STATUS

(a) Before screening controls

	nodes negative	nodes positive or distant metastases	Total
Controls	367	307	674
First screen	286	77	363
Later screens	338	68	406
Interval	144	119	263
Refusers	42	68	110
Total	1177	639	1818

(b) During screening of controls

Controls (first screen)	190	55	245
Later screen (ASP)	15	4	19
Interval	10	3	13
Refusers	3	0	3
Total	218	62	280

In Table 6 there were 141 invasive cases for which the node status was unknown.
Omitted are tumour in situ, cases detected between randomization and screening or cases
detected after screening ceased (Ages 70-74).

Figure 3 shows the cumulative rate of stage II+ cancers in ASP and PSP, and figure 4 the
cumulative rate of mortality from breast cancer.

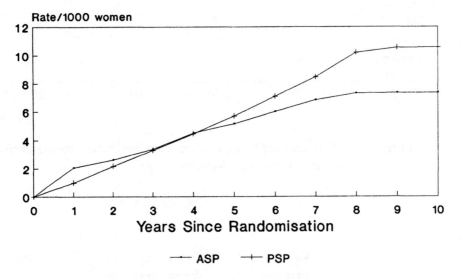

Figure 3 Cumulative Rates of Stage II+ Breast Cancer. Both counties, ASP and PSP.

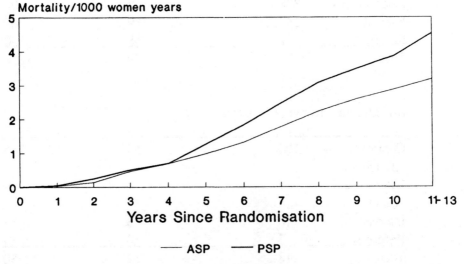

Figure 4 Cumulative Mortality from Breast Cancer. Both counties, ASP and PSP.

The risks of death from breast cancer in the ASP relative to the PSP as estimated by crude analysis after 6, 8 and 10 years of follow-up are given in Table 7. The P value for a chi-squared test for a difference between counties is shown (interaction). No such significant difference was observed.

Table 7   Results of crude analysis of the effect of screening (in fact, invitation to screening) on breast cancer mortality. W-E Trial age 40-74 at entry.

Follow up time average	Combined RR (95% CI)	x^2	significance	interaction*
6 years	0.69 (0.51, 0.92)	6.17	0.013	0.6
8 years	0.70 (0.56, 0.88)	10.40	0.001	0.5
10 years	0.70 (0.57, 0.85)	14.03	<0.0005	0.3

* Test for heterogeneity of screening effect between counties.

Table 8   Results of analysis of the effect of invitation to screening on breast cancer mortality, with adjustment for time since randomization, age and county.

(a) All ages

Factors adjusted for	RR	(95% CI)	Significance
None	0.71	(0.59, 0.87)	<0.001
Time	0.71	(0.59, 0.87)	<0.001
Age+Time	0.70	(0.58, 0.85)	<0.001
Age+County+Time	0.69	(0.57, 0.84)	<0.001

(b) Age-specific results adjusted for time and county

Age group	RR	(95% CI)	Significance
40-49	0.99	(0.61, 1.61)	0.9
50-59	0.61	(0.43, 0.87)	0.006
60-69	0.60	(0.43, 0.83)	0.002
70-74	0.84	(0.54, 1.29)	0.4

Table 8 shows the results of analysis of breast cancer mortality when adjustment is made for time since randomization, age at randomization and county. Rates of mortality per person-year at risk are the basis of this analysis. The results are similar to those of the crude analyses, with a relative mortality of about 70% (p<0.001).

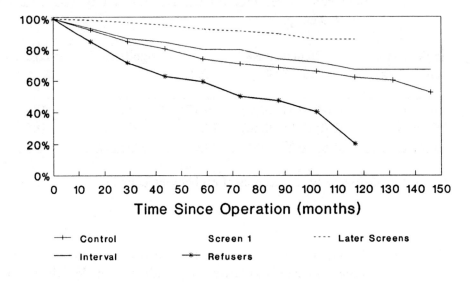

Breast cancer cases only

Figure 5   Cumulative Percentage Surviving. Grouped According to Detection Method, W-E Trial, Women age 40-74 on entry.

Table 9   Relative hazards of death from breast cancer in women in ASP subgroups, relative to controls excluding tumours diagnosed after screening of controls. W-E Trial, age 40-74.

Category	Relative Hazard*	95% CI
control	1.00	
first screen	0.25	(0.17, 0.35)
later screens	0.26	(0.18, 0.37)
interval	0.75	(0.56, 0.99)
refusers	2.09	(1.55, 2.83)

*Adjusted for age and county; estimated by Cox's proportional hazards regression.

Figure 5 shows the survival curves for the different detection subgroups, with the corresponding relative hazards, adjusted for age and county, given in Table 9. Particularly low relative hazards were observed for screen-detected cancers, and the highest relative hazard was that of the refusers. The endpoint is death from breast cancer, and deaths from other causes are censored.

4 DISCUSSION

The average 10 year follow-up of 2,454 women with breast cancer in the two county Swedish trial provides evidence that breast cancer mortality can be reduced by mass screening using mammography. The results at 6, 8 and 10 years average after randomization show consistency and are increasingly significant (Table 7). A 30% reduction in mortality from breast cancer has been achieved among women invited to screening relative to the control group (Table 8). The statistical analysis reveals no difference in the effectiveness of screening between the two counties (chi-squared test for county effect; p=0.3).

The continuous evaluation and update of the W-E trial not only serves to strengthen the evidence for a reduction in breast cancer mortality following screening with mammography, but provides the opportunity for us to gain insight into the reason for its effectiveness. Also, further detailed analysis of data enables us to deduce the practical implications for monitoring and evaluating future screening programmes.

The outcome for a breast cancer patient will be determined by a complex combination of factors, particularly the histologic grade, nodal status and tumour size. In general, the size of an invasive carcinoma will increase with time, and the nodal status is also a time related tumour characteristic. Tumour size and nodal status are therefore quantitative expressions of whether or not the time of diagnosis has been advanced. For screening to be effective, the diagnosis has to be advanced, particularly for those tumours which would lead to death if not detected and treated at an earlier stage in their natural history.

The W-E trial has clearly shown that reducing the stage of breast cancer at diagnosis is a pre-requisite for decreasing mortality (Tabar et al, 1988). There is a remarkable parallelism between cumulative rates of stage II cancers and cumulative mortality rates (figures 3 and 4). However, a significant decrease in the rate of advanced cancers can be achieved only if the size of invasive carcinomas at detection is reduced. In the W-E trial there was a significant shift in the size distribution of invasive carcinomas towards smaller sizes in the ASP compared with the PSP (Figure 1); also, significantly fewer cases with positive nodes and distant metastases at the time of diagnosis were found in the ASP (Figure 2). These indicate that an advance in the time of diagnosis has really taken place, and it is probable that this is directly related to the observed mortality reduction of 30%.

The ASP is, however, a heterogeneous population, and it is of interest to note that the hazard of breast cancer death among breast cancer cases in the different subgroups, relative to the controls, showed considerable variation (see Figure 5 and Table 10). On the beneficial side, the cases detected at the screening rounds had a reduction in risk of about 75% while at the other extreme, the risk of dying from the disease for the non-attendees was about twice that of the PSP.

One can speculate that the screening detected cases were diagnosed much earlier in their natural history relative to the controls; according to our above reasoning this should be reflected in a more favourable tumour size distribution and a reduced rate of detection of cases with metastases in this group. This is indeed the case (Tables 5 & 6).

At the other end of the spectrum, there is additional time available for tumour growth in refuser cases ("patient's delay") relative to the controls. This is reflected in the worst distribution of tumour size and nodal status among refusers as compared with any other group (Tables 5 & 6). The predominance of very advanced stage tumours led to a high mortality rate from breast cancer among refusers: 43% of all breast cancer cases among the non-attendees died from the disease. In fact, whilst only 9% of breast cancer cases in the ASP occurred in this subgroup, it accounted for 26% of all breast cancer deaths in the ASP.

There are women among the compliers who develop breast cancer in the interval between two screens. In some of these cases, diagnosis will take place at an earlier stage than in the control group, provided that increased awareness regarding breast self examination leads to earlier presentation and treatment. In other cases, diagnosis could have taken place at an earlier stage, but for different reasons does not. If the cancer is fast growing de novo, or if it is missed because of suboptimal image quality or insufficient expertise at film reading, then the opportunity to advance the time of diagnosis as much as for the screening cases is lost. The situation is even worse if, in addition, the patient consciously or unconsciously postpones diagnosis, possibly until her next screening appointment ("doctor's delay"), failing to heed symptoms between screens. The time available for tumour growth will be inadvertently extended, artificially producing an effect similar to that observed in the refusers. If a large proportion of interval cases come into this category, not only will there be no benefit but there could be harm. We thus hypothesise that poorly performed screening could be worse than no screening at all.

The proportional interval cancer incidence and the size and nodal status of interval cancers will give early indication of the extent to which this detrimental effect exists in a given screening program (Tabar et al, 1987). Should the mortality of the interval cancers substantially exceed that of the control group cases, it will then indicate that the given screening has not advanced the time of diagnosis for high risk breast cancers.

In the W-E trial, the size and nodal status were more favourable among interval cases than controls. This resulted in a reduced estimate of the hazard of breast cancer death relative to controls (Table 9).

The outcome for interval cases has shown variation between different screening trials (Tabar et al, 1987; Andersson et al, 1988). Careful comparison of size and nodal status, rather than stage, of the interval cancers relative to the control cases could give valuable insight into how a given screening program is affecting the target population.

The evidence from the W-E trial confirms that breast cancer mortality is decreased when screening results in intervention earlier in the natural history of the disease relative to the unscreened population. The size and nodal status of the tumours detected gives an indication of the extent to which the time of diagnosis has been advanced. These factors should be considered in each subgroup among those invited to screening. Recognition of this has important practical implications; for screening to work, there must be a significantly higher rate of invasive cancers, smaller in size by comparison with the unscreened population, and a significant decrease in the detection rate of cases with metastases. To achieve this, high compliance, optimal mammographic image quality and a high level of diagnostic accuracy are essential. Education of women to heed sympoms occurring between screening is also an important factor contributing to the effectiveness of screening.

Acknowledgements

We thank Ulla Brith Krusemo of Uppsala University Computing Centre for computing assitance. The research was supported by a grant from Kopparberg County Council, Sweden. The additional members of the project group in Kopparberg were A Cohen, Department of Surgery, A Gad, Department of Pathology, and U Ljungquist, Department of Surgery, Central Hospital, Falun, Sweden. Additional members in Ostergotland were L G Arnesson, Department of Oncology, O Garontoft, Department of Pathology and JC Mansson, Department of Clinical Cytology, University Hospital, Linkoping, Sweden.

REFERENCES

Anderson I, Aspergen K, Janzon L, Landberg T, Lindholm K, Linell F, Ljungberg O, Ranstam J, Sigfusson B. Mammographic screening and mortality from breast cancer: the Malmö mammographic screening trial. Brit Med J 1988; 297:943-948.

Cox DR. Regression models and life tables. J Roy Statist Soc B 1972; 34:187-220.

Fagerberg CJG, Baldetorp L, Grontoft O, Lundstrom B, Mansson JC, Nordenskjold B. Effects of repeated mammographic screening on breast cancer stage distribution. Acta Radiol (Oncol) 1985; 24:465-473.

Fagerberg CJG, Tabar L. The results of periodic one-view mammography screening in a randomised controlled trial in Sweden. I. Background, organisation, screening program, tumour findings. In Day NE, Miller AB (eds). Screening for Breast Cancer. Huber: Toronto, 1988, pp. 33-38.

Lundgren B, Jakobsson S. Single view mammography: a simple and efficient approach to breast cancer screening. Cancer 1976; 38:1124-1129.

Shapiro S, Strax P, Venet L. Periodic breast cancer screening in reducing mortality from breast cancer. JAMA 1971; 215:1777-1785.

Tabar L, Gad A. Screening for breast cancer: the Swedish trial. Radiol 1981; 138: 219-222.

Tabar L, Dean P. The control of breast cancer through mammography screening. What is the evidence? Radiol Clin North Amer 1987; 25:993-1005.

Tabar L, Fabergerg G, Day NE, Holmberg L. What is the optimum interval between mammographic screening examinations? An analysis based on the latest results of the Swedish two-county breast cancer screening trial. Brit J Cancer 1987; 55:547-551.

Tabar L, Fagerberg CJG, Day NE. The results of periodic one-view mammography screening in a randomised controlled trial in Sweden. II. Evaluation of the results. In Day NE, Miller AB (eds). Screening for Breast Cancer. Huber: Toronto, 1988, pp. 39-44.

Tabar L, Fageberg G, Duffy SW, Day NE. The Swedish two-county trial of mammographic screening for breast cancer: recent results and calculation of benefit. J Epidemiol Comm Hlth 1989; 43:107-114.

4 The Malmö Mammographic Screening Trial

L. JANZON and I. ANDERSSON

University of Lund, Malmö General Hospital, Sweden

1 INTRODUCTION

When the code was broken in the mammographic screening trial in Malmö (MMST) on December 31, 1986, there was no significant difference in mortality from breast cancer between the study group and the non-invited control group (Andersson et al., 1988). Further analysis indicated that the effect of mammographic screening was related to age. In women older than 55 at invitation, breast cancer mortality was 20% lower in the study group than in the control group. In women younger than 55 at invitation breast cancer mortality was 29% higher in the invited group. Considering the results from the W-E study in Sweden (Tabár et al., 1985) and the HIP study (Shapiro et al 1971) from New York it was concluded that invitation to mammographic screening may lead to reduced mortality from breast cancer, at least in women aged 55 or over. The effect of invitation to screening has now been updated until December 1988. The lower breast cancer mortality in the invited group remains but is still not statistically significant. (Table 1).

Table 1   <u>MMST</u>   Breast cancer deaths, Age at entry: 45 - 69 [*]

	Invited	Controls	RR	95% CI
1977 - 1986	63	66	0.96	(0.68 - 1.35)
1977 - 1988	81	90	0.90	(0.67 - 1.22)

[*] Data for 1987 - 88 are preliminary

The breast cancer mortality in the invited group of women below 55 years of age remains higher (Tables 2-3).

Table 2   <u>MMST</u>   Breast Cancer deaths, Age at entry: 55 - 69 [*]

	Invited	Controls	RR	95% CI
1977 - 1986	35	44	0.80	(0.51 - 1.24)
1977 - 1988	50	61	0.82	(0.57 - 1.19)

[*] Data for 1987 - 88 are preliminary

Table 3   <u>MMST</u>   Breast Cancer deaths, Age at entry: 45 - 54 [*]

	Invited	Controls	RR	95% CI
1977 - 1986	28	22	1.29	(0.74 - 2.25)
1977 - 1988	31	29	1.08	(0.65 - 1.79)

[*] Data for 1987 - 88 are preliminary

Important questions in the Malmö study besides the effect on breast cancer mortality have been to give valid estimates of the attendance rates in an urban population, to describe and assess the impact of interval carcinomas on the outcome of screening, to study the relationship between breast cancer and other types of cancer and to evaluate the case-control method in the assessment of mammographic screening.

2 ATTENDANCE RATE IN MMST

In the MMST 25% of the invited women did not come to the first screening examination (Table 4). The greater proportion of non-attenders among old women and the high proportion of stage II+ tumors among non-attenders indicates that age and presence of a breast tumour influence women's willingness to participate in mammographic screening. The inverse relationship between age and attendance rate seems at first hand conflicting. Since breast cancer incidence increases with age one would assume that old women would be more concerned than young women to participate. However, breast cancer is only one

Table 4   Attendance rate and prevalence of stage II+ tumours in relation to age at invitation (based on results 31 Dec. 1986)

Age at invitation	Attendance rate at 1st screening	Number of cancers in the invited group		Number of cancers among non-attenders		Percent stage II+ tumours among non-attenders
		n	rate/1000	n	rate/1000	
> 55 n=7981	79%	198	24.8	33	4.1	72.7
≥ 55 n=13107	70%	381	29.1	73	5.6	71.2

of the many diseases that are related to age and that might reduce old women's willingness and possibilities to come to the examination. The screening examination was introduced in the letter of invitation as a means to avoid death from breast cancer. Considering the fact that about 70% of the tumours among non-attenders were stage II+ it is reasonable to assume that many of the women with breast cancer already at invitation knew they had a tumour and might not expect to benefit from screening. In fact, it might be that invitation to screening in this situation causes a further delay of the diagnosis. Women attend screening with the expectation to be informed that they are healthy. Many, not to say all, of those who have a tumour or who have a fear of having one are not mentally prepared for the cancer diagnosis. Invitation to screening could in this situation be perceived as a threat of something that one still is not fully prepared for. Considering the high non-attendance rate in this urban population together with a high proportion of advanced carcinomas among non-attenders it seems urgent that more efforts are devoted to studies that can teach us more on how to convince women to participate.

Other important issues before embarking on full-scale mammographic screening programmes is to assess the magnitude of the breast cancer problem and to estimate the existing diagnostic capacities for early breast cancer diagnosis. The effect of screening is related to breast cancer mortality which varies between areas. In Sweden the number of woman-years lost due to breast cancer varies form 1.22 - 2.19/1000 woman years in the age groups below 65.

In a random sample from the non-screened control group in Malmö it was found that almost 25% of all women had been on mammography, in most cases only once. The rate varied from 13% in women aged 65-69 at entry into the study to 35% in women aged 45-49 at entry. In the two-county study 13% of women in the control group had undergone mammography. This shows that the availability of health care, in particular mammography, and women's attitudes to seeking advice for breast symptoms are quite different in different areas and that the experience from one programme cannot be used to calculate what can be expected in another population.

3 INTERVAL CARCINOMAS

One-hundred of the 588 cancers in the invited group were detected in intervals between screening. The incidence of interval carcinoma was related to age. In women below 55 years of age at invitation about 15% of all tumours were detected in intervals between screening compared to 18% among women older than 55 at entry. The proportion of carcinoma in situ was 27.1% in the older age group and 17.2% in the younger age group. The proportion of stage II+ in the corresponding age groups was 58.8% and 50% (Table 5).

Table 5 Incidence and stage of interval carcinoma in relation to age at invitation

Age at invitation	Number of interval carcinomas	Percent of all detected cancers	Rate of interval carcinoma/1000	Tumour stage (%)				
				0	I	II	III	IV
> 55	29	14.6	3.6	5 (17.2)	12 (41.4)	8 (27.6)	4 (13.8)	-
≥ 55	70	18.4	5.3	19 (27.1)	21 (30.0)	25 (35.7)	3 (4.3)	2 (2.9)

The breast cancer mortality was in each stage higher in the interval cancer group than it was in the control group (Table 6). When taking age at invitation and tumour stage into account it was found that the survival rate was lower for women in the interval cancer group than it was among cancer cases in the control group. In all, 41% of the breast cancer deaths in the younger age groups and 28% in the older age groups occurred among women with interval carcinomas. About 75% of all interval carcinomas were detected within 18 months after screening. Considering the quality of the mammographic examination in then Malmö trial it does not seem likely that the magnitude of the interval carcinoma problem can be reduced by improvement of the radiographic examination. For practical reasons it does not seem feasible to use shorter intervals than 18 months. Therefore it is urgent to develop new treatments that will improve survival for women with interval carcinoma.

Table 6 Breast cancer mortality among women with invasive interval carcinoma in relation to tumour stage. Women in the not-invited control group used for comparison.

Tumour stage	Interval carcinoma n = 75 Dead from breast cancer		Control group n = 393 Dead from breast cancer	
	n	%	n	%
I	4	12.1	5	3.1
II	9	27.3	28	16.3
III	5	71.4	9	33.3
IV	2	100.0	22	68.8
All	20	26.7	64	16.3

4 MULTIPLE PRIMARY TUMOURS

Seventy-six percent of the women with breast cancer who died underwent post-mortem examination. Of the 193 women with breast cancer who died 41 had or had previously had at least one other malignancy. The proportion of women with a second primary was 22.8% in women above 55 at entry and 18.2% in women below 55. The second primary was the cause of death in 31 patients. The most common secondary site was cancer of the ovary and endometrium (11/41). Hence one could say that many of the breast cancer victims suffer not from breast cancer but from cancer disease. How this influences on the course of breast cancer and what should constitute the optimal treatment in this group is not known but should merit further research.

5 EVALUATION OF THE MMST USING THE CASE CONTROL METHOD

In the discussions following the publication of the MMST, results from published case control studies (Palli et al., 1986; Verbeek et al., 1984; and Collette et al., 1984) were used to support the view that mammographic screening leads to reduced breast cancer mortality. From a methodological point of view it is clear that results from a controlled trial and a case control assessment (Andersson et al., 1988) are not immediately comparable. The controlled trial is an assessment of the effect of invitation to screening whereas the case control method is an assessment of the benefit for those who attend screening. Tables 7 and 8 illustrate the different results when using the clinical trial approach and the case control method. With the latter method there seems to be a significant risk reduction in the Malmö Mammographic Screening Trial. The odds ratio was in the same range as in other published studies. This risk reduction is in clear contrast to the results from the clinical

Table 7   The Malmö mammographic screening trial assessed as a clinical trial

	Invited n = 21,088	Controls n = 21,195
Proportion	50%	50%
Breast ca deaths	63	66
Mortality rate	0.299%	0.311%

| Relative risk | 0.96 (0.68 - 1.35) |

Table 8   Assessment of effect using the case-control approach

		Living controls	Women dead from breast cancer	Total
Participated in mammographic screening program	Yes	229	36	265
	No	71	24	95
Total		300	60	360

Crude odds ratio: 0.46
Adjusted (matching for age) odds ratio: 0.42 (95% C.I. 0.22 - 0.78)

trial. Thirty-one of the 63 women who died from breast cancer in the invited group were non-participants in the clinical trial. By the end of December 1986, 29% of the breast cancer cases in the group of non-attenders had died. This is in striking contrast to the 3% among women with cancer detected at screening. The higher mortality among non-attenders is explained by the high proportion of advanced carcinomas. The breast cancer incidence among non-attenders did not differ from the breast cancer incidence among women in the control group. Obviously, one cannot use a comparison of the breast cancer incidence in these two groups to get a valid estimate of the selection bias caused by non-attenders. Hence if the case control method is to be used to assess the public health effects of mammographic screening it is necessary to estimate and adjust for the selection bias caused by non-attendance.

6 CONCLUSIONS

The general impression from published mammographic screening programs is that the effect of screening is age-dependent. In post-menopausal women there seems to be a reduction of the breast cancer mortality rate associated with screening whereas no corresponding effect has been shown in pre-menopausal women.

The beneficial effect in older women is surprising considering that older women have a lower participation rate, a higher incidence of carcinoma among non-attenders and a higher incidence of advanced interval carcinoma.

The difference in effect when comparing older and younger women might be explained by differences in tumour biology but also by different detection rates. Although there was a greater proportion of interval carcinomas and a higher incidence of breast cancer among non-attenders in the older age group the detection rate, compared to the control group, increased form $20.8/10^3$ to $29.1/10^3$ in the older age group but only from $21.0/10^3$ to $24.8/10^3$ in the younger age group. The proportion of stage II+ cancers was reduced with 43% among old women but only 23% in the younger age group. The proportion of in situ carcinomas increased in comparison with the control group with 63% among old women but only with 34% among the young ones (Table 9).

Table 9   Shift of tumour stage distribution by screening
                  in relation to age at invitation

Age at invitation	Stage II+		In situ carcinoma	
	Invited group	Control group	Invited group	Control group
> 55	34.0% Reduction: 22.7%	44.0%	18.7% Increase: 34.0%	14.7%
≥ 55	32.5% Reduction: 43.0%	57.0%	14.7% Increase: 63.3%	9.0%

Hence the beneficial effects associated with screening seem to be related to the increase in detection rate and to the shift in stage distribution. It might be that a certain critical level of detection and shift of the stage distribution must be exceeded before any effects can be seen. The effect is related to time. This raises questions whether in the design and evaluation of screening programmes there should be allowance for a delay when estimating the effect. The case-control method gives a false estimate of what is really achieved by invitation to mammographic screening unless the selection bias caused by non-attendance can be adjusted for.

REFERENCES

Andersson I, Aspegren K, Janzon L et al. Mammographic screening and mortality from breast cancer: the Malmö mammographic screening trial. Br Med J 1988; 297:943-948.

Collette HJA, Rombach JJ, Day NE et al. Evaluation of screening for breast cancer in a non-randomised study (the DOM project) by means of a case-control study.Lancet 1984; i:1224-1226.

Palli D, Roselli Del Turco M, Buiatti E et al. A case-control study of the efficacy of a non-randomized breast cancer screening program in Florence (Italy). Int J Cancer 1986; 38:501-514.

Shapiro S, Strax P, Venet L. Periodic breast cancer screening in reducing mortality from breast cancer. JAMA 1971; 215:1777-1785.

Tabár L, Fagerberg CJG, Gad A et al. Reduction in mortality from breast cancer after mass screening with mammography: randomized trial from the breast cancer screening working group of the Swedish National Board of Health and Welfare. Lancet 1985; i:829-832.

Verbeek ALM, Holland R, Sturmans F et al. Reduction of breast cancer mortality through mass screening with modern mammography. Lancet 1984; i:1222-1224.

5 The Canadian National Breast Screening Study

A. B. MILLER, C. J. BAINES, T. TO and C. WALL

Department of Preventive Medicine and Biostatistics, University of Toronto, Canada

1 INTRODUCTION

The Canadian National Breast Screening Study (NBSS) is an individually randomised efficacy trial with two major objectives:

1). To determine in volunteers age 40-49 on entry to the study whether unselective annual screening with mammography and physical examination reduces mortality from breast cancer.

2). To determine in volunteers age 50-59 on entry to the study the additional contribution of routine annual mammographic screening to screening by physical examination alone in reducing mortality from breast cancer. (Miller, Howe and Wall, 1981; Miller, 1988).

All women between the ages of 40 and 59 years who had not had breast cancer, had had no mammogram in the previous 12 months and were not currently pregnant were eligible for the study if they provided informed consent to participate and completed questionnaires giving full identifying information and data on risk factors for breast cancer.

Screening centres were responsible for recruiting women and used a number of mechanisms through screening centres. Women were randomized after supplying the data on risk factors for breast cancer, signing the informed consent form and having an initial physical examination of the breast. All mammograms were performed using dedicated units and film-screen technology. There was careful monitoring of radiation dosage and quality control of technical factors and radiologists' interpretation of films. Those allocated to the comparison, non-recall (PX) group age 40-49 received only an initial physical examination and were then followed annually by mail. All other groups were rescreened annually for a total of 5 or 4 screens (4 screens only were offered to the latter third of those enrolled in the study). Half the women in the study received mammography (the MA groups), all were taught breast self-examination. The physical examinations of the breasts were given by specially trained nurses, but by physicians in the Province of Québec. If an abnormality was found either on physical examination or mammography, the woman was referred to a review clinic. Recommendations on management were made by the study surgeon to the woman's family physician.

Recruitment and screening commenced in Toronto in January 1980, in Québec in August 1980, in centres in Montréal, Hamilton and Winnipeg in May 1981, in Vancouver in

March 1983, two centres in Ottawa, a second in Montréal and a centre in London in June 1983, a centre in Halifax in August 1983, centres in Edmonton, Red Deer and Calgary in January 1984 and a second centre in Toronto in April 1984. Recruitment was completed in the first 5 centres in 1984, and in the remaining 10 in March 1985, the mid point of recruitment was in 1983. A total of 89,835 women are included in the study, 50,430 age 40-49 and 39,405 age 50-59. Screening continued to June 88. The study coordinating centre is at the University of Toronto, where the NBSS data base is maintained.

The basic endpoint on the study is mortality from breast cancer. It was originally anticipated that the first report would give 5-year results. However, as several recent studies in Europe have suggested that differences can not be anticipated much before 7 years, we plan our first report on mortality when we have a 7-year average follow-up (i.e. complete data on follow-up to 5 years, with maximum follow-up of 10 years).

Data on deaths from breast cancer are obtained in two ways: from annual follow-up of all the breast cancers identified in the study, and through linkage with the National Mortality Data Base maintained by Statistics Canada. Identification of breast cancers was through the screening centres while they were operational, and subsequently through linkage to the files of the provincial tumour registries in the provinces where the study was conducted. We have linked our files to the tumour registries of Alberta, British Columbia, Nova Scotia, Ontario and Québec, linkages are pending with the Manitoba registry, and further updates are planned with the Québec registry. The first National death linkage was conducted in 1990. In this paper data will be reported on some operational aspects of the study and intermediate outcome data relevant to the main endpoint.

2 RESULTS

The screening centres were unable to make direct referral for management of a detected abnormality. Instead, for women found abnormal on review, a report had to be rendered to the participant's family physician who decided on the surgeon to whom the woman was referred.

Table 1 Benign to malignant ratio for biopsies, by age, allocation and screening year

Year	Age at entry and allocation							
	40-44		45-49		50-54		55-59	
	MA	PX	MA	PX	MA	PX	MA	PX
1	14.9	7.8	6.3	3.9	5.5	2.6	4.4	2.7
2	13.4	-	8.9	-	4.4	3.0	3.4	2.8
3	8.2	-	5.8	-	4.6	6.3	3.8	2.0
4	5.8	-	4.4	-	2.8	3.2	2.6	3.4
5	7.6	-	8.0	-	4.1	1.4	2.9	1.6

Accordingly, women were assessed in a variety of hospitals, very few being equipped for detailed investigation, and open biopsy (usually with needle localisation for impalpable lesions) was the main diagnostic test. Hence the benign to malignant ratios were substantially higher than those reported from Europe, especially in the younger women (Table 1).

The cancer detection rates were largely as anticipated from previous studies (Table 2), and, for those allocated to mammography, were very similar to those reported for the US Breast Cancer Detection Demonstration Project (BCDDP) (Baker, 1982). The expected annual incidence in Canadian women is 0.99 per 1,000 at ages 40-44, 1.52 at ages 45-49, 1.76 at ages 50-54 and 2.10 at ages 55-59 (Statistics Canada, 1988) . Therefore the ratio of prevalence to expected incidence for the mammography allocation (MA) was 2.2 at ages 40-44, 3.8 at ages 45-49, 3.7 at ages 50-54 and 3.8 at ages 55-59. The corresponding ratio for the physical examination alone allocation (PX) was 1.7, 1.9, 1.9, and 1.5, respectively.

Table 2   Cancer detection rates (including in situ lesions) per 1,000, by age, allocation and screening year

Year	Age at allocation							
	40-44		45-49		50-54		55-59	
	MA	PX	MA	PX	MA	PX	MA	PX
1	2.18	1.72	5.79	2.94	6.48	3.41	7.96	3.14
2	1.18	1.50	2.16	1.51	3.41	1.68	3.77	2.04
3	1.64	1.50	2.29	1.85	2.38	0.80	2.48	1.93
4	2.27	1.20	2.50	1.59	3.09	0.81	3.07	0.98
5	1.70	0.60	1.68	0.59	2.06	1.74	4.19	1.99

Underlined rates are for incident cancers in non-recall women.

The excess of screen-detected cases in the MA allocation compared to the PX for women age 50-59 at each screen was somewhat unexpected, as after the prevalence screen, providing the threshold of screening remains the same and there is no overdiagnosis, the detection rates should be very similar. In part this appears to have been due to false negatives at screen 1 detected at screen 2 (Baines et al, 1986;1988) and an increase in the efficiency of mammography as the study progressed, as well as a poorer sensitivity of the physical examination at year 3 (Baines et al, 1989).

In the NBSS all cancers occurring in the 12 month period following a previous screen which were not diagnosed following a recommendation from the screening centre were regarded as interval cancers, those diagnosed after 12 months as incident cancers. The interval cancer rates were, in general, higher in the PX allocation than the MA (Table 3).

Table 3 Interval cancer rates per 1,000, by age, allocation and interval

Interval	Age at allocation							
	40-44		45-49		50-54		55-59	
	MA	PX	MA	PX	MA	PX	MA	PX
1	0.73	1.05	1.00	1.71	1.04	0.95	0.65	1.17
2	0.49	-	1.09	-	0.85	1.05	0.52	0.91
3	0.24	-	0.55	-	0.38	1.61	0.66	1.18
4	0.60	-	0.57	-	0.31	0.80	0.91	0.45

From these rates it is possible to compute the relative sensitivity of mammography plus physical examination in comparison to physical examination alone (1 - proportional incidence of interval cancers) (Day, 1989). In interval 1 for women age 40-44 this is 1 - 0.73/1.05 or 30%, for women 45-49 42% and for women age 55-59 44%. There was no apparent effect in women age 50-54. In intervals 2 through 4 for women age 50-54 and 55-59 the range is from 19% to 76%, but there was no apparent effect in interval 4 for women age 55-59. In addition one can calculate the sensitivity of the combination screen for women age 40-44 and 45-49 in comparison to the incident cancers ascertained in the control group (see Table 2), this ranges from 28% to 84%. The estimates derived from intervals 3 and 4 may be too low, however, as there may have been some underascertainment of cancers following the last screening year of the study in view of the incompleteness of the cancer registry linkages with Québec and Manitoba.

Using the data from Table 3, and the underlined incident rates from Table 2, it is possible to derive estimates of proportional incidence with Canadian national rates as the basis for expectation, making adjustments for the aging of the cohort. The results of such calculations are displayed in Table 4.

Table 4 Proportional incidence by age, allocation and interval, with Canadian national rates as basis for expectation.

Interval	Age at allocation							
	40-44		45-49		50-54		55-59	
	MA	PX	MA	PX	MA	PX	MA	PX
1	0.69	1.00	0.65	1.11	0.58	0.53	0.30	0.55
2	0.43	_1.30_	0.68	_0.94_	0.46	0.56	0.23	0.41
3	0.19	_1.20_	0.34	_1.13_	0.20	0.83	0.29	0.53
4	0.41	_0.82_	0.34	_0.95_	0.16	0.40	0.38	0.19

Underlined proportions are based on incident cancers ascertained.

The calculations confirm that both screening regimens reduce the expected incidence occurring as interval cancers, and that in general the addition of mammography results in improved sensitivity, as already demonstrated. They also suggest greater sensitivity with increasing age and duration in the programme. For the PX group age 40-49, the ascertained cancer incidence exceeds the expected rate, though there is a fall off in interval 4.

Table 5   Nodal status for screen detected invasive cancers

| Number of nodes | Screen 1 | | | | Screens 2-5 | | | |
| | 40-49 | | 50-59 | | 40-49 | | 50-59 | |
	MA	PX	MA	PX	MA	PX	MA	PX
None	51	30	68	35	77	-	94	45
1-3	13	14	21	11	21	-	24	22
4+	19	5	8	10	8	-	10	12
No data	1	3	16	5	8	-	11	2
Total	84	52	113	61	114	-	139	81

The nodal status for the invasive cancers detected in the prevalence screen is presented on the left side of Table 5. The row for no data indicates the cancers which were regarded by the operating surgeon as clinically negative in terms of axillary involvement and so small that axillary dissection was not required, hence there are no data on the nodal status pathologically. Although there was the expected excess of node-negative cancers detected in women allocated MA in both 10 year age groups, there was also an excess of node-positive tumours. The excess consisted of cancers with 1-3 nodes positive in women age 50-59, but 4 or more nodes positive in women age 40-49.

The right side of Table 5 presents the distribution of nodal status for the invasive cancers detected in the subsequent annual screens (screens 2,3,4 and 5). If the tumours with nodal involvement are considered advanced (all would be stage 2 or 3 in the UICC classification) the proportion of advanced tumours was 25 % in each age group allocated MA but 42% in the PX group age 50-59. However, this difference is due to fewer node-negative cases in the PX group compared to the MA, as the absolute numbers of involved node cancers are identical in the two groups.

The left side of Table 6 presents the nodal status of the invasive cancers ascertained in the participants other than at screening, and the right side the totals so far ascertained from all sources (the combined total from Table 5 and the left side of Table 6). Considering the left side of Table 6 the larger numbers for the PX allocation age 40-49 are due to the fact that these women only received the initial screen. The larger numbers for the PX allocation age 50-59 is due to the higher interval cancer rates as well as some "catch-up" in terms of

Table 6 Nodal status for other (interval and incident) invasive cancers, and total invasive cancers ascertained.

Number of nodes	Other (interval and incident)				Total ascertained			
	40-49		50-59		40-49		50-59	
	MA	PX	MA	PX	MA	PX	MA	PX
None	44	89	30	55	172	119	192	135
1-3	18	27	17	24	52	41	62	57
4+	19	16	14	14	46	21	32	36
No data	3	14	10	11	12	17	37	18
Total	84	146	71	104	282	198	323	246

cancers ascertained after the end of the period of screening. That the catch-up may not yet be complete is indicated by the excess of node-negative cases in both MA groups on the right side of Table 6. For node-positive cases, there is a continuing excess in the MA group age 40-49 compared to the PX, but equality for the 50-59 age groups.

Tables 7 and 8 provide corresponding information to Tables 5 and 6 for tumour size as reported to us. In interpreting these data it should be borne in mind that we are dependent on a host of pathologists in numerous community hospitals for these data. No attempt during the course of the study was made to determine tumour size in a central reference laboratory, though this process is now underway. Frequently the only measurements recorded on the pathology report forms were macroscopic, and rarely when there was a small invasive component of the tumour was this accurately recorded. Hence there are many tumours with no data on size, while even when measurements were available, they may have over-estimated the size of the invasive component as required for the UICC pTNM staging system.

Table 7 Tumour size for screen detected invasive cancers

Size (cm)	Screen 1				Screens 2-5			
	40-49		50-59		40-49		50-59	
	MA	PX	MA	PX	MA	PX	MA	PX
<1	7	8	16	1	21	-	27	4
1.0-2.0	43	30	52	37	43	-	71	45
2.1-5.0	20	9	26	18	26	-	26	24
>5.0	3	2	0	2	3	-	1	2
No data	11	3	19	3	21	-	14	6
Total	84	52	113	61	114	-	139	61

From Table 7 the proportion of tumours detected on screening that were recorded as T1 (2 cm in size or less) can be determined. These were 60% for the MA group and 73% for the PX group age 40-49 at screen 1, 60% for the MA group and 62% for the PX group age 50-59 at screen 1, while at the subsequent screens the proportions were 56% for the MA group age 40-49, 70% for the MA group age 50-59 and 60 % for the PX group age 50-59. These proportions are almost certainly underestimates, as a large proportion of the tumours with no data appear from the pathology report to be small tumours, or to have a small invasive component in a largely intraductal lesion. Even so, the numerical data suggest that at screen 1 the addition of mammography to physical examination not only increases the absolute numbers of small invasive, but also large invasive tumours, while in women age 50-59 the addition of mammography to physical examination does not result in a reduction in the numbers of large invasive tumours detected at screens 2 to 5.

Table 8 Tumour size for other (interval and incident) invasive cancers, and total invasive cancers ascertained.

Size (cm)	Other (interval and incident)				Total ascertained			
	40-49		50-59		40-49		50-59	
	MA	PX	MA	PX	MA	PX	MA	PX
<1	7	10	5	7	34	17	47	11
1.0-2.0	39	67	35	45	125	97	158	127
2.1-5.0	26	44	15	37	72	53	67	79
>5.0	4	6	4	3	8	8	5	4
No data	8	19	12	12	41	23	46	22
Total	84	146	71	104	282	198	323	246

Even for the interval or incident cancers at least half were recorded as T1 (Table 8), namely 55% in the MA group age 40-49, 53% in the PX group age 40-49, 56% in the MA group age 50-59 and 50% in the PX group age 50-59. Considering all cancers so far ascertained, although there were larger numbers of T1 cancers in the MA groups, there remains an excess of large cancers in the MA group age 40-49, and only a small reduction in the MA compared to the PX group age 50-59.

3 DISCUSSION

The NBSS is the largest study to date evaluating combination screening in women age 40-49, and the only study evaluating the effect of mammography over and above physical examination in women age 50-59. The interim outcome measures presented in this paper, especially those relating to advanced breast cancer, suggest that so far, at 7 years on average from the start of the study, there is no evidence that screening will be shown to reduce breast cancer mortality in women age 40-49, or that the addition of mammography to physical examination of the breasts has resulted in a measurable reduction in mortality.

Previous studies using more classical approaches to estimating the validity of the screening tests have suggested that our physical examinations were very efficient (Baines et al, 1989) and that the sensitivity of the mammography was not inferior to published data from other studies (Baines et al, 1986;1988). The analyses of proportional incidence, nodal status and tumour size presented here tend to confirm this. Nevertheless the quality of our mammography has been severely criticised, especially by those who have been provided with access to unselective samples of mammograms (Kopans, 1990). Indeed our very openness may have done us a disservice (Miller et al, 1990). Recently therefore we had a further random sample assessed by 3 independent experts, who confirmed a general raising of standards as the study progressed (as happened elsewhere as new technology became more widely available and experience increased) (Baines et al, 1990).

It is difficult to see how mammography of a standard achieving the detection and interval cancer rates and the sensitivity levels we have reported could be responsible for the current anomalous findings with regard to advanced breast cancer. There are several possible reasons for them:
  i. The findings are due to bias.
  ii. The findings are real.
  iii. The findings are due to chance.
Each of these explanations will now be discussed in turn.

i. The findings are due to bias. Bias could take one of two forms: underascertainment of breast cancer cases by the study procedures; some bias in the initial allocation.

While screening continued, the follow-up processes for women with identified abnormalities on screening, and for ensuring return of women to the screening centres (or for the controls age 40-49 the return of questionnaires by mail) were the main mechanisms that resulted in identification of breast cancer cases. There did not seem to be any reason to suspect underascertainment of cases during the course of the study, as the efficiency of the mail follow-up was as good as the return to the screening centres (over 90% in all groups were contacted at the end of the screening period). Since the screening ceased, however, we have been dependent on information provided by our former collaborators to identify newly diagnosed breast cancers, and this seems to be more efficient for those who were being regularly screened, many of whom made arrangements locally to continue with screening. Thus, although the efficiency of follow-up was very high and similar in all groups at the end of screening, it is possible that there has been more underascertainment of breast cancer cases in the PX group age 40-49 after the screening centres closed. Even so, this does not satisfactorily explain the excess of advanced cancers at screen 1 in the MA group age 40-49. The linkages to the cancer registries that have been conducted have not resulted in the identification of more than a few breast cancers unknown to us during the period of screening, though the linkage still has to be conducted with the Manitoba cancer registry and that with the Québec tumour registry updated.

Bias in the allocation procedures could lead to the findings if the allocation was subverted to direct women with symptoms, obvious risk factors (such as a positive family history) or a palpable mass into the mammography arm [although such subversion for those with a palpable mass was unnecessary as all women with abnormalities on the physical examination were to be referred to the study surgeon for review]. Our quality control procedures included checks on the allocation process and no errors that could have led to the findings were ever detected. There are no inequalities in the distribution of risk factors or breast symptoms by study centre nor in the proportion of women referred to review (Wall et al, 1990) The originals of the allocation sheets have been carefully checked in relation specifically to those who have died and no evidence of any falsification, erasure or other changes were found. We therefore believe that bias in allocation did not occur.

ii. The findings are real. If this is the explanation they indicate an early adverse effect of screening in women age 0-49, and no benefit so far from mammography in women age 50-59, as the cumulative rate of advanced disease appears to predict breast cancer mortality (Tabar et al, 1987). Previous studies have shown a small excess in advanced breast cancer or mortality in the screened group compared to the control in women under the age of 50 in the early years of follow-up (Tabar et al, 1985; Verbeek et al, 1985) or in one study in women under the age of 55 in the first five years (Andersson et al, 1988). Our excess of advanced cancers may be more pronounced and more persistent because our study has the largest number of women age 40-49, and all were enrolled through screening centres. In other studies randomisation was of invitations to atttend screening, and the "refusers", not present in our study, had a diluting effect on the results. For women age 50-59, it is possible that the contribution of mammography is just delayed, indicating that physical examination could provide much of the initial benefit demonstrated in many studies (Collette et al, 1984; Palli et al, 1986; Shapiro et al, 1988; Tabar et al, 1985,1989) between 3 or 4 to 7 years in women of this age group.

iii. The findings are due to chance. This is still possible, though as the difference for women age 40-49 continues to persist with continuing follow-up since it first became apparent four years ago this seems less and less likely.

Clearly continued follow-up of the total study population will be required for many years, to determine whether a benefit from screening eventually occurs in either age group. In order to facilitate this, we plan to repeat the linkage with the National Mortality Data Base in 1993, and simultaneously link with the National Cancer Incidence Reporting System which by then should be fully accessible for record linkage purposes. Even with linkage then, we shall only have reached the 9 year mean follow-up, and it will probably be necessary to continue the follow-up for a further 5 or more years before we may be in a position to fully evaluate the effect of screening in women age 40-49, and perhaps the contribution of mammography in women age 50-59. In the meantime, the current recommendations in Canada are to screen women age 50-69 with biennial mammography and physical examination, but not those age 40-49 (The Workshop Group, 1989).

REFERENCES

Andersson I, Aspergren K, Janzon L et al. Mammographic screening and mortality from breast cancer: the Malmö mammographic screening trial. Br Med J 1988; 297: 943-948.

Baines CJ, McFarlane DV, Miller AB et al. Sensitivity and specificity of first screen mammography in 15 NBSS centres. J Can Assoc Radiol 1988; 39: 273-276.

Baines CJ, Miller AB, Bassett AA. Physical examination. Its role as a single screening modality in the Canadian National Breast Screening Study. Cancer 1989; 63: 1816-1822.

Baines CJ, Miller AB, Kopans DB et al. Canadian National Breast Screening Study: Assessment of technical quality by external review. AJ R, 1990; 155:743-747.

Baines CJ, Miller AB, Wall C et al. Sensitivity and Specificity of first screen mammography in the Canadian National Breast Screening Study: A preliminary report from five centres. Radiology 1986; 160: 295-298.

Baker L. Breast Cancer Detection Demonstration Project: Five-year summary report. CA 1982; 32: 194-225.

Collette, H.J.A., Day, N.E., Rombach, J.J. et al: Evaluation of screening for breast cancer in a non-randomized study (the DOM project) by means of a case-control study. Lancet, 1984; i: 1224-1226.

Day NE. Quantitative approaches to the evaluation of screening programs. World J Surg 1989; 13: 3-8.

Kopans D. The Canadian screening program: a different perspective. AJR, 1990; 155: 748-750.

Miller AB. The Canadian National Breast Screening Study. In Day NE and Miller AB (eds). Screening for Breast Cancer. Toronto, Hans Huber, 1988, pp 51-58.

Miller AB, Baines CJ, Sickles EA. Canadian national breast screening study (letter). AJR, 1990; 155: 1133-1134.

Miller AB, Howe GR, Wall C. The National study of breast cancer screening. Clin Invest Med, 1981; 4:227-258.

Palli D, del Turco MR, Buiatti E et al. A case-control study of the efficacy of a non-randomised breast cancer screening program in Florence (Italy). Int J Cancer, 1986;38:501-504.

Statistics Canada. Cancer in Canada, 1983. Catalogue 82-207, annual. Minister of Supply and Services, Ottawa, 1988.

Shapiro, S., Venet W, Strax P, Venet L. Periodic screening for breast cancer. The Health Insurance Plan Project and its sequelae, 1963-1986. The Johns Hopkins University Press, Baltimore. 1988.

Tabar L, Fabergerg G, Day NE, Holmberg L. What is the optimum interval between mammographic screening examinations? An analysis based on the latest results of the Swedish two-county breast cancer screening trial. Brit J Cancer 1987; 55:547-551.

Tabar L, Fagerberg G, Duffy SW, Day NE. The Swedish two county trial of mammographic screening for breast cancer: recent results and calculation of benefit. J Epidemiol Commun Hlth.,1989; 42:107-114.

Tabar L, Fagerberg CJG, Gad A et al. Reduction in mortality from breast cancer after mass screening with mammography. Lancet 1985; i: 829-832.

Verbeek ALM, Hendriks JHCL, Holland R et al. Mammographic screening and breast cancer mortality: Age-specific effects in Nijmegan project, 1975-82. Lancet 1985; i: 865-866.

Wall C, Miller AB, Baines CJ et al. The National Breast Screening Study; the study participants. In preparation, 1990.

The Workshop Group. Reducing Deaths from breast cancer in Canada. Can Med Ass J 1989; 141: 199-201.

6 The USSR/Germany/WHO BSE Study and Global Strategies for the Control of Breast Cancer

V. KOROLTCHOUK*

Cancer and Palliative Care Unit, World Health Organization, Geneva
* On behalf of the WHO Study Group (Prof V Semiglazov, Dr V Sagaidak, Dr V Moiseyenko, Dr E Mikhailov, Prof A B Miller, Dr J Stjernsward, Dr K Stanley, Dr A Tsiatis, Prof K Ebeling, Dr P Nischan and Dr I Mittra).

1 INCIDENCE, MORTALITY AND TRENDS

In most developed and many developing countries, breast cancer is the most frequent cancer and the leading cause of cancer death in women (Stanley et al, 1987). Towards the end of this century, about 730,000 women a year will develop breast cancer, 362,000 of them in developed and 368,000 in developing countries. At present, more than 40% of all breast cancers are found in developing countries, but the incidence pattern is progressively approaching that of the developed countries, and it is predicted that by the year 2000 more than 50% of breast cancers will occur in developing countries (Koroltchouk et al, 1990).

Breast cancer mortality, especially in European countries, has been gradually increasing (Figures 1-3). The major exceptions among the industrialized countries are Canada, the Nordic countries and the US; in these countries in particular, the public has been educated on the value of early detection, and limited screening programmes have been conducted.

The widely discussed benefits due to advances in breast-cancer treatment, (if they exist) have not yet been seen in the national mortality statistics of Australia, Italy and the UK, although investigators in these countries were major participants in clinical research to develop them (Granroth et al, 1988).

2 STRATEGIES FOR CONTROL OF BREAST CANCER

In the development of guidelines for the early detection of breast cancer WHO emphasizes the importance of widespread coverage of high-risk groups (as opposed to repetitive screening of low-risk groups) as the key factor for early detection to be effective. Most breast cancer studies are presently done in developed countries because for many years to come few, if any, of the developing countries will be able to establish national programmes with enough coverage for screening to be effective. In the meantime, approaches are being investigated to evaluate down-staging by physical examination and BSE, and to implement efficient curative therapies.

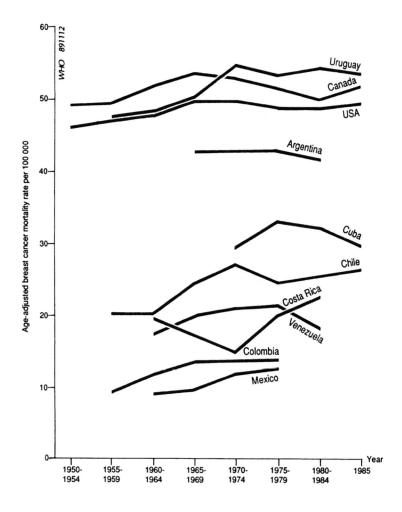

Figure 1   Breast cancer mortality trends (age-adjusted rates for ages 35-69 years): Region of the Americas.

Breast cancer mortality can be further reduced by the use of systemic adjuvant therapies to surgery or radiotherapy by at least 20-25% regardless of menopausal, nodal and/or estrogen-receptor status.

It is well known that more than two-thirds of breast cancers occur in women over age 50. This group is best served by the use of adjuvant tamoxifen, an anti-estrogen with few side effects, suitable to being administered by medical personnel with minimal training and experience. It can be taken for long periods without monitoring or frequent follow-up.

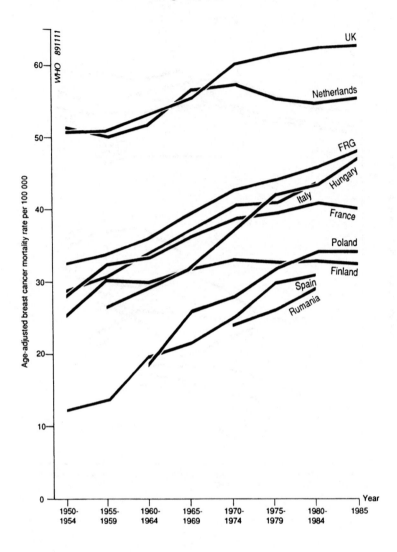

Figure 2   Breast cancer mortality trends (age-adjusted rates for ages 35-
                   69 years): European Region.

On the other hand, although chemotherapy is more toxic and its administration requires somewhat greater skills, it, too, can be readily administered at the community level in most parts of the world.

The effectiveness of tamoxifen for post-operative adjuvant therapy in the treatment of primary breast cancer with or without pathologic involvement of the axillary lymph nodes has been rather well established, so that it can be recommended as public-health policy at national and community levels.

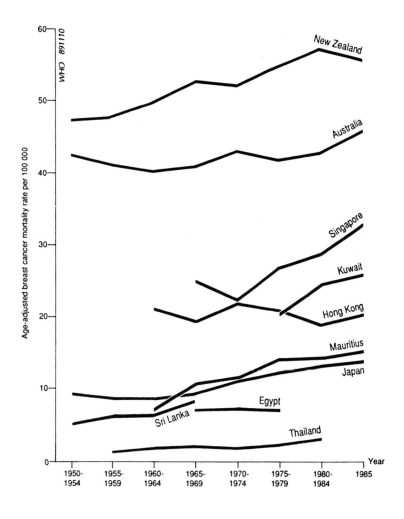

Figure 3   Breast Cancer mortality trends (age-adjusted rates for ages 35-69 years): other regions.

Further research is needed to a) more accurately identify combinations of first-generation prognostic factors (receptor status, tumour size, pathologic parameters of the high-risk group for recurrence), and for second-generation factors (DNA ploidy and S-phase, oncogene amplification and expression and other); and b) establish rational approaches for real progress in the adjuvant treatment of node-negative breast-cancer patients. Despite these research needs, we are now ready for the implementation of clear recommendations for adjuvant treatment at the community and national levels in order to obtain a worthwhile reduction in breast-cancer mortality.

Palliation, not prolongation of survival, is the principal goal of therapy for the other 50% or less of patients with cancer in advanced, incurable and metastatic disease. A response to therapy is associated with an improvement of quality of life, and this may result in a small prolongation of survival as well. Palliation of the symptoms may be achieved with the appropriate use of analgesics, with radiation to bone and brain metastases, by surgical excision of local recurrences, or by the administration of systemic therapy. The latter, including both endocrine and chemotherapy, is the mainstay of most palliative programmes.

The WHO Expert Committee Meeting on Cancer Pain Relief and Active Supportive Care (July 1989, Geneva) recommended that palliative care, cancer pain relief and terminal care should be an integral part of the national health policy of each country. They should be incorporated as a comprehensive approach into existing health-care systems of countries, in order to achieve a state of complete physical, psychological, spiritual and social well-being for the highest possible quality of life for the patient and his family. Pain relief must be made freely available – much more so than at present, when often legislative obstacles and widespread lack of symptom-management training prevent the adequate use of drugs, and thus leave terminal patients bereft of comfort or dignity.

Table 1   Breast Cancer Staging.

Countries	I	II	STAGES (%) III	IV	Unknown
China (Shanghai, 1986)	21	50	25	4	
India (Bombay, 1984)	5	14	36	24	21
Indonesia (Jakarta, 1988)			> 86 incurable		
Puerto Rico (1976)	5	38	44	7	7
Yugoslavia (Slovenia, 1986)		33	52	13	3
USA (SEER, 1987)		49	41	7	3
USSR (1986)	13	38	39	10	
New Zealand (1986)	46	25	17	7	5

3 EARLY DETECTION

Due to absence of public education programmes the lack of resources available for early detection, the great majority of all breast-cancer patients in developing countries will not be diagnosed until the disease has reached an advanced incurable stage (Table 1). Under these conditions, early detection will be the most important approach for improving the effect of therapy. The greatest decrease in breast cancer mortality is likely to derive from treatment at an earlier stage. Once a women is diagnosed as having breast cancer, her chance of surviving the next five years is approximately 75% in the US (Table 2).

Table 2   Stage and five-year survival rate (%).

| Country | All Stages | STAGE | | | | |
		I	II	III	IV	Unkn.
Egypt	46	80	52	42	14	
USSR	55	86	68	39	12	
USA	75		90	68	18	46
China	61					

However, the prognosis directly depends upon the stage of the cancer at time of diagnosis. As indicated in Table 1, about half of the cases in industrialized countries are diagnosed as having local disease (Stage I and II), where the five-year survival rate is approximately 90%. In the other half of the cases, the disease will have spread to the lymph nodes or beyond; in the US, these cases have a survival rate of 68% for Stage III and 18% for Stage IV.

In the data from the National Cancer Institute of Egypt, the corresponding five-year survival rates were found to be 80%, 52%, 42% and 14% for stages I, II, III and IV, respectively (Omar et al, 1988). In India, the five-year survival rate is 40.8%. The first-year mortality figure of 21% in Greater Bombay was more than four times higher than that of 4.7% in the United States (Mittra et al, 1989).

Three basic techniques for early detection have been developed: mammography, physical examination by health professionals and breast self-examination by women (BSE). The reported results indicate that screening with mammography with or without physical examination can reduce mortality (Table 3).

The main barriers for implementation of national screening programmes are two-fold. First, it is uncertain if the results of early detection programmes by specialized teams is reproducible at the national level. The second impediment is the high cost for imaging technologies. For these reasons, breast-cancer screening programmes involving mammography and other imaging technologies cannot be adopted in most countries as a routine public health activity.

Breast self-examination has been suggested as a practical solution. Though reported as not being as effective as mammography or an examination by a trained nurse or physician, it

Table 3 Randomized controlled studies of breast cancer screening.

Countries	Age Group	Mammography	BSE*	BPE*	Reduction in Mortality (%) 5-10 years	10 years	18 years
USA	50-64	2-view	–	+	40	32	21
(HIP)	40-49	2-view	–	+	0	0	24
Canada	50-59	2-view	+	+	–	–	–
(NBSS)	40-49	2-view	+	+	–	–	–
Sweden	70-74	1-view	–	–	–	19	–
(2-county)	60-69	1-view	–	–	–	41	–
	50-59	1-view	–	–	–	38	–
	40-49	1-view	–	–	–	6	–
Sweden	55-69	2-view	–	–	20	–	–
(Malmö)	45-54	2-view	–	–	0	–	–
USSR/Germany	40-64	–	+	–	–	–	–
(WHO)							

*BSE = breast self-examination, BPE = breast physical examination

may be a cost-effective screening method, particularly for countries which otherwise cannot afford to screen the whole female population at risk. BSE has been thought to be useful and that its practise has no significant adverse consequences. Despite this generally favourable view, the major question of the precise influence of BSE on mortality from breast cancer remains to be answered. This can only be achieved through a prospective study with careful attention to research design and methodology, evaluating the effect on mortality from breast cancer.

4 THE USSR/GERMANY/WHO BSE STUDY

The first prospective randomized controlled trial of BSE was initiated by WHO in 1985 with colleagues in Leningrad and Moscow. The major objective of the study is to determine the effect of a breast self-examination programme on mortality from breast cancer. Leningrad and Moscow were ideal sites for this study due to:

     a)   high rates of breast cancer

     b)   availability of high quality diagnosis and treatment facilities; and

     c)   very low public awareness of the value of early detection and consequently low rates of such activities.

In Leningrad, the study was implemented through 18 district polyclinics and ten large enterprise clinics. In Moscow, more than 200 factories and other institutions were randomly assigned to either BSE education or control. More than 200,000 women aged 40-64 years have been enrolled in the BSE and control groups. In Moscow, the education programme is based on a two-way communications principle with education in groups of up to 20 individuals. Feedback is through specially designed personal calendars filled out by the study participants based on the calendars pioneered by Dr G Gastrin in Finland. In Leningrad, individual and small-group instruction is provided by trained nurses or doctors. The teaching session always includes a demonstration of BSE technique on one of the women. At the end of each session, each woman fills in a questionnaire (concerned with demographic data and risk factors) and receives a leaflet and BSE follow-up calendar with the doctor's address and consulting hours. Posters and local broadcasting are employed selectively, and calendars renewed and the entries reviewed on an annual basis.

Women who detect symptoms of breast disease are referred for examination, diagnosis and treatment, if necessary. This referral is carried out according to a standard scheme which makes use of the existing health-care structure and specialized services. Since methods of treatment of cancer patients in oncological dispensaries and institutions in the USSR are rather uniform, special conditions for cancer cases from the study setting were not required. It is expected that more than 1622 patients will develop breast cancer during the study. Their follow-up will continue for ten years after their diagnosis date to determine the mortality pattern.

Table 4 USSR/Germany/WHO BSE study accrual.

Year	Moscow	Number accrued: Leningrad	Germany	Total
1985	12,535	49,802	–	62,337
1986	12,264	40,170	–	52,434
1987	22,618	19,082	–	41,700
1988	18,603	11,256	–	29,859
1989	11,553	8,700	12,000	32,253
Predicted future accrual:				
1990	8,427	–	38,000	46,427
1991	–	–	50,000	50,000
1992	–	–	50,000	50,000
Total	86,000	129,010	150,000	365,010

It was originally planned to enrol 225,000 women into the USSR/WHO BSE study to have sufficient power to answer the question as to whether a BSE programme could reduce breast cancer mortality. This was for an estimated compliance of BSE of at least 75%, but, in practice, compliance was lower than expected. The study has therefore been expanded to Germany, where another 150,000 women will be enrolled (Table 4). With an accrual of 365,000 women, the USSR/Germany/WHO study will have more then sufficient power to detect a mortality reduction of 30%, and moderate to good power to detect a 20% reduction, depending on the BSE compliance achieved.

5 PRELIMINARY RESULTS OF THE USSR/GERMANY/WHO BSE STUDY

In preliminary data from Leningrad (Semiglazov and Moiseyenko, 1987) during the first two years of the study, 89,972 women were enrolled, 44,890 in the control group. During this period, 1840 (4,1%) of the women in the BSE group and 366 (0,80%) of the women in the control group appealed to oncologists for consultation (Figure 4). The more than five-fold difference in consultation rates between the BSE and control groups shows that a wide-scale programme of BSE education is accompanied by an increase in the numbers seeking help from specialists. Breast cancer was diagnosed in 50 patients of the target group and 32 patients of the control group.

A difference in the extent of disease involvement in the cases diagnosed as breast cancer is apparent. The average size of the tumours detected was 1.3 cm smaller in the BSE group. Tumours larger than 5 cm were more than twice as common the control group (37.5% versus 16.4%). The average size of the primary tumour in the BSE group in this study was larger than that seen in other investigations (Huguley and Brown, 1981; Philip et al, 1984).

Compliance in performing BSE was monitored by interviewing 400 women selected at random from the BSE group. A total of 27.8% of the women in the feasibility phase practised BSE 12 or more times per year; this frequency was maintained by 31.5% and 55% after six months and 12 months, respectively. The compliance rate 12 months after BSE teaching were similar to those reported in other studies of BSE (Philip et al, 1984; Baines et al, 1986) and are sufficiently high to demonstrate the effectiveness of this education programme.

The study has so far demonstrated:
> a) the feasibility and effectiveness of the BSE education programme as measured by the frequency and technique of performance of BSE,
> b) a substantial increase in the number of cases of breast   abnormalities detected,
> c) a shortening of the time between detection and the visit to the   doctor, and
> d) a shift to an earlier stage of disease in the cases diagnosed with breast cancer. As this study continues, it will be possible to objectively determine the degree of reduction in breast cancer morality, if any, resulting from the practice of BSE and whether or not BSE should be incorporated into community based programmes for the early detection of this disease.

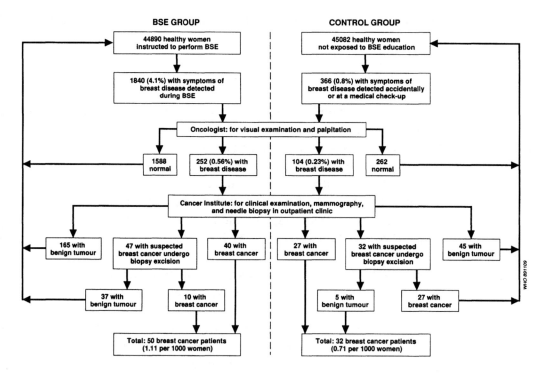

Figure 4   USSR/WHO prospective controlled trial of BSE: steps of referral and examination results of women in the BSE and control groups in Leningrad.

6 OTHER INTERNATIONAL BSE AND PHYSICAL EXAMINATION STUDIES (BPE)

A WHO multi-centre investigation has been proposed to evaluate whether physical examination of the breasts combined with the teaching of BSE reduces mortality from breast cancer. In this approach we are relying upon the evidence from the ongoing Canadian National Breast Screening Study that has suggested that a major part of the benefit in the reduction of breast cancer mortality may be derived from the physical examination, when comparing its role with mammography and BSE (Miller, 1989; Baines et al, 1989). Furthermore, with increasing expertise gained by interest, special training, and experience, clinical examination alone may detect as high a number as 80% of all breast cancers (Hansel et al, 1988).

The study would only be conducted in areas where there are good medical facilities, and a well-developed cancer registry. Participation is pending from some Latin American countries, and the Philippines. It may well be possible to include this group in a combined study. In Greater Bombay, India, a two year feasibility/a pilot study is planned on physical examination of the breast, conducted at regular intervals by trained female paramedical personnel as part of a community based public health and education programme (Mittra and Daniel, 1989).

Most breast-cancer therapy can be given at the community level, and does not require highly specialized physicians. Almost all endocrine therapy and chemotherapy can be given by surgeons, radiotherapists and family doctors. However, a network of regional cancer centres with radiotherapy units (and possibly a few national research centres as well) should be available, ideally, as back-up to community hospitals and clinics. Nevertheless, adjuvant breast cancer treatment can be efficiently given in a community setting by appropriately trained but non-specialized doctors and nursing personnel. For much of the developing world, where ideal medical infrastructure will not be available for some decades to come, tamoxifen and adjuvant chemotherapy should be given priority as a breast cancer treatment goal. They can save medical resources as well as lives.

A high priority of the WHO cancer control programme is an outreach approach that facilitates worldwide access to cancer therapies of proven value. The greatest decrease in breast cancer mortality is likely to derive from effective treatment at an earlier stage. Therefore, the first priority in national health programmes for breast cancer is to encourage patients to present for diagnosis and treatment at an earlier stage of the disease. All three main elements - public education, early detection and locally available treatment - must be part of a national comprehensive programme for the control of breast cancer.

REFERENCES

Baines CJ, Miller AB, Bassett AA. Physical examination. Its role as a single screening modality in the Canadian National Breast Screening Study. Cancer 1989; 63:1816-1822.

Baines CJ, Wall C, Risch HA et al. Changes in breast self-examination behaviour in a cohort of 8214 women in the Canadian National Breast Screening Study. Cancer 1986; 57:1209-1216.

Bonadonna G, Valagussa P. Current status of adjuvant chemotherapy for breast cancer seminars in oncology. 1987; 14:8-22.

Early Breast Cancer triallists' collaborative group. Effects of adjuvant tamoxifen and of cytotoxie therapy on mortality in early breast cancer. An overview of 61 randomized trials among 28,896 women. New Engl J Med 1988; 319:1681-1692.

Granroth H, Stanley K, Lopez AD. Time trends in mortality from cancer. In WHO Technical Document. Can/88.4. Geneva, World Health Organization, 1988.

Hansel DM et al. The accuracy of mammography alone and combined with clinical exam and cytology in the detection of breast cancer. Clin Radiol 1988; 39:150-153.

Huguley CM, Brown RL. The value of breast self-examination. Cancer 1981; 47:989-995.

Koroltchouk V, Stanley K, Stjernswärd J. The control of breast cancer. A World Health Organization Perspective. Cancer; 1990, 65:2803-2810.

Miller AB. The Canadian National Breast Screening Study. In: Day NE, Miller AB (eds). Screening for Breast Cancer. Toronto: Hans Huber, 1988, pp 51-58.

Mittra I, Bade RA, Desai PB et al. Early detection of breast cancer in developing countries. Lancet 1989; April i: 719- 720.

Mittra I, Daniel EE. A pilot/feasibility study on the effectiveness of physical examination and teaching of breast self-examination in reducing mortality from breast cancer in Greater Bombay. Tata Memorial Hospital, Bombay, 1989.

Omar Sh, Genin J, Contesso G et al. Staging of breast cancer and end results of therapy. In: Contesso G, Omar Sh (eds). Breast Cancer. London: Korba (International), 1988, pp 33-44.

Philip J, Harris WG, Flaherty C et al. Breast self-examination: clinical results from a population based prospective study. Brit J Cancer 1984; 50:7-12.

Semiglazov VF, Moiseyenko VM. Breast self-examination for the early detection of breast cancer: a USSR/WHO controlled trial in Leningrad. Bulletin of the World Health Organization 1987; 65:391-396.

Senn HJ, Barett-Mahler AR, Jungi WF et al. Adjuvant chemoimmunotherapy with LMF and BCG in node-negative and node-positive breast cancer patients: 10 years results. Eur J Cancer Clin Oncol 1989; 25:513-525.

Stanley K, Stjernswärd J, Koroltchouk V. Women and cancer. WHO Health Statistics, Quarterly 1987; 40:267-278.

7 A Cost-Effectiveness Approach to Breast Cancer Screening

J. D. F. HABBEMA, B. M. VAN INEVELD and H. J. DE KONING

Department of Public Health and Social Medicine, Erasmus University, Rotterdam, The Netherlands

1 INTRODUCTION

The decision to implement breast cancer screening should rest on the judgment that its benefits and savings outweigh its costs and risks. Such a judgment is by no means trivial. For breast cancer, we are in the comfortable position that it has been shown that screening by modern mammography is effective in reducing breast cancer mortality, at least in the age group over 50 (Andersson et al, 1988; Tabar et al, 1989). When there is no such indication of effectiveness, the answer is easy: one should not consider screening as a valuable health care service.

There are three related types of analysis for assessing relationships between costs, risks and health benefits (Drummond et al,1987; Warner and Luce,1982). All three types rest on the interdisciplinary research of medical researchers and economists. Other disciplines may contribute as well. The first type of analysis is called cost-effectiveness analysis (CEA). In this case, one effect measure is chosen, e.g. life-years gained, and the analysis tries to answer what the costs of screening are and the effects. For costs one should ideally think of social costs as "opportunity costs", i.e. benefits forgone because the resources are not used for other excellent purposes. Social costs may be quite different from financial streams. A second type of analysis is called cost-utility analysis (CUA). This type of analysis arises when one is not satisfied with expressing the health benefits and risks of screening in only one effect measure. In cost-utility analysis, several effect measures are weighted in order to arrive at one overall measure for the health effects of screening, called the utility. The best known example of a utility measure is "quality adjusted life years" or QALY's. In this case the life-years lived are weighted by the quality in which these years are spend. At the last there is cost-benefit analysis (CBA). In this case the costs and utility from the cost-utility analysis are traded off by fixing a price value for one unit of utility. Most analyses carried out thus far are cost-effectiveness analysis. We too will present a cost-effectiveness analysis. See however the discussion.

When a cost-effectiveness analysis is supplemented by a number of other considerations, like organisational aspects, impact on the health care needs and demands, legal and ethical issues, etc, it may be called a "medical technology assessment" (Institute of Medicine, 1985).

Two types of cost-effectiveness analysis calculations can roughly be distinguished. The first one considers an idealised birth cohort that is followed from birth to death. This analysis gives useful insight, and is easy to interpret from an epidemiological point of view. The second approach, the one we will follow, is a real-time, real-population approach. In this case a dynamic population is followed over time, including mortality and births. Moreover, the situation concerning the disease is assessed at the start of the screening, and future time trends are superimposed on it.

The second type of cost-effectiveness analysis is more complex than the first type (in practice, one usually starts with exploratory cohort calculations, even when real population analysis is the aim). But it has a number of advantages. The results of a real-population analysis are more readily useful for policy advise. They will provoke more discussion from people involved, because it is so close to their reality. It is also easier to assess impact on needs and demands in the health care system. Moreover it is a natural first step towards later evaluation and monitoring. Because the real-population type cost-effectiveness analysis requires extensive calculations, we have developed a computer programme MISCAN (Micro-simulation Screening Analysis) which simulates individual life histories of women according to specified assumptions, including the natural history of cancer and the impact of screening (Habbema et al, 1984; Habbema et al, 1987).

The present paper discusses the lines along which such cost-effectiveness analysis has been carried out by the technology assessment task force for breast cancer screening.[1] Organisation and decision making concerning breast cancer screening has been considered in another paper (Habbema and Koning, 1990). The main results of the cost-effectiveness analysis, as based on an interim report (Maas et al, 1988), have been reported elsewhere (Maas et al, 1989). Recently, a final report of the study has appeared (Koning et al, 1990). The present paper focuses less on results but more on the phases a cost-effectiveness analysis has to go through before it is completed, and the types of assumptions that have to be made during the analysis. If not otherwise indicated, results come from the two reports.

2 THE ANALYSIS PHASE

A cost-effectiveness analysis should in the first place be based on the current knowledge of the epidemiology and the natural history of disease, its pre-clinical stages, and the impact of screening. Therefore, a cost-effectiveness analysis can usefully be broken down into two broad phases: an analysis phase in which current knowledge is synthesized and an evaluation phase, in which costs and effects of options are calculated (Habbema, 1983). These are, A: ANALYSIS, in which validated assumptions on disease process and screening are obtained and B: PROSPECTIVE EVALUATION, in which the costs, risks and benefits of screening policies are assessed. MISCAN is the name of the computer program which is used for the calculations. (Figure 1)

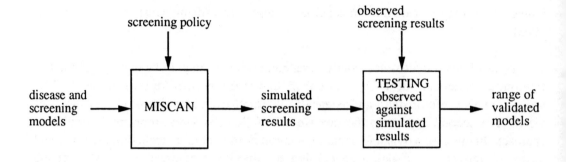

A: ANALYSIS

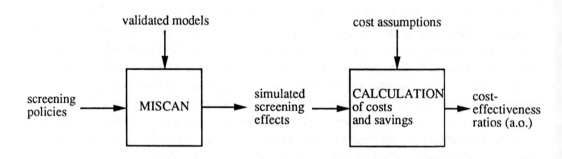

B: PROSPECTIVE EVALUATION

Figure 1. The two phases of a cost-effectiveness analysis of screening.

In the analysis phase, the results of screening trials are analyzed in order to draw conclusions on the underlying processes concerning disease and screening. In the case of breast cancer screening, use is made of the HIP randomised trial, of the mortality reduction results of the recent trials in Sweden and of the studies in Utrecht and Nijmegen in the Netherlands.

Table 1 shows some main results concerning the disease process derived from the analysis. Assumptions concerning: A. Duration of pre-clinical disease stage, B. Sensitivity of single view, oblique mammography, and C. Mortality reduction are presented. These assumptions were derived in the analysis phase of the cost-effectiveness study for breast cancer screening. For a full description of the analysis see Oortmarssen et al (1990).

Table 1   Assumptions derived in the analysis phase of the cost-effectiveness study for breast cancer screening.

A: Average duration of the total preclinical screen detectable stage

AGE	AVERAGE DURATION (years)
40	1.9
50	2.3
60	2.9
70	4.1

B: Sensitivity of mammography

dCIS	40%
< 10 mm	70%
10-19 mm	95%
$\geq$ 20 mm	95%

C: Reduction in probability of death when breast cancer is early detected

size at detection	reduction in probability
< 10 mm	64%
10-19 mm	60%
$\geq$ 20 mm	48%

3 ASSUMPTIONS FOR THE EVALUATION PHASE

In the evaluation phase, different screening policies have to be assessed for their costs, risks, benefits and other consequences. This requires a large number of other assumptions. The main ones concern:

3.1 Period of Screening

It is assumed that screening will take place during the period 1990-2017 in the Netherlands.

3.2 Base-case

The future developments in case of screening should always be compared with what would happen if there were no screening. We assumed that present age-specific rates of mammographic examination in the Netherlands will also apply during the period 1990-2017.

3.3 Situation at Start

It is assumed that age specific incidence, stage-distribution at clinical surfacing and stage-specific survival will remain at the 1988 level during the whole period of screening. We assume a population dynamics according to the middle scenario of the Dutch Central Bureau of Statistics.

3.4 Build Up Phase

It is assumed that during the period 1990-1994 the whole of the Netherlands will gradually be covered by a network of screening units. The screening units will be fixed, mobile or semi-mobile, depending on the population density in the area.

3.5 Diagnostic and Treatment Protocols

National average treatment protocols have been derived. These are based on current practice, and on opinions about changes in the near future. The protocols indicate what the chances of different treatment modalities are for each clinical stage.

3.6 Costs

Detailed cost studies have been undertaken. From a economic point of view, costs can be broken down in direct costs and indirect costs. Direct costs can again be split up in medical costs and other costs. Indirect costs have as components production losses and medical costs during life-years gained. In our cost-effectiveness analysis we only consider the medical costs of screening, diagnostics and treatment for breast cancer. In this way costs of organisation and execution of the screening programme, including evaluation, have been estimated. Costs of different diagnostic and therapeutic procedures and costs of treatment of end-stage disseminated breast cancer are also assessed. The influence of the three other cost-components has been studied in a sensitivity-analysis

3.7 Discount Rate

In accordance with several recommendations, including those of the Dutch government, a yearly discount rate of 5% has been applied to both costs and effects (Russel, 1987).

3.8 Attendance Rates

In accordance with what has been observed in the field-studies in the Netherlands, attendance is taken to be 75% for women under 50, slowly decreasing to 65% at age 70 and steeply decreasing over 70, to 45% at age 75. Attendance rates differ widely between women who did or did not attend the previous screening. Attenders attendance is 85% and non-attenders attendance 25%.

4 SOME RESULTS

A number of possible screening strategies have been evaluated prospectively, using the assumptions from sections 2 and 3. The four main policies concern screening between ages 50 and 70. They differ in the frequency of screening: 5, 10, 15 and 20 screenings during these 20 years. We will first consider the results for the 10 screenings policy which has finally been adopted in the Netherlands. Screening takes place at ages 51, 53, 55, 57, 59, 61, 63, 65, 67 and 69. Mortality reduction gradually builds up after the start of the screening. After about 20 years, mortality reduction will be greatest. There will be 700 breast cancer deaths less in the Netherlands, or about 16% of what total breast cancer mortality would have been in the case of no screening. Note that 700 is a larger number than the total cervical cancer mortality would be in the absence of screening.

Table 2 reviews all main favourable and unfavourable effects of screening. The numbers concern the total programme over the whole period of the screening programme from 1990-2017 (a), and the average numbers per million total female population per year of screening (b).

Table 2 A review of favourable and unfavourable effects induced by breast cancer screening in the Netherlands. 1990-2017.

	(a) Total number	(b) Per million women per year
Favourable effects		
less deaths	17,000	84
life years saved	260,000	1,284
less treatment advanced disease	17,000	84
less adjuvant therapies	8,300	41
less breast amputations	11,900	59
less biopsies outside screening	50,500	249
Unfavourable effects		
screening investigations	15,800,000	78,024
lead-time life-years with brst ca	275,000	1,358
negative biopsies	33,000	163
more surgical treatments	9,200	45
more radiotherapies	10,300	51
radiation deaths	60	0.3
life-years lost by radiation	400	2.0

Favourable effects are clearly dominated by the life-years saved. But a number of other effects are also non-negligible. Unfavourable effects include the large number of screening investigations, earlier labelling of cancer patients because of the lead time effect, some induced diagnostics and treatment and a relatively small number of radiation induced cancer deaths.

Table 3 gives the total costs and effects for the four screening policies. Costs refer to the total costs of screening and its induced diagnostic and treatment costs, compared to the situation of no screening. A 5% discount has been applied to costs and effects. Observe the rapid increase in marginal cost-effectiveness ratio when the screening programme is intensified to more than 10 screenings within the age range 50 to 70.

Table 3   Costs, effects, cost-effectiveness and marginal cost-effectiveness of screening for breast cancer in the Netherlands, 50 to 70 years, 1990-2017.

Invitations	5	10	15	20
Total costs (mln.Dfl.)	272	466	657	831
Life-years saved	40000	61000	70000	74000
Costs/lys	6900	7650	9390	11200
Marginal costs/lys	6900	9100	21100	41000

5 DISCUSSION

5.1 The Interpretation of Cost-effectiveness

The cost-effectiveness ratio describes the relationship between the social costs of a screening programme on the one hand and the public health effects in terms of life-years saved on the other. From Table 3, we can only compare screening options between ages 50 and 70. In this internal comparison, it is clear that the ratio between costs and effects is relatively favourable for 5 or 10 screenings, and becomes progressively more unfavourable with larger numbers. So, 10 screenings appears a reasonable choice from this internal comparison. However, breast cancer screening is only one of the very many health care procedures. And it could be that even the relatively favourable ratios for 5 and 10 screenings are far worse than those of most other health care services. Or, the other way round, the higher ratios for 15 or even 20 screenings might prove to be more favourable than those of many other services. Ideally, all health care services should be assessed on their costs, risks and benefits, in order to make a rational ordering and choice possible. This is not yet the case. Cost-effectiveness ratios have only been calculated for a few services. We ourselves did extensive studies for cervical cancer screening, liver transplantation and heart transplantation. Within this small group of 4 services, breast cancer screening was clearly the most rewarding service in terms of cost-effectiveness ratio. Even the marginal cost-effectiveness of going from 10 to 15 screenings compares favourably with efficient policies for cervical cancer screening, liver transplantation and heart transplantation.

5.2 Have We Been too Optimistic?

We have been assuming that the build up of the screening and the organisation and execution afterwards will not meet any major problems. We may have been too optimistic in these or other respects. Here, the advantages of following a real-population approach pay off: we have made predictions in such a detail that monitoring of the actual progress of the screening programme will enable us to get an early warning of too optimistic or too pessimistic assumptions. Suggestions for improvement can then be made. Also, cost-effectiveness ratios may easily be recalculated for the adjusted assumptions.

5.3 Sensitivity Analysis

Most assumptions have their associated uncertainty. Therefore we have been studying the sensitivity of our conclusions with respect to the assumptions made. Major sensitivity analyses concern the attendance rates and the improvement in prognosis with early detection: there is a considerable difference in mortality reduction between the Swedish two counties trial and the Malmö trial (Andersson et al, 1988; Tabar et al,1989). Discussing the results of the sensitivity analyses is beyond the scope of this paper, but the importance of carrying out detailed sensitivity analyses cannot be stressed enough.

5.4 Quality of Life Considerations

It can rightly be argued that not only life-years gained should be considered but also the quality of these life-years. This would lead us to calculate quality adjusted life-years, and would bring us from cost-effectiveness analysis to cost-utility analysis. Indeed, a first effort has been made to assess quality of life changes induced by a screening programme. Results will be published elsewhere. Our studies did not indicate any major change in conclusion by moving from life-years gained to quality adjusted life-years gained.

5.5 Impact on Health Care Demand

The impact of screening on the demand of different diagnostic and therapeutic procedures has been assessed (Koning et al, 1990b). The most important conclusion from this part of the study was that the already overloaded radiotherapy departments in the Netherlands will experience extra demand for breast cancer radiotherapy in the order of magnitude of 30 to 40 percent. This is caused by a shift from complete mastectomy to breast conserving therapy, and by the fact that a large number of cancers are diagnosed during the prevalence screen. Thus, after 1997, when the prevalence screen is over, the workload will be reduced somewhat.

5.6 Transfer to Other Countries/Regions

The real-time, real-population approach lends itself very well to transfer of the cost-effectiveness analysis to other countries. It can be decided for each assumption if it can be maintained or that new country/specific values should be inserted. For example, during the first half of 1990, breast cancer screening in Australia has been evaluated in a joint project with the University of Sidney and the National Institute of Health in Australia. It was decided to leave the deep assumptions on disease model, sensitivity of the screening test, and the improvement of prognosis after screening unchanged. But a number of other assumptions were changed considerably, including those on costs of screening and costs of treatment (report in preparation). Presently, the possibility of cost-effectiveness analysis in other countries is being explored.

6 CONCLUSION

A cost-effectiveness analysis in the sense described in this paper is a useful addition to other research in the field of cancer screening. Some of the advantages are the following:

1. Maybe its most importance function is that it serves as an integrative framework. Seemingly disparate facts can be connected with each other, and discussion between different disciplines involved in screening is stimulated.

2. A cost-effectiveness analysis may reveal gaps in knowledge, which have to be filled in order to evaluated screening properly. In this way, applied research can be proposed that fills these gaps most efficiently.

3. The relationship between social costs of a programme and population health effects is explored in detail. Only in this way, health services can ultimately be compared in order to chose rationally a socially most desirable package of services.

4. By making detailed predictions over the years to come, an important ingredient for a future monitoring system is provided.

The uniform approach to evaluation in the cost-effectiveness study makes a comparison between different health care services possible. In the long run, this will enhance a more rational approach to decision making in health care.

Acknowledgements
The Dutch technology assessment task-force for breast cancer screening consists of:
H.J. de Koning[1], Drs. B.M. Ineveld[1], Ir. G.J. van Oortmarssen[1], Ir. R. Boer[1], Prof.dr. H.J.A. Collette[4], Dr. A.L.M. Verbeek[2], Dr. J.H.C.L. Hendriks[3], A.E. de Bruyn[1], Drs. H.M.E. van Agt[1], Dr. J.C.J.M. de Haes[1], L. van der Zwan[1], Drs. M.A. Koopmanschap[1], Dr. J.J.M. Deurenberg[4], Prof.dr. J.D.F. Habbema[1], Prof.dr. P.J. van der Maas[1] (project-leader)

[1] Instituut Maatschappelijke Gezondheidszorg, Erasmus Universiteit Rotterdam
[2] Instituut Sociale Geneeskunde/[3] Instituut Radiodiagnostiek, Katholieke Universiteit Nijmegen
[4] Prevention, Vakgroep Algemene Gezondheidszorg en Epidemiologie, Rijksuniversiteit Utrecht

REFERENCES

Andersson I, Aspegren K, Janzon L, et al. Mammographic screening and mortality from breast cancer: the Malmö mammographic screening tiral. Br Med J 1988; 297: 943-948.

Institute of Medicine. Assessing Medical Technologies. Washington: National Academy Press, 1985.

Drummond MF, Stoddart GL, Torrance GW. Methods for the economic evaluation of health care programmes. Oxford: Oxford University press, 1987.

Habbema JDF, Lubbe JThN, Maas PJ van der et al. A computer simulation approach to the evaluation of mass screening. MEDINFO-83. JH van Bemmel, MJ Bal, O Wigertz (eds). North-Holland, Amsterdam 1983: 1222-1225.

Habbema JDF, van Oortmarssen GJ, Lubbe JThN et al. The MISCAN simulation program for the evaluation of screening for disease. Comput Meth Progr Biomed 1984; 20: 79-93.

Habbema JDF, Lubbe JThN, van Oortmarssen GJ et al. A simulation approach to cost effectiveness and cost benefit calculations of screening for early detection of disease. Eur J Oper Res 1987; 29: 159-166.

Habbema JDF, Koning HJ de. Breast cancer screening in the Netherlands. To appear in the Proceedings of the December 1988 workshop on Information Systems in breast cancer detection, M Greberman, PC Prorok and S Shapiro, eds, 1990.

Koning HJ de, Inveveld BM van, Oortmarssen GJ van, et al. The costs and effects of mass screening for breast cancer. (in Dutch) Final report, Erasmus University Rotterdam, 1990, ISBN 90-72245-50-4.

Koning HJ de, van Oortmarssen GJ, van Ineveld BM, et al. Breast cancer screening: its impact on clinical medicine. Br J Cancer 1990b; 61: 292-297.

Maas PJ van der, Ineveld M van, Oortmarssen GJ van, et al. The costs and effects of mass screening for breast cancer. Technical Report, Erasmus University Rotterdam, 1988, ISBN 90-72245-03-2.

Maas PJ van der, de Koning HJ, van Ineveld BM. The cost-effectiveness of breast cancer screening. Int J Cancer 1989; 43: 1055-1060.

Oortmarssen GJ van, Habbema JDF, Maas PJ van der, et al. A model for breast cancer screening. Cancer 1990, in press.

Russel LB. Evaluating preventive care. Washington: The Brookings Institute, 1987.

Tabár L, Fagerberg G, Duffy SW et al. The Swedish two county trial of mammographic screening for breast cancer: recent results and calculation of benefit. J Epidemiol Comm Hlth 1989; 43: 107-114.

Warner KE, Luce BR. Cost-benefit and cost-effectiveness analysis in health care. Ann Arbor: Health Administration Press, 1982.

8 Summary of the Discussion on Breast Cancer Screening

There is a problem in conveying understandable information on available knowledge to politicians and the public to ensure that appropriate decisions are made on policy. This has been exacerbated by the tendency in some countries to conduct pilot studies essentially restricted to the prevalence screen. Such studies may give an over-optimistic estimate of the effect, especially if in situ cancers are included in the count of cancers detected. At the very least the interval cancers occurring after the first screen should be identified and the proportionate incidence computed so that it can be compared with that of other programmes of known effectiveness. These problems may be particularly acute in relation to the demand for screening women under the age of 50, currently fuelled in many countries by inappropriate recommendations from prestigious bodies in the United States. Even in countries such as Canada that have taken a decision to restrict invitations to screening to women over the age of 50 it has been decided to allow women under the age of 50 who present at screening centres to be screened. This was avoided in Finland, where it was explained that funds were only available in the public system to screen women in the invited birth cohorts. The public concern over this has now largely dissipated.

In the Swedish 2-county (WE) trial publicity was used to persuade the control groups to accept no mammography, and the randomized controlled trial design. Mammography was available if judged clinically necessary for the controls, 13% had mammography. The randomization process was open in that the public knew about it and a politician was invited to perform the randomization process. Once the results were available in the first report in the Lancet a decision was taken to screen the control groups, which commenced in 1986.

The stable relative risk in the WE trial also led to some discussion. As screening had no effect for 4 years it would be expected that the contribution of those initial years of no effect would become progressively less with increasing time from entry. In part this seemed to reflect an analysis by calendar time rather than year of entry, in part a lack of a smooth widening of the separation of the cumulative mortality curves and in part the fact that they are plotted linearly and not logarithmically. The latter would make it clearer that although the absolute benefit is increasing, the relative benefit is not. In that respect it was suggested that the benefit so far seen must relate to relatively fast growing tumours, as the mean duration from diagnosis to death in most clinical series was 8 years. It was questioned, therefore, whether it might ever be possible to determine the effect on slower growing cancers. However, with a trial where there was a limited period of differential screening (in HIP where only 4 screens were offered and in the WE trial where the study group was offered screening over 10 years and the controls were then screened), an effect of screening on slower growing tumours should be demonstrable with prolonged follow-up.

It has now been recognised that small invasive cancers with extensive surrounding ductal carcinoma in situ (EIC - extensive intraductal component) do worse than cancers with a similar extent of invasion but no EIC. This causes difficulty in relation to the UICC TNM classification where only the invasive component should be measured for screening.

It was pointed out that in the UK trial as well as the Malmö trial women age 50-54 seemed to do worse than older women (there was a suggestion of a similar effect in the Utrecht case-control study for women age 50-59). Perhaps this could be related to a later age at menopause in such groups. In the UK, for example there seemed to be no difference in sensitivity of the screen between the 45-49 and 50-54 age groups. This question will be further evaluated in the planned Swedish overview analysis, though even in that analysis there might not be sufficient power for analysis by quinquennia. Although the Malmö study had low power, additional problems arose over the mortality from breast cancer in the non-compliers and the number of examinations in the control group. In a city such as Malmö the opportunity to demonstrate a major effect of screening is less than in a rural area. Even so, it was clear that the confidence intervals around the estimate for effect in women age 55-64 in Malmö was compatible with the effect seen in women over the age of 50 in the WE trial. These considerations underline the importance of achieving sufficient compliance in a population when screening is offered routinely if the expected effect is to be seen.

It was pointed out that in addition to the Canadian trial there are several other studies which show a possible adverse effect in the younger age group. Although these effects could be due to chance it would be appropriate to evaluate further the characteristics of those women who died and identify the factors responsible for the poor outcome. This is underway in the Canadian trial but could be extended to the other studies also. One factor that might explain poor prognosis for mammography detected cases could be delay in presenting until a subsequent screen for those women with false negatives after a previous screen. This factor, if present, cannot explain all of the effect in the Canadian trial as a similar excess of deaths have occurred in those with cancers detected on the first screen as for those detected on later screens combined with the interval or incident cancers Although the Canadian trial had a learning curve for mammography, this has been documented for other programmes as well.

In considering the simulation of the programme in the Netherlands, some surprise was expressed over the fact that the peak benefit was not reached until shortly before the planned screening stopped. One possible reason was that until then the programme was continuous whereas in the HIP study, where the peak benefit was reached early, only 4 annual screens were used. In addition, in the HIP study the stage distribution of the screen detected cancers was much worse than now experienced, and considerably worse in the control group. Thus much of the effect with screens of low sensitivity was in detecting advanced disease earlier, an effect that may not be seen in many countries today where the stage distribution in the absence of screening is much better than in the HIP study. In programmes now, therefore, the effect may be delayed but longer lasting.

Although in the simulation there was a parity between the life years saved and the lead time gained, the former must apply only to the much smaller number of women who receive the benefit of mortality reduction, though lead time is gained for nearly all screen-detected cancers.

It was noted that the marginal cost-effectiveness of moving from the 3-yearly frequency of screening in the Swedish two-county trial to a programme of two-yearly screening was currently assessable only through simulation. Although, as demonstrated in the Netherlands simulation analysis, this may be judged to be appropriate, it seemed unlikely that in a population there would be a major effect of moving from biennial to annual screening. Such considerations, after an informal analysis, have resulted in the decision to screen women age 50-69 every two years in Canada.

State of the Art on Screening for Colorectal Cancer

The current trials will eventually give an answer on the effect of screening for occult blood in the stool on colorectal cancer mortality, but each trial alone will not be definitive and most will still take several more years. It will also take several more years of follow-up before it can be determined if removal of adenomas has an effect on cancer incidence.

In the mean time screening for colorectal cancer or its precursors is not justified as public health policy.

Recommendations for Research
Evaluate the validity of new screening tests for faecal occult blood.
Develop approaches to increase compliance with screening.
Conduct combined analyses of the currently ongoing faecal occult blood test trials.
Evaluate the efficacy of flexible sigmoidoscopy performed every three years.
Evaluate cost-effectiveness of different aspects of colorectal cancer screening, eg specificity, compliance, frequency vs effectiveness issues.

9 Colon Cancer Control Study: Status and Current Issues

T. R. CHURCH[1], J. S. MANDEL[1], J. H. BOND[2], F. EDERER[3],
D. C. SNOVER[4], G. M. BRADLEY[4], S. E. WILLIAMS[5], and
L. M. SCHUMAN[6]

[1] Division of Environmental and Occupational Health, School of Public Health, University of Minnesota; [2] Department of Medicine, School of Medicine, University of Minnesota; [3] The Emmes Corporation, Washington, D.C.; [4] Department of Laboratory Medicine and Pathology, School of Medicine, University of Minnesota; [5] Department of Surgery, School of Medicine, University of Minnesota; and [6] Division of Epidemiology, School of Public Health, University of Minnesota.

1 INTRODUCTION

The Colon Cancer Control Study is a clinical trial designed to test whether periodic screening for occult blood using a commercially available guaiac-impregnated slide (Hemoccult ™, Smith-Kline Diagnostics) can result in significantly reduced colorectal mortality. The study began in 1975; by April 1978 46,550 living subjects residing or employed in Minnesota had been randomized into one of three treatment groups: a biennially screened group (screen every two years, survey every year), an annually screened group (screen and survey every year), and a control group (yearly survey only). The original plan was to screen for five years and follow the subjects for another five years. However, in 1986 screening was reinitiated for an indefinite period to compensate for the considerably lower-than-expected event rate observed up to that time. The initial five-year screening period is referred to as Phase I and the reinitiated screening as Phase II.

Figure 1 shows the design of the study in schematic form. In brief, the annually screened and biennially screened groups are mailed six guaiac slides yearly or every two years, respectively. The returned slides are tested, and the subjects returning at least one positive slide are invited for examination by a study colonoscopist; those who decline are strongly encouraged to receive an examination including colonoscopy. All cancers and polyps found during colonoscopy are noted and removed for biopsy, and complete records obtained. Yearly surveys are conducted on all three groups to ascertain health and vital status. Records of deaths and reported gastrointestinal cancers are pursued vigorously. All deaths are reviewed blindly to determine the cause by a panel of four physicians. The design of the study is presented in more detail in Gilbertsen et al. (1980).

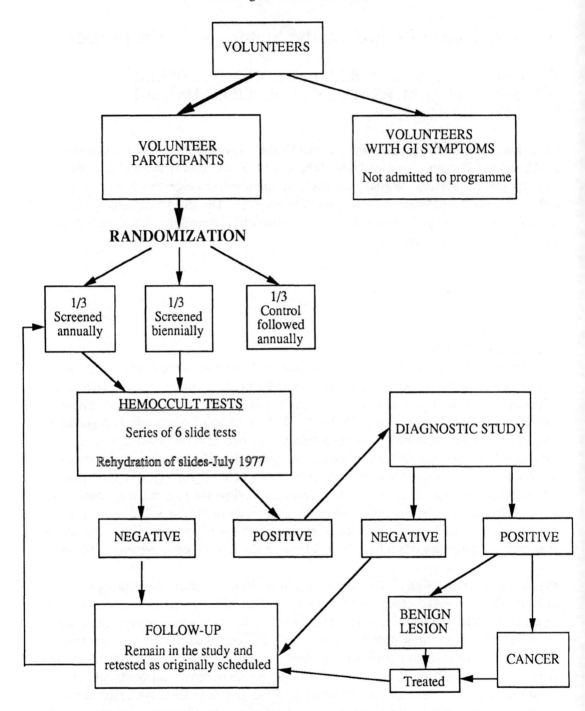

Figure 1 Design of the study

This paper will address several areas of interest related to the design of screening studies. Although some of the areas – compliance and variability – affect all studies, most are specific to prevention studies, screening studies or colorectal cancer in particular. The results of the screening test itself will be assessed in terms of sensitivity, specificity and predictive value. Projecting the mortality rate is a particular issue with prevention trials (Ederer et al, 1990), and the relationship of polyps to colorectal cancer is an interesting sidelight to this study. Because the trial is ongoing, no treatment group comparisons are possible. Results reported herein are current through 1989.

A Policy and Data Monitoring Group assembled in 1982 meets periodically to thoroughly review the status of the study and the analysis of the data to date. The group then makes recommendations to the National Cancer Institute and to the study investigators regarding the conduct, analysis, and continuation of the study.

2 STATUS OF THE STUDY

The 36,853 subjects still living have a median age of 73 years and 55.3% of them are female. Over 400,000 annual surveys have been returned, over 150,000 screens completed and nearly 10,000 colonoscopies performed as a result of positive tests. A total of 9,697 deaths have occurred with all but 426 classified as to cause of death. Fewer than 1,200 (3.3%) subjects have not been contacted in the last 16 months. Only 299 (0.8%) subjects have refused all further contact; the current location of 2 is not known.

2.1 Compliance

Perhaps the most universal difficulty in running large clinical trials is compliance. Compliance will be addressed in three main areas: annual followup by mail or telephone to determine vital status; utilization of the screening test; and the diagnostic evaluation of test positives.

Periodic Followup. A questionnaire is sent each year to all participants. It is the primary means of ascertaining whether a subject has died or had colorectal cancer and, if so, provides information to begin gathering medical records necessary to accurately determine the incidence of and mortality from colorectal cancer. Table 1 shows that few (~3%) of the subjects have not been seen in the previous 16-month period and that the completeness of followup is very similar between groups. The compliance decreases slightly with increasing age (but even at ages 85 or more 91.7% of the females and 94.2% of the males had been contacted in the last 16 months); female and male compliance are similar (the detailed findings are not presented here). The high degree of compliance was accomplished primarily by a rigorous schedule of mailing, reminder letters and telephone tracing.

Table 1   Length of time since last contact with surviving subjects by experimental group (percentage distribution)

Experimental group

Time since last contact (months)	Biennnial	Annual	Control
Less than 16	96.9	97.0	97.0
16-19	1.7	1.7	1.5
over 19*	1.5	1.4	1.6
Total	100.0	100.0	100.0

*Includes 299 participants considered withdrawn from the study.

Guaiac Slides. Table 2 shows the compliance with the screening protocol in the annual and biennial groups by the percent of attempted screens completed. The two groups have similar completion rates and in both about 90% have completed at least one screen. Figure 2, showing the compliance rate for the most recent screen by age and sex, illustrates the higher compliance for females and the lower compliance for subjects older than 80 years of age.

Table 2 Compliance with Hemoccult slides by experimental group

Percentage of slide sets returned	Biennial			Annual		
	Number	%	Cumulative %	Number	%	Cumulative %
100	10,136	64.6	64.6	9,387	59.6	59.6
75-99	1,546	9.9	74.5	1,577	10.0	69.6
50-74	1,090	6.9	81.4	1,515	9.6	79.2
25-49	1,096	7.0	88.4	892	5.7	84.9
1-24	0	0.0	88.4	708	4.5	89.4
0	1,822	11.6	100.0	1,678	10.6	100.0
Total	15,690			15,757		

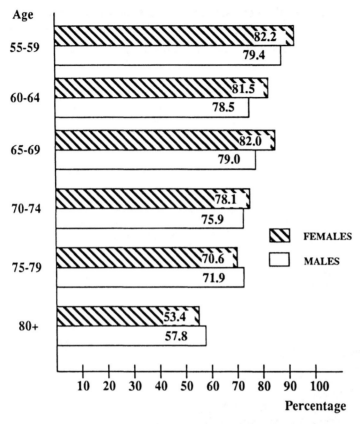

Figure 2 Compliance with Hemoccult testing by sex and age

Table 3 Compliance with screening by outcome of prior screen and examination
status

Screening test outcome and examination status on prior screen	Participated in next screen	Did not participate in next screen	Total
Negative test	61,534 (90)*	6,983 (10)*	68,517
Positive and examined	3,564 (81)	863 (19)	4,427
Positive and not examined	108 (51)	103 (49)	211

*Percentage

Table 3 gives the percentage complying with Hemoccult testing by prior screening compliance and outcome. Ninety percent (90%) of those who yielded a negative test on the

previous screen participated in the next screen, whereas only about half (51%) of those testing positive and refusing diagnostic workup on the previous screen did so. Those receiving a diagnostic workup for a positive result on the previous screen complied with next screen 81% of the time.

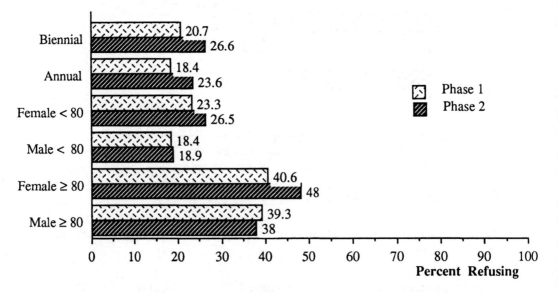

Figure 3 Percentage refusing diagnostic workup by phase by group and by age and sex

Colonoscopy. Figure 3 shows the compliance with the diagnostic examination by age and sex. Besides equivalent compliance for both screening groups, it shows that men tend to comply slightly better than women and that subjects over age 75 comply less well than younger ones. Other characteristics affected compliance with examination; specifically, more education, a participating spouse, and living in the metropolitan area resulted in better compliance, while being widowed or divorced and working in farming or fishing led to worse compliance. Although the compliance with the CCCS diagnostic procedure was around 70%, overall 80% underwent colonoscopy, and about 90% had some diagnostic workup of the colon or rectum.

2.2 Results of Guaiac Screening

The rate of positive tests greatly affects the ability of diagnostic services to deal with mass screening, since a higher rate increases the examination workload. There are two types of positives: the true positives, who have the disease, and the false positives, who do not. Without sufficient numbers of true positives, the disease can not be appreciably attenuated; with too many false positives, the cost per case becomes prohibitive. Often, increasing the number of true positives will increase the number of false positives (Morrison 1985), so the two categories must be balanced in assessing the test.

Table 4 Positive Hemoccult ™ slide sets by year and hydration status

Year	Percentage Positive		Percentage of
	Rehydrated	Not Rehydrated	Slides Rehydrated
1976	---	2.0	0.0
1977	3.9	1.8	42.7
1978	8.4	1.8	78.2
1979	8.7	1.4	93.6
1980	11.9	4.0	73.8
1981	12.4	5.3	84.0
1982	11.7	---	100.0
1986	12.1	---	100.0
1987	12.4	---	100.0
1988	12.8	---	100.0
1989	15.4	---	100.0

Positivity Rates. The overall positivity rate was 7.4% for Phase I and 13.1% for Phase II. Table 4 shows the positivity rate by calendar year for rehydrated and non-rehydrated slides. The rate for non-rehydrated slides varies from 1.4% to 5.3%, whereas that for rehydrated slides varies from 11.7 to 15.4. By year, the ratio of the rehydrated to non-rehydrated rate varies from 2.2 to 6.2. The positivity rate for the non-rehydrated slides shows more relative variability than the rehydrated rate, but in absolute rates, their variability is similar. However, without 1989, the rehydrated rates would seem to be fairly homogenous, both relatively and absolutely. This apparent anomaly is discussed in Section III.

Table 5   Percentage of subjects with positive Hemoccult ™ slide sets
by hydration status, age and sex

a)

Age	Slides Rehydrated	Slides not Rehydrated
<50	6.7	0.7
50-59	8.0	1.6
60-69	9.8	2.4
70-79	11.6	3.0
80-89	14.4	3.5
90+	20.4	14.3*
All ages	10.2	2.1

*Based on one positive out of 7 slide sets

b)

| | Percentage Positive | | |
	Males	Females	Total
Slides Rehydrated	11.3	9.1	10.2
Slides not Rehydrated	2.7	1.8	2.1

Table 5 shows that the positivity rate for the guaiac test increases with age and is higher for men than women regardless of rehydration. For positive tests (Table 6) the number of positive slides among the set of 6 is not uniformly distributed; most often, 1 or 2 slides are positive (with similar frequency), with decreasing percentages for 3 and 4 slides, 5 with the smallest frequency, then an increase for 6 slides. So far, no satisfactory model has been offered to explain this pattern, although a mixture of at least two mechanisms of positivity is strongly implied by the observed bimodal results.

Table 6 Percentage of slides positive in sets of six (among positive tests) returned

Number of slides positive in set of six	Positive slide sets (%)
1	30
2	28
3	13
4	10
5	4
6	15

Figure 4 shows the outcome and compliance of the diagnostic workup by the results of the immediately preceding screen. Subjects negative on the preceding screen yielded a positive result only 8% of the time, whereas those positive and not examined on the preceding screen yielded a positive result 34% of the time. The previously negative subjects with positives on the subsequent screen complied with the diagnostic workup almost 100% of the time, whereas those previously positive subjects who had refused a diagnostic workup complied with the diagnostic workup about two thirds of the time (66%).

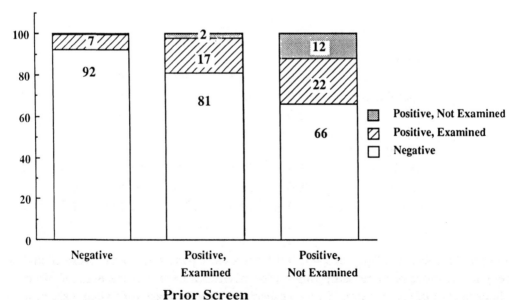

Figure 4 Outcome of screening test and compliance with diagnostic examination by results from prior screen

Sensitivity, Specificity, Predictive Value.   The sensitivity, specificity and positive predictivity were estimated by assuming that cancers diagnosed within one year of a negative test were missed by the screen. Sensitivity is higher for rehydrated than nonrehydrated slides, whereas the specificity and consequently the predictive value are lower (Table 7).

Table 7   Sensitivity, specificity and positive predictive value for colorectal cancer by hydration satus of slides

	Hydration Status		
	Not Rehydrated	Rehydrated	All Slides
Sensitivity (%)	80.8	92.2	89.3
Specificity (%)	97.7	90.4	92.7
Positive Predictive Value (%)	5.8	2.0	2.3

This pattern is clear regardless of age and sex of the subject, with the exception of men less than 60 years of age (Table 8). However, the estimates for this category are based on a small number of cases.

Table 8   Sensitivity, specificity and positive predictive value (PPV) by hydration status, age and sex

	Not Hydrated			Rehydrated		
	<60	60-69	70+	<60	60-69	70+
MEN						
Sensitivity	33.3	81.3	85.7	94.4	100.0	93.3
Specificity	98.0	96.9	96.6	90.4	89.3	88.5
PPV	0.9	6.7	5.9	1.8	2.3	3.2
WOMEN						
Sensitivity	66.7	87.5	86.7	91.7	92.3	81.3
Specificity	98.6	98.0	97.4	92.8	90.2	89.8
PPV	2.4	4.5	12.1	1.5	1.7	2.7

Rehydration, Age and Sex. In Table 9 there is a clear pattern in both rehydrated and non-rehydrated slides of increased positive predictivity for cancer as the number of positive slides in a set of six increases, with an especially large increase for five and six positives. The ratio between the non-rehydrated and rehydrated predictivities is fairly constant and around 3.

Table 9a Percentage of subjects diagnosed with colorectal cancer among those with at least one positive slide in a set of six by hydration status

Number of Slides Positive in Set	Slides Rehydrated	Slides Not Rehydrated	All Slides
1	1.1	4.4	1.5
2	1.4	3.2	1.5
3	1.6	5.4	1.8
4	1.8	5.4	1.9
5	3.8	14.3	4.5
6	5.1	16.4	5.7
Total	2.0	5.8	2.3

Table 9b Percentage of subjects diagnosed with neoplastic polyps among those with at least one positive slide in a set of six by hydration status

Number of Slides Positive in Set	Slides Rehydrated	Slides Not Rehydrated	All Slides
1	17.4	25.1	18.2
2	18.5	17.0	18.7
3	19.8	27.6	20.3
4	19.2	32.2	19.9
5	21.0	27.8	21.5
6	21.0	31.6	21.6
Total	18.9	26.2	19.4

Table 9 also suggests a pattern of increasing positive predictivity with the number of positive slides for polyps, as well, but for neither rehydrated nor unrehydrated slides is the increase large. The lack of a strong correlation between number of positive slides and positive predictive value for polyps may suggest that most of these lesions are found incidentally, not because they bled and caused a positive test. If this is the case, the prevalence rate for polyps in this population is around 20%.

2.3 Results of Diagnostic Workups (Colonoscopies)
Figure 5 compares the results of diagnostic workups at the University of Minnesota (UM) CCCS clinic to those done elsewhere on subjects unwilling or unable to come to the UM

clinic in response to a positive guaiac result, for both phases of the screening, both for colonoscopies and for all examinations.

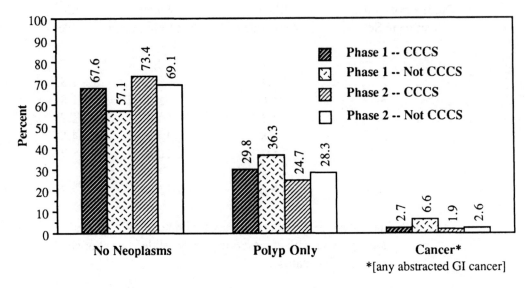

Figure 5a   Percentage distribution of findings by where examined and screening phase for all positive results where colonoscopy was performed

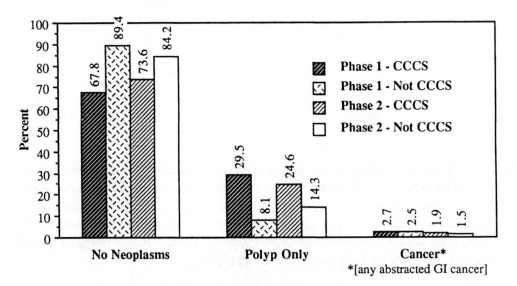

Figure 5b   Percentage distribution of findings by where examined and screening phase for all positive results

For colonoscopies (Figure 5a), there is an apparent increase in positive predictivity for those done outside the UM clinic, but this difference is reversed when all examinations are considered (Figure 5b). One possible explanation is that colonoscopy is attempted in all subjects attending the UM clinic, whereas it is most commonly attempted in the community only when another test such as a barium-enema X-ray or flexible sigmoidoscopy has revealed potential pathology.

2.4 Death

Table 10 shows that the status of ascertained and reviewed deaths is the same for each study group, with approximately 96% of all cases completely reviewed. Likewise, the numbers ascertained dead as a proportion of the group are nearly identical, indicating no bias exists in either the death ascertainment or review processes.

Table 10 Deaths to date by processing status

Status	Biennial	Annual	Control
Complete	3116 (96.0%)	3132 (95.6%)	3023 (95.5%)
In Process	130 (4.0%)	143 (4.4%)	143 (4.5%)
Total	3246 (100.0%)	3275 (100.0%)	3116 (100.0%)

Table 11 summarizes the agreements and discordances between the ICD-8 coding of the death certificates and the final classification from the review process, collapsing each into three categories. Although there are relatively few discrepancies overall, as a percentage of deaths from colorectal cancer they are large (e.g., 37/262=14%), demonstrating that careful review of the colorectal cancer deaths can considerably alter the observed mortality rate.

Table 11 Comparison of cause of death from death certificate with cause ascertained by death review committee

Death Certificate Diagnosis	Death Review Committee Decision			
	Died from Colorectal Cancer	Died with Colorectal Cancer	No Colorectal Cancer	Total
Died from Colorectal Cancer	225	5	32	262
Died with Colorectal Cancer	11	11	27	49
No Colorectal Cancer	11	12	8330	8353
Total	247	28	8389	8664

3 GUAIAC TESTING VARIABILITY

As mentioned in the previous section, there is an apparent and unexplained increase in the rate of positives in 1989 compared to previous years for rehydrated slides. After eliminating the possibility that changes in the age and sex components of study population explained the increase, two hypotheses present themselves: either a change in the lab processing which occurred about the middle of 1989 had a profound effect or the slides themselves had changed in reactivity. Figure 6 shows that the positivity rate rises sharply beginning in mid-1989, then drops near the end of the year.

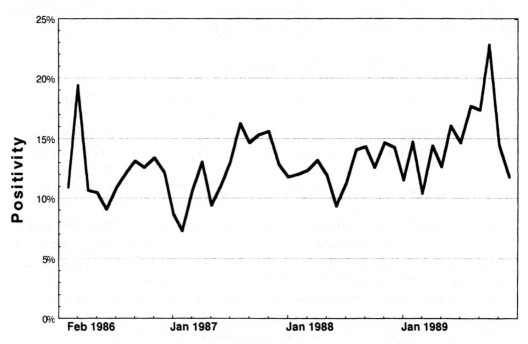

Figure 6 Slide set positivity by month

Table 12 Positivity rates by lot numbers

| | Lot Numbers of Slide Sets Received in Laboratory * | | | | | | | |
	#1	#1&#2	#1	#1&#2	#2	#3	#4	Total
Sets Received	7005	8777	5377	1734	7374	20605	3982	54752
Number Positive	817	1035	562	208	1061	2746	767	7196
Percent. Positive	11.7	11.8	10.5	12.7	14.4	13.3	19.3	13.1

* Each column represents a contiguous time period with either a single lot or mixture of lots received during that time period. Column headings identify the lot numbers.

Table 12 suggests the positivity rate varies considerably by lot number during Phase II, especially noticeable for lot #4. This lot started to arrive in the laboratory around 1989. A small change in a tray stacking procedure which had inadvertently crept into the processing, was reversed near the end of 1989 and closer supervision was instituted, possibly explaining the decrease near the end of the year. Further research will illuminate the separate contributions of laboratory procedures, lot-to-lot differences, and subjective reading in the variability of slide results.

4 POLYPS AND CANCER

It is widely believed that neoplastic polyps are precursors to cancer, not merely markers of increased risk. Because of current practice, clinicians are reluctant to leave polyps in place and observe their course, hence no ethical method of directly measuring the effect of polyp removal is available. However, some light may be shed on this hypothesis by observations from the study.

Table 13 Cases with neoplastic polyps greater than 2 cm by group screen and age as a percentage of cases with neoplastic polyps

	Screen number	Percentage of Polyps >2cm	
		Age ≤ 60	Age > 60
Biennial Group			
Phase I	1	19.0%	20.0%
	2	14.7%	12.8%
	3	4.9%	5.6%
Phase II	1	18.2%	8.7%
Annual Group			
Phase I	1	15.6%	30.0%
	2	6.1%	8.1%
	3	0.0%	10.9%
	4	7.5%	5.0%
	5	3.8%	10.8%
Phase II	1	0.0%	8.4%
	2	0.0%	6.1%
	3	0.0%	6.2%

4.1 Size, Age and Location

The distribution of polyps by age is an important clue to the relationship with cancer. The average age at diagnosis of large polyps is expected to be lower than that of cancer if polyps are precursors; although one can devise models which allowed the reverse, these would require more restrictive assumptions. A positive association between polyp diagnosis and age which mimics that for cancer and age is expected from the polyp-precursor hypothesis. Table 13 shows that the percentage of large (>2cm) polyps decreases with age for biennial screening, but shows no consistent relationship to age for annual screening. This result makes it unclear whether the polyp-to-cancer sequence is supported.

Table 14 shows that the most frequent location of lesions found on colonoscopy is the sigmoid colon. Over 50% are found in the rectum or sigmoid colon, well within reach of the flexible sigmoidoscope. If one can reach the top of the descending colon as well, a full 65% of lesions can be detected. Since cancers alone follow a similar distribution in the study (not shown) and since another 10% of cancers have associated benign lesions in the lower part of the large bowel, about 75% of all colorectal cancers would be detectable by means of a flexible sigmoidoscopy and following positive findings by colonoscopy.

Table 14   Location of lowest lesion (cancer or polyp)

	Number	%	Cumulative %
Rectum	288	14	14
Sigmoid Colon	786	39	53
Descending Colon	241	12	65
Transverse Colon	198	10	75
Splenic Flexure of the Colon	38	2	77
Hepatic Flexure of the Colon	65	3	80
Ascending Colon	166	8	88
Caecum	242	12	100
Total	2024	100	

5 INCIDENCE AND THE ROLE OF POLYPS

If polyps are precursors to cancer and not just markers of risk, then removal of polyps should reduce the incidence of cancer. Since the CCCS has performed and continues to perform colonoscopy on a large number of individuals, of whom nearly 20% have polyps found and removed during the procedure, it may be possible to study the effect of polyp removal in this group. However, colorectal cancer incidence in a screening trial may be affected by other factors, thus confounding the relationship between polyp removal and colorectal cancer incidence.

5.1 Factors Influencing Incidence Rates during Screening

Without screening, incidence rates in three randomized groups should be equal. However, screening generally affects the incidence of disease in two ways. First, the time of detection is moved back from clinical surfacing to when the screen detects disease. This change in detection time is called the lead time (Hutchison and Shapiro, 1968). Second, screening may detect disease that would have gone undetected without screening, what will be called "over diagnosis." The size of the first effect depends upon the average lead time (time from screen detection to eventual clinical surfacing) over all screen-detected cases and the sensitivity (probability of detection) of the test; the second effect depends upon the number of detectable lesions which go undetected in the control group.

5.2 Possible Effects on Incidence

Advancing the diagnosis date through screening serves to increase the incidence of disease in the screened group relative to the control group for the duration of screening. When screening ceases, cumulative diagnosis in the screened groups should eventually return to the level of the control group, so that, ultimately, there is no effect on colorectal cancer incidence.

The over diagnosis of lesions also increases the cumulative incidence relative to the control group. It is conceivable that these two effects could mask the effect of prevention due to removal of polyps, so that failure to detect a difference in colorectal cancer incidence between the screened and unscreened groups would be difficult to interpret. Without some upper bound on these confounding effects, it is only meaninfgul if a difference is observed.

5.3 Data Derived from Screening

The mean lead time and its standard error can be estimated from the study data and an upper bound placed on the increase due to over diagnoses. For example, the first-year incidence in the control group is 2.9/1000 and the initial screen prevalence is 2.8/1000, so a crude estimate of the average preclinical duration would be 2.8/2.9=.97 (Zelen and Feinleib 1969). These estimates have large standard errors because of the small number of cases used to estimate them. However, a reasonable estimate based on the data is a mean lead time of 1 year. This estimate would lead to an increase equal to the annual incidence, which averages about 2/1000 or 9% of the total over an 11-year period.

A crude estimate of the number of undetected cases in the control group can be derived by assuming that those cases discovered at autopsy are a proportion of all cases undiscovered prior to death among deaths from a given death certificate cause. Since the number of cases from the control group is small, we utilize the further assumption that the proportion of such cases which actually would have been discovered by screening is small. This justifies pooling data from all three groups. One can then project a total from the formula

$$D_p = \sum_{i=1}^{k} \frac{d_i}{r_i}$$

where D_p is the number of cases undiagnosed before death, d_i is the number of cases diagnosed at autopsy and r_i is the autopsy rate defined as a_i / m_i, where a_i is the number of autopsies and m_i is the number of deaths due to cause i, i=1,...,k. The estimated number of undetected cases is

$$D_p - \sum_{i=1}^{k} d_i$$

From the 11-year data, this turns out to be 66 over-diagnosis cases for the whole study, or 22 for the control group. If this number is accurate, this amounts to a maximum possible over diagnosis of 22/334 or 7%. Depending upon the sensitivity of the screening test and upon the sensitivity of autopsy to discover these cases, however, this number could be smaller or larger. For example, if the sensitivity of the Hemoccult for such cases is 50%, then of the 66 cases, one would expect 33 cases in the control group. Likewise, if the sensitivity of the autopsy is only 70%, then the total number expected would be 95 instead of 66. Further research will elucidate the accuracy of the various estimates. However, 7% is a reasonable estimate for the present illustration.

5.4 Confounding of Effects
If the observed difference in incidence between a screened group and the control is zero, then the true size of the effect of polyp removal in preventing colorectal cancer could be as great as the sum of 7%+9% = 16%. Of course, sampling variability will increase the minimum detectable effect above even this limit. Over time, the relative effect of earlier diagnosis will become smaller and the power to detect a prevention effect will increase. There is no reason to believe the relative effect of over diagnosis will decrease, however, so the minimum upper limit on the sum of the confounding effects is 7%.

6 PROJECTING THE COLORECTAL CANCER MORTALITY RATE
Continuing the study depends upon observing an adequate number of deaths from colorectal cancer in the control group within a reasonable time. The number of deaths from colorectal cancer depends upon the age and sex structure of the sample, which changes with time, and on the age-sex-specific mortality rates for both all causes and colorectal cancer. Information solely from past study experience would lead to unreliable estimates of age-sex-specific rates. Even if reliable estimates could be obtained, time-varying selection effects can render these internal estimates inaccurate (Ederer, Church, Mandel 1990).

6.1 Selection Effects in Recruitment of Subjects
Population-based estimates of age-sex-specific mortality could be used were it not for the fact that recruitment of volunteers is subject to two types of selection effects: constant and time-varying. An example of a constant effect is the selection of healthy volunteers, those with easy medical access to medical care and a life-long interest in healthy behavior, including utilizing medical care when necessary. Regardless of the length of the study, this effect would be expected to exert itself. In contrast, the exclusion of subjects known to have the disease of interest would be expected to diminish over time, as the incidence and subsequent fatality of incident cases pushed the rate back up to the mortality rate in the population. These effects make it unsuitable to apply the rates from the population to the sample without adjustment.

However, the assumption that these effects act on the ratio of the sample rates to the population rates (the standardized mortality ratio or SMR) allows a reasonable method of projecting mortality as the sample changes.

6.2 Using SEER Data to Model SMRs

The Surveillance, Epidemiology, and End Results (SEER) Program of the National Cancer Institute publishes relative survival rates computed from data supplied from several areas of the country, providing a set of reasonable approximations to the disease-specific interval survival for different diagnosis dates. These relative survival rates are used to construct an annual index proportional to the mortality in a group from which all prevalent cases have been removed and experiencing both constant colorectal cancer incidence and the rates given in the SEER data as in Church et al. (1991). A hyperbolic model was selected for theoretical reasons and its excellent fit to the index curve computed from the SEER data (Figure 7 plots the computed SEER Index and the fitted equation against followup year). This hyperbolic model, given as

$$SMR = \alpha + \beta/t$$

where t is the study followup year, was fitted to the actual age-sex-adjusted SMRs for both all-cause and colorectal cancer mortality in the CCCS sample (see Figure 8). This allowed for both a constant effect (α) and a time-varying effect (β/t).

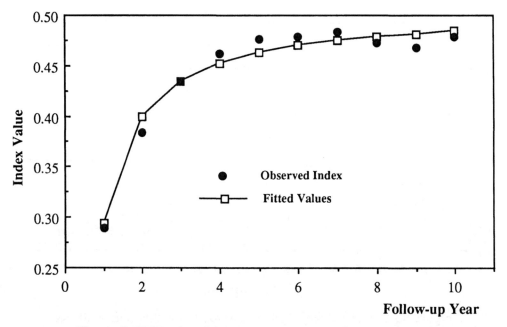

Figure 7 SEER mortality indices versus follow-up year and fitted hyperbolic model

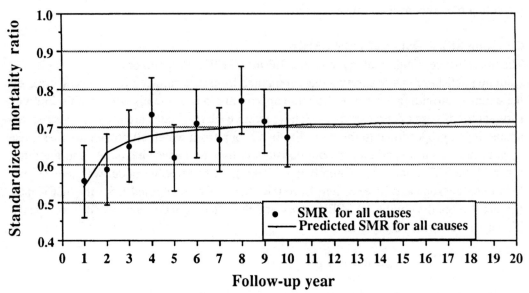

Figure 8a Actual and projected Standardized Mortality Ratios (SMRs) for All
Causes of Death. Error bars indicate 95% Confidence Intervals

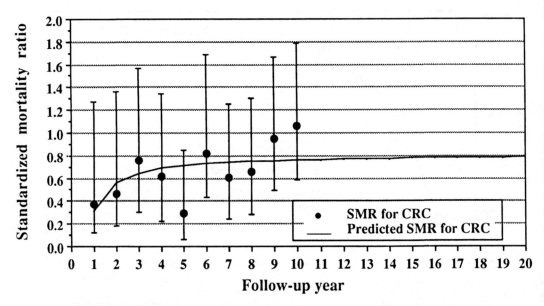

Figure 8b Actual and projected Standardized Mortality Ratios (SMRs) for
Colorectal Cancer. Error bars indicate 95% Confidence Intervals

6.3 Projecting SMRs

The estimated values of α and β specific to all-cause and colorectal cancer mortality were used to project the SMR for future followup years, and this projected SMR was multiplied by age-sex-specific rates to get the adjusted age-sex-specific rates; these results were applied to the corresponding stratum for that year, yielding the number of deaths and the number of colorectal cancer deaths in the control group, respectively. Subtracting the number of deaths from the current stratum and adding one year to the age yields the stratum for the next year at the next highest age.

6.4 Extrapolation of Mortality

Summing the number of deaths due to colorectal cancer and due to all causes in each stratum across all strata for a given year yields the projected mortality for the entire sample; accumulating these yearly projections gives the number of colorectal cancer deaths expected by the end of any given followup year. These calculations lead to the expected total number of deaths from all causes in the control group given in Table 15.

Table 15 Observed and projected deaths from all causes in the control group by sex and year

Observed Deaths

					Follow-up Year					
	1	2	3	4	5	6	7	8	9	10
Males	39	47	64	70	67	81	95	120	122	122
Females	96	107	119	151	132	163	147	177	168	165
Total	135	154	183	221	199	244	242	297	290	287
Cumulative Total	135	289	472	693	892	1136	1378	1675	1965	2252

Projected Deaths

					Follow-up Year					
	11	12	13	14	15	16	17	18	19	20
Males	138	146	155	164	173	181	190	198	206	213
Females	185	193	200	206	212	217	221	225	227	229
Total	323	339	355	370	385	398	411	423	433	442
Cumulative Total	2575	2913	3268	3638	4022	4421	4832	5255	5688	6130

Table 15 shows a steady increase in projected deaths through the end of the study period and beyond. Since colorectal cancer mortality is the primary outcome and the results are confidential, colorectal cancer mortality can not be reported at this time, but the number of deaths per year are expected to continue to increase through the 23rd year of the study, and then decline.

7 CONCLUDING OBSERVATIONS AND DISCUSSION

7.1 Current Status

Over the last 15 years, the CCCS has either screened with the guaiac test for occult blood or followed a population of nearly 46,551 individuals over the age of 50. Substantial knowledge of the positivity, sensitivity, specificity and predictivity of and compliance with the screening test gleaned from this experience can be applied to other screening tests and studies. In particular, it has been shown that compliance with the test can be as great as 80% and compliance with evaluating positive results as high as 90%. With an estimated sensitivity of over 90%, the test is being given an excellent chance of demonstrating a reduction in mortality by this study.

Each death in the study is being carefully reviewed and the results to date show that the causes of death not related to screening or colon cancer and the percentage of completed reviews are equally distributed among the study groups.

7.2 Compliance

Excellent compliance with followup, screening, and diagnosis has been accomplished through rigorous mail and telephone contact schedules, in a labour-intensive effort, involving computer-generated letters and worklists. This compliance gives screening an opportunity to function. However, such compliance is unlikely to be observed in the general population under non-research conditions. Any effects seen in this study probably will be attenuated in general use.

7.3 Polyp Removal

Not only does the test find over 90% of colorectal cancers, but also about 20% of diagnostic workups find and remove polyps, which are believed by many to be precursors of colorectal cancer. Though it is too early for definitive results, so far no large effects on incidence from the removal of these polyps has been detected. The potentially confounding effects from screening in this study could be in the range of 7% to 16%. Since the removal of polyps potentially affects only about 25% of the polyp-bearing subjects, any eventual effect on incidence would be less than that. As more subjects have positive screens, a larger proportion potentially will be affected. Although this study was not designed to answer questions about the relationship between polyps and cancer, it may indicate further research in this area.

7.4 Test Variability

The rehydration of Hemoccult ™ slides prior to testing increases the positivity rate in a way that increases sensitivity and decreases specificity (Mandel, Bond, Bradley et al. 1989). In the study, rehydration has led to a decrease in the positive predictive value of the test. As the population ages, the positivity rate increases, as does the incidence of colorectal cancer. Other sources of variability in the test outcomes are the processing methods, (e.g., how long a test is allowed to stand between rehydration and adding developer), and perhaps, lot-to-lot variability in the reactivity of the slides. Although no other study has reported this latter effect, most do not rehydrate and so get a positivity rate of around 1% to 3%. With such low rates, a doubling due to lot-to-lot variability would not be readily apparent, but when the rate is above 10%, a doubling is quite noticeable. Further study is necessary to delineate different components of the observed variability in positivity.

7.5 Mortality Projections

In order to determine how long the study might continue, projections were made based upon a hyperbolic model of selection effects validated using SEER colorectal cancer relative survival rates and simulating the removal of previously diagnosed cases from the population. The model predicts the standardized mortality ratio (SMR) of the study mortality rates to the population rates for future years, and these SMRs are used to adjust the age-sex-specific population rates. The results indicate how long the study is likely to continue before the required number of events occurs. Since the study is being sequentially analyzed and the results kept confidential, the actual projections can not be given here. Current plans will continue screening through December 1991 and followup beyond that.

REFERENCES

Church TR, Ederer F, Mandel JS, Watt GD, Geisser MS. Duration of prevention trials. In preparation, (1991).

Ederer F, Church T, Mandel J. Are sample sizes for prevention trials too small? Manuscript submitted for publication (1990).

Gilbertsen VA, Church TR, Grewe FA, Mandel JS, McHugh RM, Schuman LM, Williams SE. The design of a study to assess occult-blood screening for colon cancer. J Chron Dis 1980; 33:107-114.

Hutchison GB, Shapiro S. Lead time gained by diagnostic screening for breast cancer. J Natl Cancer Inst 1968; 41:665-681.

Mandel JM, Bond JH, Bradley M, Snover D, Church TR, Williams S, Watt G, Schuman L, Ederer F, Gilbertsen V. Sensitivity, specificity and positive predictive value of the hemoccult test in screening for colorectal cancers: the University of Minnesota's Colon Cancer Control Program. Gastroenterology 1989; 97:597-600.

Morrison AS. Screening in chronic disease. New York: Oxford University Press, 1985.

Zelen M, Feileib M. On the theory of screening for chronic disease. Biometrika 1969; 56:601-614.

10 An Update on the Nottingham Trial of Faecal Occult Blood Screening for Colorectal Carcinoma

W. M. THOMAS and J. D. HARDCASTLE

University Hospital, Queen's Medical Centre, Nottingham, UK

1 INTRODUCTION

A randomized trial of faecal occult blood screening for colorectal neoplasia, funded by the Medical Research Council, was instigated in Nottingham in 1984 following the completion of a successful pilot study (Hardcastle et al., 1983). Within the next 12 months the trial will have completed recruitment of over 160,000 asymptomatic subjects between the ages of 50 and 74 years. The protocol allows for a minimum 7 years follow up following recruitment. At the present time 142,690 subjects have been recruited, screened and investigations completed.

2 METHOD OF RECRUITMENT

Eligible subjects are identified from the records of participating general practitioners. Following stratification by age and sex, individuals are randomised, by household, into test and control groups. Subjects in the test group are sent faecal occult blood tests, with a personal letter of invitation from the general practitioner. Members of the control group are not approached but are followed up for the development of colorectal carcinoma. Screen acceptors are re-screened at two-yearly intervals.

Careful scrutiny of all participants has been necessary to detect neoplasia in the control group, those who refused the test, and in those with negative tests in whom neoplasia may have been missed. This scrutiny has been by a regular check of the histopathology reports in all hospitals serving the trial population, and of local death registers. Further information has been provided by the Trent Cancer Registry and the National Health Service Central Register. Records of all subjects moving out of the trial area have been flagged and information regarding the development of colorectal carcinoma, and cause of death, has been provided to the study.

3 DIETARY RESTRICTION

In the Nottingham study dietary restrictions have not been imposed at the initial screen. It has been found that the request to omit certain foods liable to result in false-positive reactions results in a significant decrease in compliance (Thomas and Hardcastle, unpublished data), although this phenomenon has not been observed in the other major

European series. Individuals found to have positive Haemoccult tests are however retested with dietary restrictions in an attempt to reduce the rate of negative colonoscopy.

The effect of this policy has been reported in a cohort of 18,925 subjects and has been found to decrease the rate of positive reactions (and thus colonoscopy) by 56.4% (Thomas et al., 1989). However it was found necessary to perform a further test, delayed for three months, on those who were negative on a restricted diet. In this group of 317 people a further 4 carcinomas and 20 adenomas were identified, emphasizing the caution required if a dietary-retest policy is not to be associated with an unacceptable number of missed cancers. In the future consideration must be given to the use of a sensitive, human-specific, immunological faecal occult blood test as the second line investigation.

4 SECONDARY INVESTIGATION

Subjects with persistently positive test results are seen in a designated early diagnosis clinic. Following a full clinical examination, which includes rigid sigmoidoscopy, they are referred for colonoscopy. Subjects thought unsuitable for colonoscopy (in particular those with severe chronic obstructive airways disease) are referred in the first instance for a double contrast Barium Enema examination and flexible sigmoidoscopy.

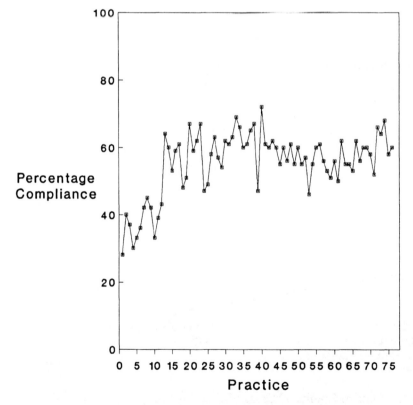

Figure 1   Compliance according to General Practice Number (numbered consecutively from the start of the pilot study until the present).

5 COMPLIANCE

At the present time compliance in the Nottingham study compares favourably with that from the other European series, with over 60% of participants completing the Haemoccult tests. However, in the early years of the study and in particular in the pilot study, when the first practices were included, the compliance was poor (Figure 1). The method of invitation has proved to be a particularly important factor in maximising participation rates; in the U.K., with its established system of General Practice, a personal letter of invitation from the family doctor results in a higher acceptance rate than that achieved by invitations sent from Health Service departments (Hardcastle et al., 1983).

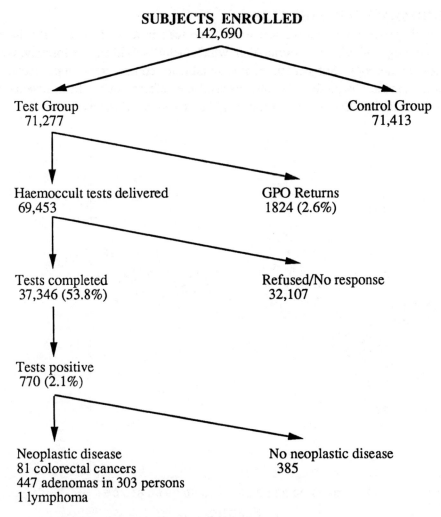

SUBJECTS ENROLLED
142,690

Test Group
71,277

Control Group
71,413

Haemoccult tests delivered
69,453

GPO Returns
1824 (2.6%)

Tests completed
37,346 (53.8%)

Refused/No response
32,107

Tests positive
770 (2.1%)

Neoplastic disease
81 colorectal cancers
447 adenomas in 303 persons
1 lymphoma

No neoplastic disease
385

Figure 2   The Nottingham Colorectal Cancer Screening Study
                  Initial Screen

It is perhaps not surprising that subjects with positive health attitudes are more likely to comply with Haemoccult screening than those who may be considered as having little regard for their general health (Farrands et al., 1983). The use of a reminder letter 6 weeks after the initial invitation results in an improvement in compliance of up to 5%. We are currently evaluating the role of a second reminder letter and also of personal telephone calls (which have been used in the Danish study to good effect), as the uptake of the tests is likely to be of critical importance in the long term outcome.

6 DETECTION OF NEOPLASIA

6.1 Initial Screen
Of the 71,277 subjects in the test group 69,453 received a screen invitation; of these 37,346 (53.8%) returned completed tests (Figure 2).

770 (2.1%) of the tests were positive and further investigation of these individuals revealed 81 cancers and 447 adenomas in 303 persons. (2.3 cancers per 1,000 screened, and 8.3 persons with adenomas per 1,000 screened).

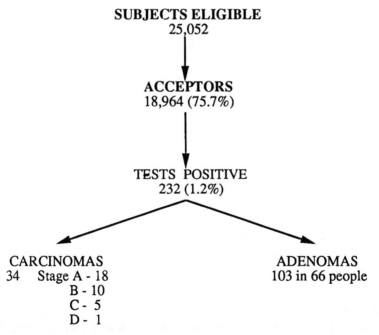

SUBJECTS ELIGIBLE
25,052

ACCEPTORS
18,964 (75.7%)

TESTS POSITIVE
232 (1.2%)

CARCINOMAS
34   Stage A - 18
              B - 10
              C - 5
              D - 1

ADENOMAS
103 in 66 people

Figure 3   The Nottingham Colorectal Cancer Screening Study
First Rescreen

6.2 First Rescreen

Compliance at the first two year rescreen was 75.7%, reflecting the motivation of the individuals who have already completed one screening test (Figure 3). Of these 232 (1.2%) had positive tests, 34 cancers (1.8 per 1,000 screened) and 103 adenomas in 66 people were diagnosed.

6.3 Second Rescreen

At the second rescreen 4,269 (81.5%) of the 5,237 eligible subjects completed the tests. Only 21 (0.5%) were positive (Figure 4). A further 6 carcinomas and 11 adenomas in 5 people were diagnosed.

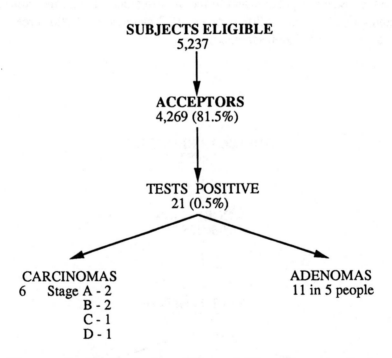

SUBJECTS ELIGIBLE
5,237

ACCEPTORS
4,269 (81.5%)

TESTS POSITIVE
21 (0.5%)

CARCINOMAS   ADENOMAS
6   Stage A - 2   11 in 5 people
        B - 2
        C - 1
        D - 1

Figure 4   The Nottingham Colorectal Cancer Screening Study
                Second Rescreen

6.4 Interval Cancer

Cancers diagnosed in the interval between a negative test and a retest are assumed to have been missed at the time of the Haemoccult screen. Thus by calculating the proportion of interval cancers in relation to the total number of cancers diagnosed in the group completing the Haemoccult test one may estimate the sensitivity of the test for asymptomatic carcinoma. Using this method, and allowing a minimum 2 year follow up, a sensitivity of 68% has been achieved for asymptomatic carcinoma in the Nottingham study (Thomas and Hardcastle, unpublished data).

6.5 Non-responder Group

In the end analysis it is essential to include the pathological findings, and mortality rates, of those who refused the screening test in the comparison with the control group. Only in this way will an allowance be made for the volunteer bias which would be expected to influence the results in favour of those who accepted screening. To date 33,931 subjects have failed to complete the tests. Amongst these 164 patients have presented with symptomatic carcinoma.

7 ANALYSIS OF CANCERS IN THE TEST AND CONTROL GROUP

7.1 Tumour Stage

The proportion of Stage A cancers is significantly higher in the screen detected group than in the control group ($X^2 = 66.07$, p <0.001) (Table 1). The difference is also seen when the whole test group is compared with the control group ($X^2 = 23.76$, p <0.001).

Table 1   Test and Control Group Cancers – Stage

	Test group (n=71,277)				Control group (n=71,413)
	Screen detected	Interval cases	Non-responders (n=33,931)	Total	
DUKES A	63 (52.1%)	13	23	99 (29.9%)	33 (12.9%)
DUKES B	29 (24.0%)	8	56	93 (28.1%)	88 (34.5%)
DUKES C	23 (19.0%)	18	32	73 (22.1%)	77 (30.2%)
Distant spread	6 (4.9%)	9	51	66 (19.9%)	57 (22.4%)
Unstaged	-	-	2	2	6
Total	121	48	164	333	261

The proportion of Stage D cancers is significantly lower in the screen detected group than the control group ($X^2 = 17.80$, p <0.001); however this difference is not maintained for the test group as a whole which has a similar proportion of advanced cancers to the control group ($X^2 = 0.51$).

7.2 Cancer Differentiation

The emergence of a length bias has previously been noted in the analysis of the first 107,000 subjects (Hardcastle et al., 1989), when a significantly higher proportion of cancers in both the screen detected (90%; $X^2 = 10.26$, p <0.001) and the whole test group (81% ; $X^2 = 5.22$, p <0.05) were well or moderately differentiated than were those in the control group (70%).

The present analysis (Table 2) maintains this trend. Currently tumour differentiation is being reviewed and a more comprehensive assessment of length bias is planned.

Table 2   Test and Control Group Cancers - Differentiation

	Test group				Control group
Differen-tiation	Screen detected	Interval	Non-responders	Total	
Good/Moderate	94	35	98	227	167
Poor	7	7	21	35	42
*Not Classified	20	6	45	71	52
Total	121	48	164	333	261

* Includes cancers currently under review

7.3 Treatment by Endoscopic Polypectomy Alone

Twenty one (17.3%) of the screen detected invasive cancers have been treated by endoscopic polypectomy alone; in contrast only 6 (2.3%) of the control group cancers have been amenable to this form of treatment ($x^2 = 28.22$, p<0.0001).

The difference from the control group is maintained for the whole test group where a total of 26 (7.8%) of the 333 cancers have been endoscopically treated ($X^2 = 8.71$, p<0.01).

In addition to the obvious advantage to individual patients this finding is also likely to represent a considerable financial saving to the Health Service if one assumes that many of the screen-detected malignant polyps would have eventually required colonic resections.

7.4 Adenomatous Polyps

A total of 571 polyps in 374 people have been detected by screening, a detection rate of 8.3/1,000 subjects screened at the initial screen, 3.5/1,000 subjects at the first rescreen and 1.2/1,000 at the second rescreen (Table 3).

Table 3 Test and Control Group Polyps – Distribution by Size

	Test group			Control group
Size (cm)	Screen detected	Interval	Non-responder	
0 – 0.9	204	19	38	65
1.0 – 1.9	249	21	28	65
> 2.0	118	9	16	42
Number of Polyps	571	49	82	172

The distribution according to histological type is given in Table 4.

Table 4   Histology of Screen-detected Polyps

Histological Type	Number
Tubular	275
Tubulovillous	204
Villous	15
Not retrieved	77
Total	571

As expected there is a clear correlation between adenoma size and degree of dysplasia. Considering only those screen detected adenomas in which the degree of dysplasia has been reviewed 20.8% of those 2cms or larger demonstrated severe dysplasia, compared with 10.5% of those between 1 - 1.9cms and only 1.7% of those smaller than 1cm.

8 FUTURE DEVELOPMENTS

It remains too early to demonstrate a mortality reduction, attributable to screening and independent of the screening biases. The large number of Stage A cancers in the screen detected group would suggest that a mortality reduction may be shown in the future. If this is achieved, consideration must be given to the introduction of mass population screening to the 'at risk' age group. In this situation cost will inevitably prove a determining factor.

The Nottingham study has incorporated a comprehensive economic assessment. Initial estimates suggest that the cost of detecting a cancer using the Haemoccult test, according to the present protocol, is approximately £3,000 sterling, a figure which compares favourably with that of cervical and breast cancer screening.

The other major contribution of the screening programme is the number of adenomas excised, especially the large, severely dysplastic adenomas. Given the well established malignant potential of such polyps it is possible that a reduction in the incidence of invasive cancers may be achieved although clearly this is a long-term objective and evaluation will require many years of follow-up.

8.1 Compliance

Compliance will possibly prove the critical factor in the success or otherwise of this study. Encouraging advances have already been made and one would expect that outside the confines of a screening study, and with the benefit of mass population education, compliance could be increased further.

International variations must be taken into account. Whereas the natural history of colorectal cancer may be expected to be very similar throughout the Western World, compliance may differ markedly, reflecting cultural differences.

Table 5   Yield of Neoplasia for 3 Day or 6 Day Haemoccult Testing

	3 Day	6 Day
Number offered test	17,616	17,568
Number completing test	10,176 (57.8%)	9,461 (53.8%)
Number postitive	131 (1.29%)	160 (1.69%)
Pathology detected	20 carcinomas	24 carcinomas
	112 adenomas	123 adenomas

8.2 Sensitivity of Faecal Occult Blood Tests

Although the sensitivity of Haemoccult appears to be higher in the Nottingham study than in the other worldwide studies, it must be considered a major limitation of the screening technique. We have examined the role of extended Haemoccult testing in an effort to improve sensitivity in a large study comprising 35,184 subjects randomly allocated to complete tests over 3 or 6 days (Thomas et al., 1990) (Table 5). There was an increased yield for both carcinoma and adenoma for 6 day testing; however this did not reach statistical significance, and the expected increase in sensitivity, derived from studies in symptomatic patients (Farrands and Hardcastle, 1983) was not attained.

The use of a combined faecal occult blood test with immunological test (Feca EIA) has previously been reported (Armitage et al., 1985). Again the yield of carcinoma was higher but this was associated with an unacceptable decrease in the specificity of the test for neoplasia, resulting in an unmanageable rate of colonoscopy.

In the Nottingham study we have not introduced test card rehydration although this has been found necessary elsewhere. In particular Kewenter et al (1988), found that if rehydration of tests slides was not employed the sensitivity for cancer was only 22.2%.

9   CONCLUSION

The Nottingham study continues to demonstrate the ability of the Haemoccult test to detect asymptomatic, early-stage carcinomas, and potentially malignant adenomas. The recruitment phase of the trial is now approaching completion; during the follow up phase it will become apparent whether the favourable pathological findings in the study group are translated into a mortality reduction and possibly a decrease in cancer incidence.

REFERENCES

Armitage NC, Hardcastle JD, Amar SS, Balfour TW, Haynes J, James PD. A comparison of an immunological faecal occult blood test Fecatwin Sensitive/Feca EIA with haemoccult in population screening for colorectal cancer. Br J Cancer 1985; 51:799-804.

Farrands PA, Chamberlain J, Hardcastle JD. Factors affecting compliance of screening for colorectal cancer. J Exper Clin Cancer Research 1983; 2:45.

Farrands PA, Hardcastle JD. Accuracy of occult blood tests over a six-day period. Clin Onc 1983; 9:217-225.

Hardcastle JD, Farrands PA, Balfour TW, Chamberlain J, Amar SS, Sheldon MG. Controlled trial of faecal occult blood testing in the detection of colorectal cancer. Lancet 1983; i:1-4.

Hardcastle JD, Thomas WM, Chamberlain J, Pye G, Sheffield J, James PD, Balfour TW, Amar SS, Armitage NC, Moss SM. Randomised, controlled trial of faecal occult blood screening for colorectal cancer: results for first 107,349 subjects. Lancet 1989; i:1160-1164.

Kewenter J, Bjork S, Haglind E, Smith L, Svanvik J, Ahren C. Screening and rescreening for colorectal cancer. A controlled trial of faecal occult blood testing in 27,700 subjects. Cancer 1988; 62:645-651.

Thomas WM, Pye G, Hardcastle JD, Chamberlain J, Charnley RM. Haemoccult screening for colorectal cancer - the role of dietary restriction and selective three month rescreening. Br J Surg 1989; 76:976-978.

Thomas WM, Pye G, Hardcastle JD, Mangham CM. A randomised trial of three and six day haemoccult screening for asymptomatic colorectal carcinoma. Br J Surg 1990; 77:277-279.

11 A Randomised Trial of Faecal Occult Blood Testing for Early Detection of Colorectal Cancer.
Results of Screening and Rescreening of 51325 Subjects.

J. KEWENTER [1], M. ASZTELY [2], B. ENGARÅS [1], E. HAGLIND [1], J. SVANVIK [1] AND C. ÅHRÉN [3]

Departments of Surgery [1], Radiology [2], and Pathology [3] .
Sahlgrenska Hospital, Göteborg, Sweden.

1 INTRODUCTION

The prognosis for subjects with colorectal cancer has improved during the last few years (Jeekel, 1987). This may partly be due to an increased survival after surgery but this is probably not the only factor. Population screening by faecal occult blood testing might be one way to reduce the mortality in this disease, which is among the most common types of carcinoma in western countries (Chamberlain, 1988). Prospective randomised trials are the only way to determine the value of this type of screening and five such studies are underway, two in the United States (Winawer et al, 1980; Gilbertsen et al, 1980) and three in Europe (Kewenter et al, 1988; Hardcastle et al, 1989; Kronborg et al, 1989).

The controlled trial of faecal occult blood screening described in this paper was started in 1982 and includes 27,700 inhabitants of Göteborg, Sweden, who were then between 60 and 64 years of age. Five years later, in 1987, 23,822 inhabitants who were then between 60 and 64 years of age were included in the study. This means that the whole population born between 1918 and 1927 participated in the study. Parts of this study have been presented previously (Kewenter et al, 1988).

2 MATERIAL AND METHODS

Although the two cohorts were studied at different times, the methods used were the same and the results are therefore pooled (Fig 1). Subjects were randomly allocated to a control group (25,670 persons) or to a test group (25,655 persons). In the first cohort, 13,759 test group subjects were offered screening between August 1982 and December 1983, with rescreening 16 - 22 months later (mean 20 months after the first screen). Rescreens were completed in December 1985.

In the second cohort, screening was offered to 11,896 persons in the test group between January 1987 and May 1988. The rescreening was started 14-17 months (mean 15 months) after the first screen and finished in May 1989.

Entire test population	Invitation and Hemoccult II slides + instruction
4 weeks	↓
Remaining test population	Reminder letter one
4 weeks	↓
Remaining test population	Reminder letter two and Hemoccult II slides + instructions

↓

Individuals with blood in the Hemoccult tests
investigated by sigmoidoscopy and
double contrast barium enema
Adenomas and cancers removed

14-22 months later

Entire test population	Invitation to rescreening and Hemoccult II slides + instruction
4 weeks	↓
Remaining test population	Reminder letter one
4 weeks	↓
Remaining test population	Reminder letter two and Hemoccult II slides + instructions

↓

Individuals with blood in the Hemoccult tests
investigated by sigmoidoscopy and
double contrast barium enema
Adenomas and cancers removed

Figure 1   Protocol for Screening

A letter of invitation and instruction together with three Hemoccult II tests (Smith Kline Diagnostic, Sunnyvale, CA) and a reply-paid envelope were mailed to the subjects in the test group The subjects were asked to perform Hemoccult II testing with two samples from each of three consecutive stools and to mail the slides back immediately after the last test. Two reminder letters were sent out to subjects who did not answer. In the last letter, another set of Hemoccult II slides were included All subjects were offered screening 14 - 22 months later in exactly the same way. The subjects were asked to avoid fresh fruit and vegetables, meat, food made of blood, and vitamin C tablets two days before and during the testing. All tests but those from persons in the first cohort born between 1 January, 1918 and 30 June 1920, were rehydrated before development. All tests were analysed within 5-6 days after stool collection. Individuals with one or more positive tests were called to the hospital for work-up including digital rectal examination, proctoscopy, rectosigmoidoscopy (60 centimeter) and a double contrast barium enema (DCE). Proctoscopy was performed as it is almost impossible to diagnose anal diseases e.g. haemorroids with rectosigmoidoscopy. Before work-up, the subjects were asked about abdominal symptoms during the last six months. It was also noted whether they had observed blood in the faeces during the last six months.

The statistical calculations were performed using Fisher´s exact test and the test for trend in contigency table.

3 RESULTS

3.1 Compliance and Prevalence of Positive Tests
Sixty-five per cent (16,711 persons) of the 25,655 subjects completed the test; 74% (12,305) of all responders returned the slides after the first mailing, 18% (2,994) after the second and 8% (1,412) after the third letter (Table 1).

Table 1   Distribution of subjects in the test groups at screening and rescreening.

	Number
Test group at the start of the initial screening	25655
Test group at the start of the rescreening	25048
Participants in the initial screening	16711
Participants in the rescreening	14917
Died in the interval between screenings	571
Lost to follow-up after the initial screening	36
Participated in both screenings	13924
Participated in the initial screening only	2716
Participated in the rescreening only	993

Sixty per cent (14,917 persons) of the remaining 25,048 subjects completed the test at the rescreening. Seventy per cent of those (10,416) returned the slides after the first mailing, 22 % (3,314) after the second and 8 % (1,187) after the third letter. Ninety-three per cent of those who submitted the slides at the second screening had also performed the first testing; 7% (993) had not participated in the first screening.

Of the subjects in the unhydrated test group, 1.9% (84/4,436) had a positive test compared to 6.1% (751/12,275) of the subjects in the group where the slides were rehydrated before development in the initial screen. At the rescreening 6.0% (895/14,917) were positive. Among those where the slides were also rehydrated in the first screening, 5.3% (588/11,097) were positive on rescreening.

Seven hundred and twelve of the 835 (85%) subjects with a positive test at the first screening had a complete work-up, 47 (6%) a limited work-up with proctoscopy and sigmoidoscopy and 76 subjects (9%) refused work-up. In the rescreening, 783 of the 895 (87%) had a full work up, 41 (5%) a limited work-up and 71 (8%) refused work-up. Sixty-one subjects had a positive test in both the first and second screening and fifty-six of these had a full work-up on both occasions.

3.2 Carcinomas
Initial screen   Thirty-eight subjects with carcinomas were diagnosed at the initial screening, which corresponds to 2.3 per 1000 who performed the test (0.9 per 1000 subjects with unhydrated and 2.7 per 1000 subjects with rehydrated slides). The stages of all carcinomas are shown in Table 2 and the sites of the carcinomas in Table 3.

Table 2   Subjects with diagnosed carcinomas in the test and control groups, and distribution according to Dukes' classification.

Stage	No.(%) in the test group						No.(%) in the control group
	Screening-detected			Non-			
	Initial	Re-screened	Interval*	responders	Total		
A	19 (50)	8 (31)	0	1 (8)	28 (30)		4 (12)
B	7 (18)	7 (27)	6 (33)	2 (17)	22 (23)		8 (24)
C	11 (29)	6 (23)	8 (45)	4 (33)	29 (31)		13 (38)
D	1 (3)	5 (19)	4 (22)	5 (42)	15 (16)		9 (26)
Total	38	26	18	12	94		34

* Two subjects with a carcinoma and positive test overlooked at the work-up are included in this group.

Rescreening   Twenty-six subjects with carcinomas were diagnosed at the rescreening, which corresponds to 1.7 per 1000 persons who performed the test.

Nineteen of the screening-detected carcinomas were adenomas with foci of invasive cancer. Fifteen of these subjects had a large bowel resection. In four subjects polypectomy was the only treatment.

Interval carcinomas   Sixteen carcinomas were diagnosed in the time period between first screening and rescreening among subjects with a negative Hemoccult II test. Thirteen of these belonged to the initial group (4,436 individuals) where the slides were unhydrated. In two subjects with positive tests (one with unhydrated and one with rehydrated slides), the carcinomas were overlooked at DCE. Half of the carcinomas were located in the right colon and half in the left colon including the sigmoid colon and the rectum (Table 3).

Table 3   Site of carcinomas

Site	Screen detected (n=64)	Interval (n=18)	Non-responders (n=12)	Control group (n=34)
Rectum	19 (30%)	2 (11%)	5 (42%)	18 (53%)
Sigmoid	29 (45%)	7 (39%)	4 (33%)	5 (15%)
Descending	5 (8%)	1 (5%)	1 (8%)	3 (9%)
Transverse	3 (5%)	3 (17%)	2 (17%)	2 (6%)
Caecum/ ascending	8 (12%)	5 (28%)		6 (17%)

Non-responders   Twelve carcinomas were diagnosed among the refusers (8,944 individuals) during the same period. The incidence of colorectal carcinomas was 0.8 per 1000 person-years. These persons had on their own initiative undergone investigation due to symptoms.

Control group   Thirty-four subjects with carcinomas have been diagnosed in the control group corresponding to an incidence of 0.7 per 1000 person - years. These persons had on their own initiative consulted a doctor due to symptoms. Two of these carcinomas were adenomas with foci of invasive cancer. Both these subjects had a large bowel resection.

3.3 Adenomas
Initial screen   204 benign adenomas were diagnosed in 159 subjects, which corresponds to 9.5 per 1000 subjects screened; 113 of the adenomas in 95 subjects were one centimetre or more in diameter (5.7 per 1000 subjects screened) (Table 4).

Table 4   Numbers of subjects with diagnosed adenomas in the test and control groups, and the number of adenomas in the two groups.

	Test group					Control group
	Screen detected		Interval	Non-responders	Total	
	First screening	Rescreened				
Number of subjects	159	153	10	11	333	40
Number of adenomas	204	209	14	13	440	50
Number of adenomas 1.0 cm or more	113	107	6	8	234	21

Rescreening   209 adenomas were diagnosed in 153 subjects at the rescreening, which corresponds to 10.3 per 1000 subjectss screened; 107 of the adenomas in 90 subjects were one centimetre or more in diameter (6.0 per 1000 subjects screened) (Table 4).

Interval adenomas   Fourteen adenomas were diagnosed in 10 subjects (Table 4). Six of the adenomas were one centimetre or more in diameter. These subjects represent the number of persons with a negative test in the first screening who, on their own initiative, consulted a doctor due to gastrointestinal symptoms. The investigation then revealed an adenoma.

Non responders   Thirteen adenomas were found in 11 subjects (8,944 individuals), which corresponds to an incidence of 0.7 per 1000 person-years (Table 4). Eight of the adenomas had a diameter of one centimetre or more (0.3 per 1000 person-years). All these persons had consulted a doctor on their own initiative, and the adenomas were found at that investigation.

Control group   Fifty adenomas were diagnosed in 40 subjects during the same period, which corresponds to an incidence of 0,8 per 1000 person-years (Table 4). Twenty of the adenomas in fourteen subjects were one centimetre or more in diameter (0.3 per 1000 person-years). All these subjects underwent investigation on their own initiative.

3.4 Comparison of Carcinomas in Different Groups

The distribution according to Dukes' stage was more favourable in the whole test group compared to the control group ($p < 0.05$), in the screening detected carcinomas compared to the control group ($p < 0.001$) and in the screening-detected carcinomas compared to the interval carcinomas ($p < 0.01$). There was a significantly increased number of Dukes' A carcinomas among the screening detected carcinomas compared to the control group ($p < 0.01$).

4 DISCUSSION

The compliance was 65% at the initial screening and dropped to 60% at the rescreening. These figures were reached after two reminder letters. To send out these letters was costly, time-consuming and demanded a lot of work. However, if this had not been done the compliance would have been as low as 48% and 43% respectively. The compliance figures are, together with those from Denmark (Kronborg et al, 1989), the highest reported for this type of screening. It is possible that the compliance can be further increased by advertising in the press. However, we have not used the mass media and not discussed the study in public, in order to avoid any contaminating effect on the control group.

In contrast to the Nottingham and Funen studies all subjects were invited to participate in the rescreening regardless of whether they had participated in the first study or not (Hardcastle et al, 1989; Kronborg et al, 1989). Nine hundred and ninety-three (7% of the participants in the rescreening) persons sent in the slides for the first time at the rescreening. Five carcinomas were diagnosed in five subjects and an adenoma one centimeter or more in diameter in five more subjects. Four of the subjects with a carcinoma were asymptomatic, that is, they reported no bleeding or other gastrointestinal symptoms at the interview.

The compliance for a full work-up was eighty-six per cent of the 1,730 subjects with a positive test and five per cent more underwent rectosigmoidoscopy only. These figures were obtained after repeated telephone calls to those with positive tests who did not come for examination after the first call. No neoplasm has up to now been diagnosed among the 147 subjects who refused work-up.

The interval cancer rate, which is an expression of the number of false negative tests for carcinomas, differed markedly depending on whether the slides were rehydrated or not. In the small part of the study with unhydrated slides, the rate of interval carcinoma was 77% (14 of 18 subjects with a carcinoma) but it dropped to 11% (4 of 36) with rehydrated slides. One of the four carcinomas was overlooked at the work-up, so that the true rate of false negative tests was 8% (3/36). The corresponding figures for the English and Danish studies with unhydrated slides were 22% and 44% respectively (22/98, 40/90) (Hardcastle et al, 1989; Kronborg et al, 1989). The test group contains more screening-detected carcinomas in Göteborg compared to the English and Danish studies.

The prognosis according to Dukes' classification for the interval carcinomas seemed to be less favourable than for the screening-detected carcinomas in the Danish study but this did not seem to be the case in the English study (Hardcastle et al, 1989; Kronborg et al, 1989). In the present investigation, the distribution according to Dukes' classification showed significantly more unlocalised tumours among the interval carcinomas compared to the screening-detected carcinomas, indicating that the number of Hemoccult false negative carcinomas (i.e. interval carcinomas) must be kept to a minimum.

Among the screening-detected carcinomas, there was a significant increase of Dukes' A carcinomas (42%) compared to the control group, which is in accordance with the English and Danish trials (Hardcastle et al, 1989; Kronborg et al, 1989). Nineteen of the sixty-four screening-detected carcinomas were pedunculated and initially removed endoscopically, compared with two carcinomas of 34 in the control group. Without further resection, these carcinomas would all have been classified as Dukes' A, which has been the case in the other trials, 19 in the English and 9 in the Danish study, as their policy has been polypectomy alone without resection (Hardcastle et al, 1989; Kronborg et al, 1989). In our material, fifteen of the nineteen subjects with a malignant polyp underwent a colonic resection. On examination of the resected specimens, twelve were found to belong to Dukes' A, one to Dukes' B and two to Dukes' C; 47% would have been misclassified as Dukes' A if resection had not been performed. Both Dukes' C carcinomas fulfilled the criteria outlined by Morson for endoscopic polypectomy only (Winawer et al, 1980).

The number of carcinomas among the refusers constitute 13% of the carcinomas in the test group in our study, compared to 46% and 30% respectively in the English and Danish studies (Hardcastle et al, 1989; Kronborg et al, 1989). The difference between the English and the Scandinavian studies can at least partly be explained by the difference in compliance. The difference between the Swedish and the Danish study, where the compliance was the same, is difficult to understand. It might partly be explained by the fact that all subjects were offered rescreening in the Swedish study but only those who participated in the first study in Denmark. Five of the twenty-six carcinomas diagnosed at the rescreening in the Göteborg study belonged to this group.

The vast majority of the slides were rehydrated as the number of false negative tests with unhydrated slides was found to be too high (Kewenter et al, 1988). The increased sensitivity obtained with rehydration occurs at the cost of decreased specificity (Mandel et al, 1989). It has been argued that the increased number of subjects with a positive Hemoccult test obtained by rehydration would necessitate a less accurate examination than colonoscopy in order to deal with all subjects with a positive test (Kronborg et al, 1989). We have clearly shown that double contrast barium enema combined with flexible sigmoidoscopy is as accurate as colonoscopy (Jensen et al, 1990). Nevertheless, it is desirable to increase the specificity on rehydration with no or only a small change of the sensitivity. Elliot et al (1984) suggested retesting of those with a positive Hemoccult test combined with dietary restriction and work-up of only those who were positive on retesting

(Jensen et al, 1990). We have investigated the value of a similar approach, where participants with a positive initial Hemoccult test were asked to perform another series of six Hemoccult tests. In a cohort of 3,561 individuals, the rate of positive Hemoccult tests dropped from 5.9% to 1.9% on retesting. Ten of eleven subjects with diagnosed carcinomas and 15 of 21 with adenomas with a diameter of one centimetre or more were positive on retesting. The specificity increased from 95% to 98%, which means a large reduction of the number of subjects to be worked-up in a population based screening. One way to reduce the negative effects that such a method could have, due to the slightly decreased sensitivity, is probably to shorten the intervals between the screenings.

Cancers found at repeated screening are also relevant in calculating the false negative rate of guaiac testing in the initial screen. Using a denominator of 26 cancers from rescreening (assuming they were present at first screen) + 18 interval cancers + 38 initial cancers + n (undetected cancers in the remainder) the maximum guaiac sensitivity was 46 per cent (if n = 0). The corresponding figures for unhydrated and rehydrated slides were 12+14+4=13% and 14+4+34=65%, respectively. The need to increase the sensitivity of the unhydrated Hemoccult II in order to detect more colorectal neoplasms has obviously been recognised by the manufactures (Smith Kline Diagnostic) as they have recently released a more sensitive test, Hemoccult Sensa[R].

In conclusion, this screening programme for early detection of colorectal neoplasms shows that such screening can be performed using fecal occult blood testing. If the Hemoccult II is used, the slides must be rehydrated in order to achieve high enough sensitivity. The results in terms of neoplasms found and their classification are encouraging as the percentage of localised tumours increased significantly in the screened population.

Acknowledgement

This work was supported by the Swedish Cancer Society (1765-B89-08XC) and the Assar Gabrielsson Foundation. The authors acknowledge the considerable assistance provided by Kristina Gustavsson, Elisabet Lindholm,R.N., Christina Svensson, R.N. and the staff of the Department of Radiology, Pathology, the Out-patient clinic, the Operation of Surgery I and Prof Kock's laboratory. We are grateful to Anders Odén for the statistical analysis.

REFERENCES

Chamberlain J. Discussion on screening for colorectal cancer. In Chamberlain J, Miller AB (eds). Screening for gastro-intestinal cancer. International units against cancer. Hans Huber Publishers, Toronto, 1988, pp. 53-61.
Elliot MS, Levenstein JH, Wright JP. Fecal occult blood testing in the detection of colorectal cancer. Br J Surg 1984; 71:785-786.
Gilbertsen VA, Church TR, Grewe FJ. The design of a study to assess occult blood screening for colorectal cancer. J Chron Dis 1980; 33:107-114.

Hardcastle JD, Chamberlain J, Sheffield J, et al. Randomised,controlled trial of feacal occult blood screening for colorectal cancer. Results for first 107349 subjects. Lancet 1989; i:1160-1164.

Jeekel J. Can radical surgery improve survival in colorectal cancer? World J Surg 1987; 11:412-417.

Jensen J, Kewenter J, Asztely M, Lycke G, Wojciechowski J. Is double contrast enema and rectosigmoidoscopy a reliable diagnostic combination for detection of colorectal neoplasms? Brit J Surg 1990; 77:270-272.

Kewenter J, Björk S, Haglind E, Smith L, Svanvik J, Åhrén Ch. Screening and rescreening for colorectal cancer. A controlled trial of fecal occult testing in 27700 subjects. Cancer 1988; 62:645-651.

Kronborg O, Fenger C, Olsen J, Bech K, Söndergaard O. Repeated screening for colorectal cancer with fecal occult blood test. Scand J Gastroenterol 1989; 24:599-606.

Mandel JS, Bond JH, Bradley M, et al. Sensitivity, specificity and positive predictivity of Hemoccult test in screening for colorectal cancers. Gastroenterology 1989; 97:597-600.

Morson BC. The polyp cancer sequence in the large bowel. Proc Roy Soc Med 1974; 67:451-457.

Winawer SJ, Andrews M, Flehinger B, et al. Progress report on controlled trial of fecal occult blood testing for the detection of colorectal neoplasia. Cancer 1980; 5:2959-2964.

12 Interim Report on a Randomised Trial of Screening for Colorectal Cancer with Hemoccult-II

O. KRONBORG, C. FENGER and J. OLSEN

Department of Surgical Gastroenterology and Pathology, Odense University Hospital and Institute of Social Medicine, Aarhus University.

1 INTRODUCTION

The Funen randomized controlled trial included 30,970 persons allocated to screening with a faecal occult blood test (Hemoccult-II) every 2 years and 30,968 persons allocated to a control group, both groups being selected from a population between 45 and 74 years of age in 1985. The study has been described in detail previously (Kronborg et al, 1987; Kronborg et al, 1989). The first screening was completed in 20,672 persons and 18,779 of these completed re-screening 2 years later. Of those screened, 215 had a positive Hemoccult-II test on the initial screen and 159 on the second screen. The third screening began in August 1989 and so far 6,700 have participated.

2 THE GOALS OF THE TRIAL

Seven goals were set up at the beginning of the trial (Kronborg et al, 1988), and this contribution presents provisional answers to the questions arising from these goals.

2.1 Question 1

Does screening improve the distribution of colorectal cancer according to Dukes' classification?
If so, by how much?

Answer: Probably yes, since the proportion of Dukes' A cases has increased considerably (P=0.00001); the proportions of Dukes' C (P=0.02) as well as (Dukes' C + distant spread) cases have decreased (P=0.01). The evaluation is based upon a comparison between the whole test group (including interval cases, non-responders and those diagnosed with cancer before being invited to screening) and the controls (Table 1). Dukes' A cancer has been found in 52 of 190 persons with cancer in the test group (27%) and in 15 of 166 controls (9%). More advanced cancers including Dukes' C, those with distant spread and unclassified cancers, were found in 81 of the cancers in the test group (42%) and in 94 controls (56%).

Table 1 Colorectal cancers classified according to Dukes' staging

Group (n)	Dukes A	Dukes B	Dukes C	Distant Spread	Unstaged
Test group					
Initial screen (37)	19	11	5	2	0
Second screen (13)	7	3	3	0	0
Third screen (7)	3	2	1	0	1
Interval cases (56)	10	15	15	12	4
Non-responders:					
to initial screen (56)	6	17	7	23	3
to second screen (3)	2	0	0	0	1
Before invitation (18)	5	9	1	3	0
Total (190)	52	57	32	40	9
Control group (166)	15	57	46	39	9

2.2 Question 2

Will precancerous lesions (adenomas) be different in the test group compared to controls, according to size, degree of dysplasia and amount of villous structures?

Answer: More adenomas and more large adenomas have been removed in the test group (Table 2).

Table 2   Distribution of adenomas during two screenings according to size of largest adenoma

Group	Size of largest adenoma (mm)			
	< 10	10-19	20 or more	Total
Test group				
Initial screen	18	49	19	86
Second screen	15	42	19	76
Interval cases	18	15	7	40
Non-responders*	14	7	9	30
Total	65	113	54	232
Control group	47	36	26	109

*Including adenomas diagnosed after randomization but before invitation to screening

Tubular adenomas were more common in the test group, but mild dysplasia was less common compared to controls. Furthermore screen-detected adenomas were more frequent in males and were located more frequently in the sigmoid colon compared to controls having the majority of adenomas in the rectum.

2.3 Question 3
Will the incidence rate of colorectal carcinoma be reduced?

Answer: Colorectal cancer was detected during the 4th year of study in 14 out of the 20,672 persons having the Hemoccult-II test performed at least once, in contrast to 38 out of 30,968 controls during the same period of time (P=0.07). However, colorectal cancer was detected in 34 persons in the whole test group (30,970) during the 4th year.

2.4 Question 4
Can the mortality from colorectal cancer be reduced by 25% or more by screening with Hemoccult-II in asymptomatic persons between 45 and 74 years of age?

Answer So far, 58 have died from colorectal cancer in the test group and 71 in the control group (Table 3), a reduction of 18% (95% confidence limits 10%-29%). Six deaths in the test group occurred among the 18 patients diagnosed with colorectal cancer after randomization but before the invitation for screening could be made.

Table 3   Cases and Deaths from colorectal cancer

Group	Number of cancers	Number of deaths
Test group		
Initial screen	37	4
Second screen	13	0
Third screen	7	0
Interval cases	53	24
Non-responders	59	24
Before invitation	18	6
Total	187	58
Control group	162	71

2.5 Question 5
Will the overall mortality be reduced by screening with Hemoccult-II?

Answer: The mortality figures up to the present time are seen from Table 4; 2221 is not significantly less than 2317 (P=0.14).

Table 4 Cumulative number of deaths from all causes during the first 52
months

Months	Test group	Control group
2	53	57
6	175	194
12 (end of initial screening)	394	435
24	882	902
36 (end of second screening)	1445	1472
48	1994	2049
52 (4 months into third screening)	2221	2317

The overall mortality among non-responders (1,268/10,273) is significantly higher than among those having performed Hemoccult-II test at least once (953/20,672), and also higher than among controls (2,317/30,968). Questions relating to prolonged survival and socioeconomic consequences of screening cannot be answered at the present time.

3 DISCUSSION
Screening with Hemoccult-II increases the proportion of early cancers. This is an advantage, since radical surgery may be less extensive and followed by a lower post-operative mortality. Even endoscopic removal of small cancers may represent radical surgery. A reduction in mortality from colorectal cancer can only be achieved, if the number of more advanced cancers decreases. The figures suggest that this might happen in the future but the present reduction from 94 to 81 is not significant.

Hopefully, removal of more large adenomas within the test group will result in decreasing number of colorectal cancers, but so far this has not happened. However, the adenoma-carcinoma sequence is supposed to take several years, and a significant decrease in number of cancers cannot be expected to take place before the year 1995.

The preliminary figures suggest that mortality from colorectal cancer will be reduced by screening, but it is too early to guess the size of the reduction. Unfortunately, it was not possible to invite 30,970 people for screening and examine those with positive tests within a shorter period than one year. Since the random allocation to screening or control was performed on one day for all 61,938 persons, some developed cancer within the test group before they could be invited for screening. Exclusion of these from the final evaluation, is not possible without selection bias, and they have been included in the present comparisons. The mortality figures for non-responders did not differ form those in controls, whereas the number of the deaths from colorectal cancer in persons having had at least one negative Hemoccult-II test (24/20,457) was significantly lower than among controls (71/30,968) (P=0.005).

The reduction in mortality from colorectal cancer within the whole test group (58) compared to controls (71) is not significant (P=0.29). It is therefore not surprising that no significant effect on overall mortality from screening can be demonstrated at the present time.

The high overall mortality among non-responders is due to other severe diseases than colorectal cancer. Attempts to increase acceptability of screening beyond the present 67% may therefore not have the same expected beneficial effect on overall mortality as among the 67%.

It should be kept in mind that other severe diseases, not necessarily malignant diseases, will increase the small risk of the screening strategy itself, which includes colonoscopy and polypectomy in persons with a positive Hemoccult-II test. The present study only excluded persons with other incurable malignant diseases, because it was not possible to evaluate severity of cardiopulmonary diseases from the patient file of the county. However, patients with positive Hemoccult-II tests were examined at the clinic, and a small number with severe cardiopulmonary disease were not subjected to full colonoscopy.

Acknowledgement
Support was given by the Danish Cancer Society, Sygekassernes Helsefond, The Danish Medical Research Council, The county of Funen, Astrid Thaysens foundation and several others.

REFERENCES
Kronborg O, Fenger C, Søndergaard O, et al. Initial mass screening for colorectal cancer with fecal occult blood test. A prospective randomized study at Funen in Denmark. Scand J Gastroenterol 1987; 22:677-686.

Kronborg O, Fenger C, Olsen J, et al. Repeated screening for colorectal cancer with fecal occult blood test. A prospective randomized study at Funen, Denmark. Scand J Gastroenterol 1989; 24:599-606.

Kronborg O, Fenger C, Olsen J, et al. Preliminary report on a randomized trial of screening for colorectal cancer with Hemoccult-II. In: Chamberlain J, Miller AB, (eds). Screening for gastro-intestinal cancer. Hans Huber Publishers: Toronto, 1988, 41-44.

13 Case-control Evaluation of Colorectal Cancer Screening in the Federal Republic of Germany

J. WAHRENDORF

Institute of Epidemiology and Biometry, German Cancer Research Center
Heidelberg, Federal Republic of Germany

1 INTRODUCTION

There is not yet conclusive epidemiological evidence about the efficacy of screening programmes for colorectal cancer based on occult blood tests (Chamberlain et al., 1986). Some prospective studies are underway (Hardcastle et al., 1986, 1989; Kronborg, 1987, 1989) but it is unlikely that conclusive evidence from these studies will emerge in the immediate future. Evaluation of screening programmes by case-control methods (Sasco et al., 1986) have proven to be very efficient for cervical cancer (Clarke & Anderson, 1979; McGregor et al., 1985) and breast cancer (Collette et al., 1984; Verbeek et al., 1984). It is therefore compelling to look out for possibilities for the retrospective evaluation of colorectal cancer screening programmes.

The occult blood test was introduced as a component of the screening activities under the statutory health insurance system in the Federal Republic of Germany in 1977 and is offered to all men and women at age 45 and above. Records of all screening examinations are kept in a central institute of the health insurance system. This system was unfortunately set up without maintaining the identification of the person on the record. Consequently, only cross-sectional analyses have been carried out so far (Robra & Schwartz, 1984) and have indicated that the annual participation rate of the eligible proportion of the population is about 10 to 15%. However, it has been estimated that the cumulative participation rate (ever participated) is of the order of 50% in the German population of appropriate age.

With this high prevalence of "exposure" in the general population it seemed worthwhile to investigate whether a case-control evaluation of the colorectal cancer screening programme would be feasible in the Federal Republic of Germany. Such a case-control evaluation would have to address the question whether individuals dying of colorectal cancer have on average a history of less screening compared to appropriate healthy controls. In such a study one would therefore need to have:
    (a) access to deaths of colorectal cancer in a given population,
    (b) access to appropriate population controls and
    (c) access to the complete screening history of the cases and controls.

Following a request by the International Agency for Research on Cancer (World Health Organisation) as to whether such an investigation would be feasible in the Federal Republic of Germany a pilot study was undertaken to explore possible avenues of investigation. In this paper a description of the insights gained from this pilot study and the approaches taken for the main study, which was later supported by the European Community (Europe against Cancer) as well as the Federal Ministry of Research and Technology in the Federal Republic of Germany, will be discussed.

2 STUDY AREA AND APPROACHES TAKEN
It was decided to conduct such a feasibility study in a well defined geographical region. The Saarland is one of the ten essential administrative areas (Länder) of the Federal Republic of Germany. It covers a population of about one million and is of particular interest since the only functioning population-based cancer registry in the Federal Republic of Germany is operating in that area. In addition, the situation in the Saarland was found to be particularly suitable since its size would give rise to an appropriate number of colorectal cancer deaths and since the administrative requirements were deemed to be sufficiently manageable in a population of one million. The engagement of the Director of the Institute of Pathology of the University of the Saarland in issues such as cancer registration and cancer epidemiology, together with his broad professional experience and commitments (Chairman of the Saarland Society for Cancer Control) were felt to be particularly important for the success of an investigation in the Saarland.

In discussion with health officials in the Saarland it became apparent that the statistical office of the Saarland which collects mortality records and also runs the cancer registry is prohibited by law to release lists of individuals who died of colorectal cancer. These institutions would therefore not be able to serve as a case-finding system and alternative approaches had to be considered.

Under the current German legislation a pathologist who is analysing biopsy material from a cancer patient is considered as a co-treating physician and allowed to retrieve further individual-based information about his patients. It was therefore considered that the four pathology departments in the Saarland together with the one pathology department in nearby Trier would hold in their collection of biopsied cases a nexus of potential deaths of colorectal cancer among inhabitants of the Saarland and, thus, represent a valuable starting point.

In the feasibility study the possibility of retrieving biopsied cases from pathological institutes was explored in two such institutes and proved to be possible. Furthermore, the approach to residential registries in order to assess each individual's vital status was developed and proved feasible. The importance of getting concrete information about the referring physician from whom later the screening history was supposed to be retrieved was identified. Several inquiries to the treating hospitals who sent in the biopsy cases to the pathological departments were necessary to establish a referring physician for each index case.

During this work-up of cases possibilities for identifying appropriate controls were explored. It was felt that selecting controls from among the patients of the practitioner of an index case was a very feasible procedure. This ensures a certain degree of matching for socio-economic status and equality of the quality of information. The information for the controls was to be given anonymously to the study centre.

3 STATE OF THE MAIN STUDY

In the second half of 1988 the main study was started. From the files of the pathological institutes 2809 bioptsied cases of colorectal cancer were identified which had been diagnosed between 1979 and 1985 in the age range 45 to 74 years. An individual-based follow-up for the vital status of these cases through residential registries led to the identification of 676 individuals who died between 1983 and 1986 in the age-range 55 to 74 years. The latter age- and time-window was defined to be most important for the evaluation of the effect of colorectal cancer screening by occult blood tests, which started in 1977, on colorectal cancer mortality.

A comparison with the records of the Saarland cancer registry identified that the corresponding figures of reported cases of colorectal cancer in the cancer registry for the time period 1979 to 1985 in the age-range 45 to 74 years was 2938 and the numbers of deaths among these cases occurring in the time period of 1983 to 1986 in the age-range 55 to 74 was 685. Therefore, the results obtained by our step-by-step retrieval can be viewed to be very complete.

For all 676 deaths, contacts to a referring general practitioner were attempted in order to get concrete information about cause of death and the screening history of these cases. This procedure is currently underway and will lead also to the identification of a suitable number of controls from the files of the general practitioner. It is considered appropriate to ask the practitioner to enlist the potential age-sex-matched controls from his files, the study center will select randomly four controls for which the practitioners will then give details about their screening history.

4 DISCUSSION

The project has to take a very involved approach due to the complicated situation around cancer registration, data privacy and secrecy of medical records in the Federal Republic of Germany. Much easier linkage procedures could be devised which would facilitate answering this important question more efficiently. However, as the situation in the Federal Republic of Germany is the only one where a retrospective evaluation of colorectal cancer screening can be carried out, it seems worthwhile to undertake the efforts described above.

The contacts to the various institutions and physicians require very intensive support by staff and computing facilities. A special study centre was established at Homburg/Saar for this purpose. The retrieval of the screening history is currently underway and burdened with many day-to-day problems. However, we hope a useful answer towards an important public health question will be developed using this approach.

REFERENCES
Chamberlain J, Day NE, Hakama M, Miller AB and Prorok PC. UICC workshop of the Project on Evaluation of Screening Programmes for Gastrointestinal Cancer. Int.J.Cancer 1986; 37:329-334.

Clarke EA and Anderson TW. Does screening by 'pap' smears help prevent cervical cancer? Lancet 1979; ii:1-4.

Collette HJA, Day NE, Rombach JJ and de Waard J. Evaluation of screening for breast cancer in a non-randomised study (the DOM-Project) by means of a case control study. Lancet 1984; i:1224-1226.

Hardcastle JD, Armitage NC, Chamberlain J, Amar SS, James PD, and Balfour TW. Fecal occult blood screening for colorectal cancer in the general population: results of a controlled trial. Cancer 1986; 58:397-403.

Hardcastle JD, Chamberlain J, Sheffield J et al. Randomised, controlled trial of faecal occult blood screening for colorectal cancer. Lancet 1989; i:1160-1164.

Kronborg O, Fenger C, Sondergaard O, Pedersen KM, and Olsen,J. Initial Mass Screening for Colorectal Cancer with Fecal Occult Blood Test. A Prospective Randomized Study at Funen in Denmark. Scand.J.Gastroenterol. 1987; 22:677-686.

Kronborg O, Fenger C, Olsen J, Bech K, and Sondergaard O. Repeated Screening for Colorectal Cancer with Fecal Occult Blood Test. A Prospective Randomized Study at Funen in Denmark. Scand.J.Gastroenterol. 1989; 24:599-606.

Mac Gregor JE, Moss SM, Parkin DM, and Day NE. A case-control study of cervical cancer screening in north east Scotland. Brit.Med.J. 1985; 290:1543-1546.

Robra B-P and Schwartz FW. Experiences with a nationwide screening program for colorectal cancer in the Federal Republic of Germany." In: Hardcastle, J.D. (ed.). Haemoccult screening for the early detection of colorectal cancer: a workshop held at the XII. Internat. Gastroenterology Congress (ADNEMGE), Lisboa, Portugal, September 16-22, 1984. Stuttgart, New York: Schattauer, 1986, pp.13-20.

Sasco AJ, Day NE, and Walter SD. Case-control studies for the evaluation of screening. J.Chron.Dis. 1986; 39:399-405.

Verbeek ALM, Hendriks JHCL, Holland R, Mravunac M, Sturmans F, and Day NE. Reduction of breast cancer mortality through mass screening with modern mammography - first results from the Nijmegen Project, 1975-1981. Lancet 1984; i:1222-1224.

14 Summary of the Discussion on Colo-Rectal Cancer Screening

It was questioned whether the population in the control group in the Minnesota trial was continuing to show 70% of the mortality from colorectal cancer expected from the general population. The last three years in fact show a rise above the asymptote that could be related to the "wearing-out" of the healthy screenee effect that seems to have affected the earlier years of the trial. However, it was noted that so far there had been no difference in the cumulative incidence of advanced cancer in the three groups in the trial.

It was also suggested that the low specificity in the trial and the use of colonoscopy for diagnosis might be resulting in the situation that the assessment would be of colonoscopy rather than faecal occult blood tests. In practice, currently about 20% of the annual screen group have received a colonoscopy at least once, this proportion is expected to reach 30% within the next 5 years.

The interval cancer experience in the colorectal screening trials shows the maximal rate in the first year, falling off in the second year, which is the reverse of that seen in the breast cancer screening trials. No explanation was forthcoming for that effect.

The compliance level in the Nottingham trial, and a lower than expected colorectal cancer mortality in the control group, suggests that it may not be possible to detect the 25% mortality reduction originally sought. It is not clear why at present the number of colorectal cancers seen in the refusers is more than in those who complied with the test. Currently, to compensate for these effects, an evaluation is underway to assess the power of the trial to detect a 10% mortality reduction, with longer follow-up. Although there is some concern over a relatively low sensitivity of the test in the Nottingham trial, the investigators have decided that they could not cope with the level of false positives seen in the Minnesota trial. Although another test was tried for a while, the level of false positives was too high so they resumed the use of the Haemoccult ™ test without rehydration.

There was some discussion over the approach to improve the specificity in the Göteborg trial, involving a second test for those who test positive on the first. Two effects might be operating to explain the reduced positivity on the second test; a greater compliance with the dietary restrictions recommended before the test and a regression towards the mean phenomenon.

The very low sensitivity of the unhydrated tests in the early part of the Göteborg study appeared to be due in part to a rate of interval cancers greater than the rate in the control group. This suggests that chance variation in occurrence of interval cancers was in part responsible for this. It was also pointed out that the cancer detection rate in the Göteborg study was only marginally superior to that in Nottingham, where in addition the rate of interval cancers was low, raising the question as to whether rehydration was justified (though some of the difference in detection rates could be due to the different age groups studied).

In the Göteborg study there were far more early stage cancers in the study group than in the control group resulting in a more favourable stage distribution in the study group. However the absolute number of advanced cancers has so far not been reduced in the study group compared to the control. Part of this may be due to a lead time effect for advanced disease, or too short a follow-up time to see the expected effect.

A difference between the Danish and the Nottingham studies was the equal number of interval cancers in the study group as at the initial screen in Denmark, whereas in Nottingham there were three times as many screen detected as interval cancers. One explanation could be that not all interval cancers that will occur have been identified in the Nottingham study, as the initial round of screening still continues, whereas in the Danish study the second round is already half way through.

The question arose as to whether it will be possible to identify the date of diagnosis of all cancers, so that those who die who were diagnosed before the trial commenced could be identified and excluded. That would be an accepted practice, if possible, though in some trials it has been felt that all those randomized should be retained in the analysis even if it became apparent that they were initially ineligible because of a preexisting colorectal cancer. Comment was also made over the inequality currently of all cause mortality in the Danish trial in the two groups. As the trial was based on individual randomization of spouse pairs such an imbalance would not be expected. This should be assessed to ensure that some standardisation of results for initial inequalities was not required.

There was some discussion on the differences in approach used for review of deaths in the various trials. In the Minnesota trial the initial survey is performed by staff. If there is no indication of colorectal cancer and definitely another underlying cause of death there is no death review. If, after review of all records by a nurse there appears to be any hint of the presence of colorectal cancer, and a primary adenocarcinoma is confirmed, a formal review is performed. Reviews are conducted blind as to allocation by a four member committee who perform the reviews independently and meet every two to three months to resolve any disagreements. In the Danish trial any suspicion of colorectal cancer on the death certificate leads to a review, blind as to allocation. In the Nottingham trial, however, Drs Chamberlain and Hardcastle review the records informally, and are not blind as to allocation.

It was questioned whether extensive formal review processes were really worth the effort and expense. In the US lung trials every death was reviewed, but it was subsequently accepted that such an extensive death review process was not required. It was noted that the main problem that occurred in the HIP death review process was the increasing difficulty in deciding as the follow-up proceeded whether a second primary or an earlier diagnosed breast cancer resulted in death. Even so, there were little differences between the two primary reviewers who always worked independently and were blind as to allocation. A further difficulty in death reviews was the extent of information on the primary tumour that was provided. If stage at diagnosis was revealed there was a possibility of unblinding the reviewers as stage was associated with screening detection.

One approach that should be adopted analytically to confirm no bias in cause of death attribution was to calculate the death rate from all other causes than the cancer of interest in the compared groups. This should be equivalent. It was important that the death rate should be computed as the person-years at risk will be different and therefore the numbers of deaths from other causes will be greater in the screened group with earlier diagnosis as a result of screening.

For colorectal cancer screening there were particular difficulties over the fact that many gastroenterologists were advocating screening even though trials demonstrating mortality reduction were not yet reported. This was an ethical issue, especially as some of the advocates were associated with trials that appear to be negative but had not yet been reported as such, including the Memorial Sloan Kettering Trial in New York. This trial had been apparently ready for reporting at the time of our last meeting in Göteborg in 1985 but the mortality results had still not appeared. Part of the difficulty with individual trials was that they were almost invariably planned with over-optimistic assumptions of the numbers of outcome events that would occur in the planned period of follow-up. This was because of the assumption that population mortality rates could be expected in the participants in the trials. All trials designed in the 1970s had this error. Even for the Nottingham trial, where the fallacy of such an approach was recognised in advance of planning the sample size, there had still been an overestimate of the expected number of events as no correction had been possible for the selection bias associated with health consciousness of those who responded to the invitation to be screened (the healthy volunteer effect). Further, the influence of the non-responders in contributing to mortality in the screened group (a dilution effect) was enormous. If the trial failed to show a benefit it would relate to the compliance pattern in that population at that time. This particular effect will not be seen in the Minnesota trial, which was an efficacy as distinct from an effectiveness trial (ie the trial was planned to evaluate the efficacy of screening in those who accepted the invitation to be screened). One approach that could be adopted to overcome these difficulties was a combined analysis of the trials at an appropriate time following their initiation. This was planned for the European studies. It would be helpful to include findings from the longer running Minnesota trial in the results. In fact at present only the Minnesota trial has long enough follow-up time to use mortality as an endpoint. The average follow-up in the Nottingham and Danish trials is only 3 years. The current trials may require another 5 years follow-up before mortality results could be expected. It was at that stage that a combined analysis might prove most profitable.

Part of the difficulty over the premature recommendation of colorectal cancer screening is the over-reliance on intermediate endpoints, and the belief in the polyp-cancer hypothesis, neither of which have been validated. Pressure was nevertheless building from clinicians for colorectal cancer screening policies. However, it was a disservice to base policy on premature and potentially misleading reports. The argument that mortality results might never be forthcoming from the trials and that therefore policy decisions should be based on other considerations should be resisted. In Canada the pressure had been resisted largely by advocating primary prevention rather than screening as the prime cancer control measure for the disease. It should be noted that preliminary results available are not encouraging over an eventual mortality reduction as so far in none of the trials has a reduction in advanced disease been reported. Clinicians need to be educated over the importance of this intermediate endpoint and informed over the bias associated with relying on shifts in the stage distribution.

It was noted that since the 1985 meeting agreement had been reached that the Kaiser Permanente Trial was non-informative over the benefit of rigid sigmoidoscopy. If the planned PLC trial went ahead, flexible sigmoidoscopy to 60 cms could be expected to identify of the order of 60% of detectable colorectal cancers. For some of those at risk of cancer beyond the reach of the flexible scope, the presence of polyps could be a marker that could lead to their identification following colonoscopy. Individuals with polyps should preferably be placed on special surveillance, an approach that did not occur in the Minnesota trial where those with polyps but negative findings for cancer on colonoscopy were returned to routine screening.

State of the Art on Screening for Cancer of the Cervix

Screening for cancer of the cervix is effective in reducing the incidence and mortality from the disease, and is applicable as public health policy.

For screening to be effective, it is important that the programme be organized according to an agreed policy, the essential elements of which are:

- the target population has been identified
- individual women are identifiable
- measures are available to guarantee high coverage and attendance, such as a personal letter of invitation
- there are adequate field facilities for taking the smears and adequate laboratory facilities to examine them
- there is an organized programme for quality control of the taking of smears and of interpreting them
- adequate facilities exist for diagnosis and for appropriate treatment of confirmed neoplastic lesions and for the follow-up of treated women
- there is a carefully designed and agreed referral system, an agreed link between the women, the laboratory and the clinical facility for diagnosis of an abnormal screening test, for management of any abnormality found and for providing information on normal screening tests
- evaluation and monitoring of the total programme is organized in terms of incidence and mortality rates among those attending, and among those not attending, at the level of the target population. Quality control of these epidemiological data should be established.

Almost maximal effectiveness is achieved by an organized programme with high coverage that initiates screening at the age of 25 and continues with 3 or 5-yearly screening to the age of 60. Variations from this approach should only be considered if maximal coverage has been obtained, the resources are available and the marginal cost-effectiveness of the change recommended has been evaluated.

In developing countries, high priority should be placed on a single smear at age 40, and the programme extended to that recommended above only when high coverage has been achieved and the necessary resources are available.

Recommendations for Research

Methods to ensure high coverage of the at risk population.

The benefit from screening previously screened women at ages older than 60.

The cost-effectiveness of repeat cytology versus immediate referral to colposcopy for women with mild dysplasia.

Follow-up studies to determine the long-term effect of localised therapy for dysplasia and carcinoma in situ.

Development of appropriate screening strategies for developing countries.

Determination of the role in screening of markers for human papilloma virus infection.

15 The Natural History of Cancer of the Cervix, and the Implications for Screening Policy

A. B. MILLER, J. KNIGHT and S. NAROD

Department of Preventive Medicine and Biostatistics, University of Toronto, Toronto, Ontario, Canada

1. INTRODUCTION

Screening frequency, as well as age to start and stop screening, are critically dependent on our understanding of the natural history of preclinical states of the cervix. Although there have been a few studies in which individuals were followed to determine directly the probability of progression or regression of biopsied abnormalities (Kinlen and Spriggs, 1978), this has generally been considered unethical and in any case the process of diagnosis may have affected the natural history. We are therefore dependent on inferences derived from the follow-up of women with cytologic abnormalities, and the study of the incidence and prevalence of well characterised lesions in a defined population, preferably followed longitudinally rather than cross-sectionally (Boyes et al, 1982).

Previous studies have suggested that there is a substantial probability of regression of precancerous abnormalities of the cervix, even of carcinoma in situ (Boyes et al, 1982; Coppleson and Brown, 1975). However, doubt has remained on the propensity for the milder forms of dysplasia to progress to cancer, and the natural history of the disease in younger birth cohorts. This paper provides preliminary data on two recent studies conducted by our group that have addressed these issues.

2 THE TORONTO STUDY

The first study was conducted in a large laboratory in Toronto, with a tradition of uniform classification of cytologic abnormalities over a long period. The laboratory processed a large proportion of the cervical smears performed in women in Metropoliton Toronto. The period of study coincided with the decline in the use of cervical conisation and was largely prior to the widespread acceptance of diagnostic colposcopy. The cases were therefore generally monitored cytologically by repeat smears at approximately 6 months to annual intervals until progression to a more severe cytologic abnormality had been demonstrated. It has therefore been possible to assess the propensity for lesions classified as having different degrees of dysplasia to progress cytologically (Narod et al, 1990).

A sample of 75,585 records in the laboratory were extracted for the years 1962 through 1981. All with a cytological diagnosis of dysplasia or worse were sampled, together with a probability sample of 3% of all records. The probability sample was based on the terminal digits of the Ontario Health Insurance number which was included in the large majority of the records for the same woman at least once. For a few women with records from the early years of the laboratory when the Health Insurance number was not available, sampling was based on the terminal digits of the first laboratory smear number. The laboratory had attempted through the years to bring together all the records pertaining to the same woman, and these are the records that were extracted. Subsequently we performed an internal computer record linkage eliminating some duplicate records not identified by the laboratory staff. However, it seems likely that some duplication still exists in the file, especially for women who changed their names through marriage. As a result of the linkage the study file was reduced to a sample of 70,236 women (comprising the records of 176,808 smears). Of these 20,461 women were from the probability sample and 49,775 had been selected because of a mention of dysplasia on one or more cytology report.

The terminology used by the laboratory was that of the Canadian Task Forces (Task Force 1976,1982). The terms for cytologic atypia used were "Abnormal cells consistent with dysplasia", categorised as mild, moderate or severe. However, in addition a special term "minimal dysplasia" was used in the laboratory for the group characterised by the Task Force "Abnormal cells consistent with benign atypia (non-dysplastic)". We have retained this term, though recognising that others would regard it as only indicating a cytologic abnormality that required no more than therapy for any infection that may be diagnosed. The laboratory did not use the CIN terminology. Therefore, a cytologic diagnosis of "Abnormal cells consistent with malignancy" could be characterised as "consistent with in situ squamous carcinoma" or "consistent with invasive squamous carcinoma". Such diagnoses were almost invariably followed by further investigation and the histologic diagnosis was then entered on the file. For this analysis we have used the term "carcinoma in situ or worse" to indicate this grouping irrespective of the final outcome as we were interested in the probability of progression from the various degrees of dysplasia to more severe abnormalities.

The prevalence of dysplasia rose during the study period, from 40 per 1000 in 1965-69 to nearly 100 per 1000 in 1980-81, though much of this was due to the increase in the "minimal" category. The prevalence was highest in women under the age of 40 (over 60 per 1000), largely due to higher rates for the minimal and mild categories (each approximating to 30 per 1000), though the prevalence of severe dysplasia was highest in women age 60 or more (5 per 1000).

The incidence of dysplasia among women with normal smears initially rose to a peak at ages 20-29, falling to a low point at ages 50-59 and then rising at older ages (Table 1).

The incidence of carcinoma in situ or worse among women with dysplasia was low and relatively uniform up to the age of 50, but then rose to over 700 per 100,000 at age 70 or more (Table 2).

Table 1 Incidence of dysplasia among women with normal smears

Age group	Cases observed	Women-years at risk	Rate (per 1000/year)
15-19	11	341	32.3
20-29	242	4418	54.8
30-39	181	3738	48.4
40-49	145	3471	41.8
50-59	71	2689	26.4
60-69	29	1016	28.5
70+	10	280	35.7
Total	689	16,053	42.9

Table 2 Incidence of carcinoma in situ or worse among women with dysplasia

Age group	Cases observed	Women-years at risk	Rate (per 10,000/year)
20-29	17	14,957	11.4
30-39	36	15,743	22.9
40-49	24	13,315	18.0
50-59	14	7,650	18.3
60-69	6	2,204	27.2
70+	5	660	75.8
Total	102	54,529	18.7

The relative risk for a manifestation of carcinoma in situ or worse in a subsequent smear was greatest for those with severe dysplasia, low for those with mild dysplasia and intermediate for those with moderate dysplasia (Table 3).

Table 3 Incidence of carcinoma in situ or worse

Type of smear	Number of cases	Rate/10,000* women-years	Relative risk (95% CI)
All controls	5	2.4	1.0
Minimal dysplasia	8	4.8	2.0 (0.66-6.18)
Mild dysplasia	17	9.7	4.0 (1.50-11.0)
Moderate dysplasia	29	34.7	14.5 (5.62-37.5)
Severe dysplasia	23	111.7	46.5 (17.8-123)

* With lead in time of 10 months

The majority of the women with mild dysplasia showed normal cytology at the next smear (upper half of Table 4). Indeed, the majority of women with any type of dysplasia showed no evidence of progression cytologically, even those with severe dysplasia (lower half of Table 4).

Table 4 Regression and progression of abnormalities

Degree of dysplasia	Inter-screen interval (months)	Next smear Normal (%)	Worse (%)
Minimal	13	66	12
Mild	12	66	9
Moderate	7.5	22	8
Severe	5.5	13	(36)*
			*still severe

	Final smear Normal (%)	Less (%)	Stable (%)
Minimal	74	-	12
Mild	61	22	6
Moderate	30	45	12
Severe	16	54	17

We are planning to extend the follow-up period of this study both through the laboratory and through linkage to the Ontario Cancer Registry. In the meantime, the results confirm that the degree of dysplasia is related to the risk of progression, and that the majority of cases of mild dysplasia on cytology are likely to regress with no therapy.

3 THE BRITISH COLUMBIA STUDY

The second study was an extension of the previously reported British Columbia cohort study (Boyes et al, 1982). The originally studied birth cohorts (born in 1914-18 and 1929-33) had their follow-up extended from 1969 to 1985. In addition we have obtained data on relatively young women, those born in 1944-48 (Knight, 1989). The major concentration of the analysis was on prevalence and incidence of dysplasia and carcinoma in situ and incidence of invasive cancer in the three cohorts. Unlike the Toronto laboratory, the British Columbia laboratory is the only one in a province of over 2 million people, and has been operational since 1949. It moved from an initial phase of providing a diagnostic service to a population-based screening programme in the early 1950s. It did not distinguish the grades of dysplasia for the early period of study and thus we have chosen not to differentiate by grade for the present analysis. The categories analysed are all histologically confirmed.

The tape we obtained for study was extracted from that used to manage the screening programme. Subsequently we learnt that it had been purged three times of "inactive" records. So far we have not received the missing data and therefore we have substituted the data from the original report (Boyes et al, 1982) for the period up to 1969 for the two oldest cohorts where it was apparent that data was missing from our tape. For more recent years, corrections to the denominators have been made to attempt to compensate for missing data. These corrections have infact made little difference to the conclusions initially derived from the study tape (Knight, 1989) though it is clear that the results presented here still have to be regarded as preliminary.

There are over 75,000 women in Cohort 1, studied for this analysis from 1951 through 1985, covering the age range 35-69. Cohort 2, comprising just over 100,000 women, was studied over the same time period covering the age range 20-54. Cohort 3, comprising nearly 140,000 women, was studied from 1961 through 1985 and covered the age range 15-39. In fact there were hardly any women years under the age of 20 so the present report refers only to the age range 20-39.

For dysplasia, there is evidence of a major diagnostic bias, introduced by the provincial colposcopy programme in the 1970s. This affects all three birth cohorts, but the youngest (Cohort 3) maximally (Figure 1).

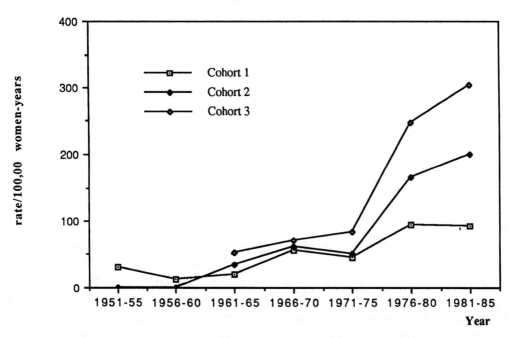

Figure 1 Incidence of dysplasia by year

There is no evidence from the data that this major increase in diagnosis of presumed precursors resulted in a similar artefactual increase in the incidence of carcinoma in situ (Figure 2).

Incidence of Carcinoma in situ by year

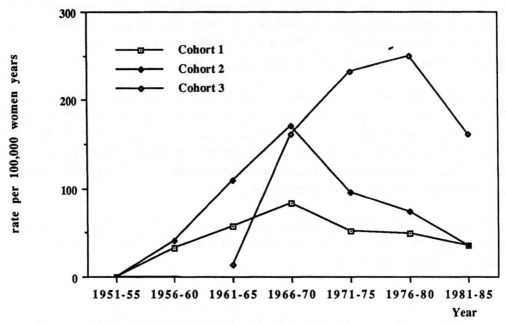

Figure 2 Incidence of Carcinoma in situ by year

The data for the prevalence and incidence (Table 5) of carcinoma in situ (CIS) by age do not suggest any major difference in natural history for the three cohorts. Thus the rates are similar at overlapping ages, even though separated by 15 calendar years, especially bearing in mind the current uncertainty over the actual values. The data confirm the previous conclusions that the incidence of CIS now peaks at about 30-34, but also shows that new disease continues to occur to an appreciable extent even in women in their 60s.

The determination of the incidence of invasive carcinoma of the cervix is complicated by the fact that women who have defaulted from screening but who then develop symptoms of invasive cancer return to "screening" as part of the process of diagnosis. Although theoretically it should be possible to identify such women, this is not possible in the British Columbia data as the tape contains no information that distinguishes those with invasive carcinoma truly identified following screening and those diagnosed with symptoms. Figure 3 indicates the solution previously adopted (Boyes et al, 1982) to this problem. The area bounded by the entries and exits to the program (the "fish") represents the surveillance years for the preclinical abnormalities diagnosed during screening. The area below and to the right of the curve for entries represents the denominator for the incidence of invasive carcinoma, providing corrections are made for death from any cause,

Table 5 Prevalence (per 10,000 women) and incidence (per 10,000 women-years) of Carcinoma in situ by Age

Age	Prevalence Cohort 1	Cohort 2	Cohort 3	Incidence Cohort 1	Cohort 2	Cohort 3
20-24		77.8	30.5			16.1
25-29		81.8	76.7		6.0	23.1
30-34		115.4	101.2		13.5	24.9
35-39	207.9	150.7	76.0		17.0	16.1
40-44	171.0	112.2		5.2	9.5	
45-49	119.6	57.7		6.7	7.4	
50-54	105.1	34.5		8.3	3.4	
55-59	82.0			5.2		
60-64	33.0			4.9		
65-69	8.0			3.6		

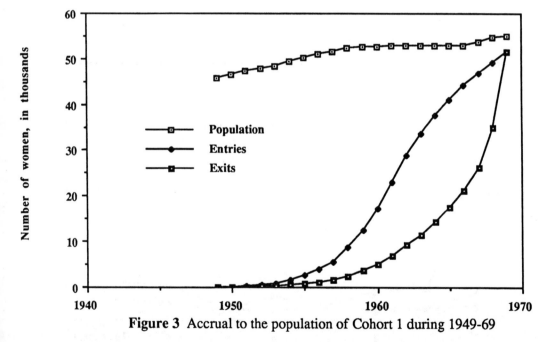

Figure 3 Accrual to the population of Cohort 1 during 1949-69

hysterectomy and out-migration from the province. Table 6 shows the estimated incidence of invasive carcinoma in women who have ever been screened after such corrections to the denominator of cumulative entrants. It seems that the incidence was less at comparable ages for cohort 2 than 1, and roughly similar for cohorts 2 and 3.

Table 6 Estimated incidence of Invasive Carcinoma of the Cervix (per 100,000 women-years) by Age

Age	Cohort 1	Cohort 2	Cohort 3
20-24			2.2
25-29			9.4
30-34		8.9	12.4
35-39		8.7	6.1
40-44	7.9	6.5	
45-49	15.1	9.5	
50-54	17.3	7.0	
55-59	21.6		
60-64	22.8		
65-69	15.9		

However, there appears to be a continuing risk of invasive cancer in older women, though this may largely represent those women who had previously defaulted from screening. That this may be so is indicated by evidence of a substantial protective effect of a negative smear for 5 years (data not presented here), even greater if there had been 2 previous negative smears (Figure 4).

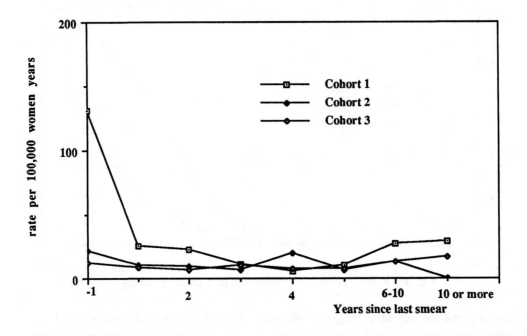

Figure 4 Incidence of Invasive Cancer for those with two negative smears

Further in each cohort, there is evidence of a substantial protective effect of 4 or more smears (Figure 5).

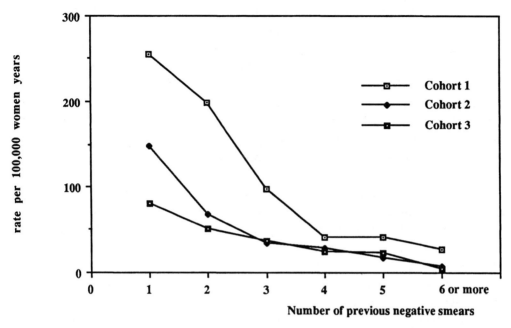

Figure 5 Incidence of Invasive Cancer by number of previously negative smears

DISCUSSION

In general, the findings from these studies are compatible with those previously reported, including the protective effect of two or more smears (Hakama et al, 1985). The preliminary findings from the British Columbia Cohort Study update are important in showing that the protective effect of two or more negative smears applies to younger as well as older birth cohorts, thus confirming the validity of the conclusions drawn by the IARC Working Group (1986) as applying to younger cohorts than those studied in that cooperative investigation. There is no indication from these data that rescreening should be more frequent for younger birth cohorts than older.   Concerning age to start screening, cohort 3 provides relevant data. At ages 20-24, although the incidence of invasive cancer was low, that for carcinoma in situ was already appreciable, and these findings have reinforced the previous recommendations in Canada to start screening by the age of 20 (Workshop Group, 1990).

In the first British Columbia Cohort Study estimates of the proportion of cases of carcinoma in situ that regress were made (Boyes et al, 1982). It was pointed out that these were minimal estimates, as to the extent that regression occurs, the regression estimated from observed data will not include the cases that have occurred, but were not detected in the time interval that they were detectable. A similar exercise has been performed in the update of the study, with estimates of regression over the age range during which each cohort was followed. For cohort 1, 61% of cases of carcinoma in situ were estimated to have regressed during ages 40-64, for cohort 2, 70% over ages 25-54 and for cohort 3 77% over ages 15-39 (Knight, 1989). The implication is as concluded before (Boyes et al, 1982), the natural history of carcinoma in situ involves a dynamic process, with regression most likely to occur at younger ages, but still occurring at a significant rate at older ages. The effect on screening frequency is to emphasise the importance of screening at older ages, at a sufficient frequency to ensure that significant disease does not slip through the screening "net". Empirical studies, however, (IARC Working Group, 1986; Yu et al, 1982) and practical experience (Hakama et al., this volume) show that screening as infrequently as every 5 years results in reduction in a high proportion of the expected incidence and therefore screening every year is not necessary.

Both of the studies summarised in this paper confirm the relative lack of progression of milder forms of dysplasia, while the British Columbia Cohort Study shows that even in a province where the policy is to follow cytologically the minor forms of dysplasia until there is evidence cytologically of progression, a major diagnostic artifact coinciding with the introduction of the colposcopy programme (Figure 1) has not been prevented. These findings influenced the Workshop Group (1990) in Canada to make very specific recommendations concerning the management of such lesions:

"In the management of women with cytological abnormalities, note should be taken of the degree of abnormality as reported by the cytopathologist.

a) For women with cytologic evidence of mild dysplasia (CIN I), with or without HPV effects, a repeat cytology smear should generally be recommended in six months. If there is no evidence of cytologic progression, repeat smears at six month intervals are appropriate for a period of up to two years, after which colposcopy should be arranged for all women with persistent abnormalities.

b) For women with cytologic evidence of moderate or severe dysplasia (CIN II or III) or malignant cells in the smear, referral to colposcopy should be arranged."

This recommendation coincides with the approach Ellman (this volume) concludes is appropriate for the UK.

The apparent continuing high rate of incidence of invasive carcinoma in the oldest birth cohort in previously screened women in the British Columbia Cohort Study needs further evaluation. Although part of the excess could be due to denominator error, it seems more likely that it is real though associated with women who were previously screened many years before who had defaulted from screening and who returned to the screening "net" because of symptoms of disease. It has been well documented in both British Columbia and Ontario, Canada that the majority of women who develop invasive carcinoma of the cervix had either not been screened at all, or had not been screened for 5 years or more (Anderson et al,1988; Carmichael et al, 1984). The protective effect of two or more negative smears appears almost as great for older as for younger women (Figure 4). Nevertheless, the data in Table 6 led the Workshop Group (1990) in Canada to recommend continuation of three-yearly screening to the age of 69, though at the same time they recommended further study into the issue of the appropriate age to stop screening in previously screened women. It is perhaps relevant that the Office of Technology Assessment have concluded that screening older women in the United States under Medicare is cost-effective (Muller et al, 1990).

Previous and continuing analyses (Miller, 1986; Arraiz et al, 1990) have confirmed that the screening programmes for cancer of the cervix have not been as successful in Canada as in other countries with organised programmes. Accordingly the Workshop Group (1990) recommended as a high priority in Canada "Governments should encourage and support the development or enhancement of organized cervical cytology screening programmes designed to reduce the morbidity and mortality from carcinoma of the cervix." It remains to be seen whether there is the political will to incur the expenditure now to undertake the necessary changes to bring this recommendation into effect. Unfortunately it already appears that certain professional groups will concentrate on our recommendations for three-yearly screening and cytological surveillance of mild dysplasia to emphasise their beliefs in annual screening and immediate referral to colposcopy for all women with any degree of dysplasia. In making the latter demand they raise issues such as the lack of consistency in subclassifying squamous epithelial dysplasia across laboratories that has led to the recommendation of a simpler reporting system in the US (National Cancer Institute Workshop, 1989). However, this appears to be particularly related to poor laboratory quality over much of the US. Yet all our recommendations were tied to the preamble:

"The recommendations should be considered as a whole. In particular the recommended frequencies should only be established as formal policy when the following are in place:
a) high quality laboratory services for the reading of cytology smears with adequate and functioning quality control systems, both internal and external;
b) information systems to monitor the frequencies and to issue reminders to attend at the recommended intervals."

The next few years will be critical in determining whether we can be successful in making the necessary changes and securing the appropriate impact on the disease that still seems possible by the year 2000 (Tomatis et al, 1990).

REFERENCES

Anderson GH, Boyes DA, Benedet JL et al. Organisation and results of the cervical cytology screening programme in British Columbia, 1955-85. BMJ, 1988; 296: 975-978.

Arraiz GA, Wigle DT, Mao Y. Is cervical cancer increasing among young women in Canada? Can J Pub Hlth, 1990; 81:396-397.

Boyes DA, Morrison B, Knox EG et al. A cohort study of cervical cancer screening in British Columbia. Clin Invest Med 1982; 5: 1-29.

Carmichael JA, Jeffrey JF, Steele HD, Ohlke ID. The cytological history of 245 patients developing invasive cervical carcinoma. Am J Obstet Gynecol 1984; 148: 685-690.

Coppleson LW and Brown B. Observations on a model of the biology of carcinoma of the cervix: a poor fit between observation and theory. Am J Obstet Gynecol 1975; 122: 127-136.

Hakama M, Chamberlain J, Day NE, Miller AB, Prorok PC. Evaluation of screening programmes for gynaecological cancer. Br J Cancer, 1985; 52:669-673.

Kinlen LJ and Spriggs AI. Women with positive cervical smears but without surgical intervention. Lancet 1978; ii: 463-465.

Knight JA. Screening for cervical cancer. A cohort study in British Columbia. MSc Thesis, University of Toronto, 1989.

IARC Working Group. Summary chapter. In Hakama M, Miller AB, Day NE, eds. Screening for cancer of the uterine cervix. IARC Scientific Publications no 76. Lyon, International Agency for Research on Cancer, 1986, pp 133-144.

Miller AB. Evaluation of the impact of screening for cancer of the cervix. In Hakama M, Miller AB, Day NE, eds. Screening for cancer of the uterine cervix. IARC Scientific Publications no 76. Lyon, International Agency for Research on Cancer, 1986, pp 149-160.

Muller C, Mandelblatt J, Schechter CB et al. Costs and effectiveness of cervical cancer screening in elderly women. US Congress, Office of Technology Assessment, OTA-BP-H-65, Washington DC, Government Printing Office, February, 1990.

Narod S, Thompson DW, Jain M et al. Dysplasia and the natural history of cervical cancer: results of the Toronto cohort study. In preparation, 1990.

National Cancer Institute Workshop. The 1988 Bethesda system for reporting cervical/vaginal cytological diagnoses. J Am Med Ass, 1989; 262:931-934.

Task Force. Cervical Cancer Screening Programs. Can Med Ass J 1976; 114:1003-1033.

Task Force. Cervical Cancer Screening Programs 1982. Ottawa, Health Services and Promotion Branch, Health and Welfare Canada, 1982.

The Workshop Group. Report of a National Workshop on screening for cancer of the cervix. In preparation, 1990.

Tomatis L, Aitio A, Day NE et al.,eds. Cancer: Causes, occurrence and control. IARC Scientific Publications no. 100. Lyon, International Agency for Research on Cancer, 1990, pp 313-315.

Yu SZ, Miller AB, Sherman GJ. Optimising the age, number of tests, and test interval for cervical screening in Canada. J Epid Comm Hlth, 1982; 36:1-10.

16 Effect of Organized Screening on the Risk of Cervical Cancer in the Nordic Countries

M. HAKAMA[1,2], K. MAGNUS[3], F. PETTERSSON[4], H. STORM[5] and H. TULINIUS[6]

1Department of Public Health, University of Tampere, Tampere, Finland;
[2]Finnish Cancer Registry, Helsinki, Finland;
[3]The Cancer Registry of Norway, Montebello, Oslo, Norway;
[4]The Swedish Cancer Registry, The National Board of Health and Welfare, Stockholm, Sweden;
[5]The Danish Cancer Registry, Danish Cancer Society, Copenhagen, Denmark;
[6]Icelandic Cancer Registry, Reykjavik, Iceland

1 INTRODUCTION

In the early 1980s an overview on the incidence trends for cervical cancer in the Nordic countries indicated a close correlation between the intensity of organized screening and reduction of risk (Hakama, 1982). This conclusion was confirmed by an analysis based on trends for mortality from cervical cancer (Läärä et al., 1987). This report updates the Nordic data and discusses the benefits of the organized programmes as practised in most of the Nordic countries.

2 THE PROGRAMMES

Most of the Nordic countries have nationwide screening programmes for cervical cancer which fulfil the general prerequisities of an organized programme (Hakama et al., 1985) and make it possible to follow up each woman for the occurrence of intraepithelial cervical neoplasia and for cervical cancer. The programmes define the ages and the frequencies of screening, use personal invitations with times and places for screening and give personal information about the results of screening even when the smear is negative.

Within the organized programmes, there are differences in cervical cancer screening policies between the Nordic countries. In Finland (Hakama and Louhivuori, 1988), Iceland (Johannesson et al., 1982) and Sweden (Petterson et al., 1985), a nationwide population-based organized programme has been in operation at least since the early 1970s, whereas only a few counties in Denmark, including the most populous ones, had organized screening programmes (Lynge, 1983; Lynge et al., 1989). The programmes are run by voluntary cancer organizations in Finland and Iceland, and by the counties in Denmark and Sweden. The recommended age groups to be covered are 30-55 years in Finland, 25-69 years in Iceland, and 30-49 years in Sweden. The screening intervals recommended are two to three years in Iceland, four years in Sweden and five years in Finland. In Denmark the practice varies by county, but the National Board of Health recommendation is to have a smear every three years from the age of 23 to 59 and every five years from 60 to 75. In Norway (Pedersen et al., 1971; Magnus et al., 1987) only 5 per cent of the population was covered by an organized programme. Cytological smears are, however, frequently taken outside the organized system by private gynaecologists and elsewhere. Such smears are taken more often than the smears in the organized programmes in all the Nordic countries with the exception of Iceland.

All the Nordic countries have a cancer registry. The Danish Cancer Registry was established in 1942. The Swedish Cancer Registry, founded in 1958, is the newest. The incidence data presented in this paper are based on the notifications to the nationwide population-based cancer registries. The mortality rates were derived from the cancer registry in Finland and from the official statistics in Denmark (National Board of Health, 1968-1987) and Norway (Central Bureau of Statistics of Norway, 1967-1986).

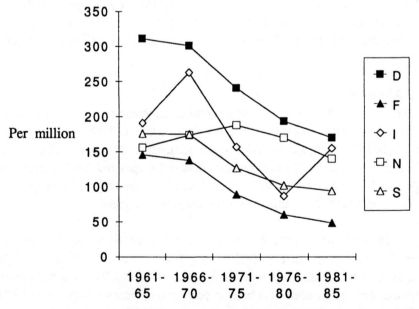

Figure 1   Trends in the age-adjusted (world standard) incidence rates of
invasive cervical cancer in 1961 to 1985 in Denmark (D),
Finland (F), Iceland (I), Norway (N) and Sweden (S)

3 EFFECT OF THE PROGRAMMES ON THE RISK OF CERVICAL CANCER

In the Nordic countries about 2,500 new cases of cervical cancer were diagnosed annually before the screening programmes were initiated. Since the early 1980s the annual number of new cases has been about 1,700. Denmark had a high incidence, in the early period the age-adjusted (world standard) incidence being about 30 per 100,000 women-years, whereas in the other Nordic countries it was about 15 with somewhat increasing trends before the screening programmes started. In the early 1980s the rates ranged from 15 (Denmark) to 5 (Finland).

There was a strong correlation between the extent of the organized screening programme and changes in the incidence of invasive cervical cancer (Figure 1). The relative reduction in the risk was steepest in Finland and Sweden, and intermediate in Denmark. In Norway the incidence rates of cervical cancer increased up to the 1970s. During the 15-year period from 1966-70 to 1981-85, the incidence rates fell by 65 per cent in Finland and 20 per cent

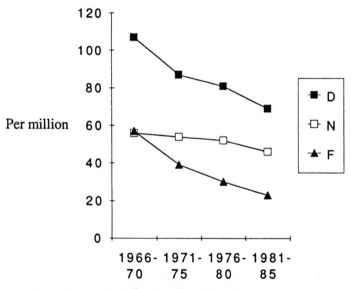

Figure 2   Trends in the age-adjusted (world standard) mortality rates from cervical cancer in 1966 to 1985 in Denmark (D), Finland (F) and Norway (N)

in Norway. The substantial decrease in incidence from the 1960s to 1970s in Iceland is partly because prevalent microinvasive lesions were diagnosed during the first round of screening in the late 1960s more frequently than in the other Nordic countries. Preliminary figures for Iceland since 1985 do not support a consistent increase in the rates in the 1980s. The rates in Iceland are subject to large random variation owing to the small population and relatively few cases of cancer. The mortality trends for cervical cancer confirmed the results based on new cases of cancer (Figure 2).

The most substantial reduction in the risk of cervical cancer occurred in the age group 40-49 years (Hakulinen et al., 1986), which probably came under the most intensive screening by the organized programme. Again, the reduction was highest in Finland (80 per cent) and lowest in Norway (50 per cent). Figures 3 to 5 demonstrate the general pattern of incidence by age. The rates were somewhat increasing at young ages, sharply decreasing for the middle-aged and were relatively stable for the elderly. The rates for women in Iceland were unstable owing to the small numbers.

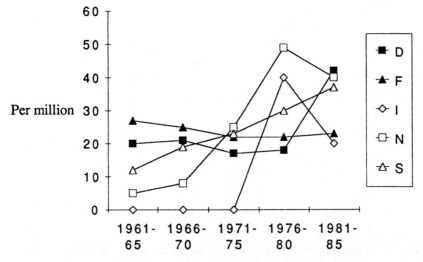

Figure 3   Trends in the incidence rates of cervical cancer, age 20-24
in Denmark (D), Finland (F), Norway (N) and Sweden (S)

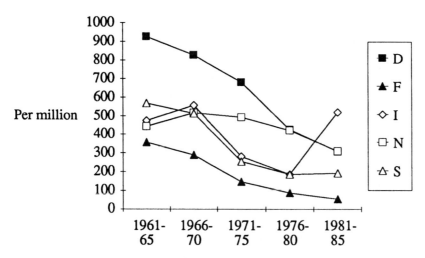

Figure 4   Trends in the incidence rates of cervical cancer, age 40-44, in the Nordic countries in 1961 to 1985

4 DISCUSSION

Three points that can be learned on the basis of the Nordic experience are discussed:
- the effect of specific determinants of an organized programme on the risk
- whether incidence trends are appropriate means of evaluation
- the effect of changes in risk at young ages on the programme

It seems that the differences in the trends can not be accounted for by the biology of the disease but that the most significant determinant of risk reduction is how well the programme is organized. A comparison of the Nordic countries shows very little relation between the interval between the screening rounds and reduction in risk, or very little relation between the target age range and reduction in risk. The IARC working group (1986a, 1986b) estimated on the basis of several large scale screening programmes that the protective effect of screening is high for screening intervals up to five years and for lower age limits up to 30 years. Organized programmes in contrast to opportunistic ones promote high attendance (e.g. by personal letters of invitation and of response). High coverage and attendance seem to be the single most important determinant of successful screening. Opportunistic screening has problems in catching those who would benefit most from screening.

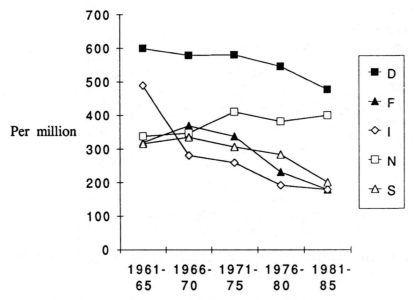

Figure 5   Trends in the incidence rates of cervical cancer, age 60-64, in the Nordic countries in 1961 to 1985

The purposes of screening for cancer are to prevent deaths from the disease subjected to screening and to improve the quality of life of patients whose cancer has been detected through screening by means of changes in the effectiveness of their treatment. Cervical cancer is an exception. Because preinvasive lesions are detected at screening, a reduced incidence of invasive disease is the objective of screening for cervical cancer. Because of length-biased sampling, screening is likely to detect more slow-growing tumours; the fast-growing ones are likely to surface as interval cancers. The speed of tumour growth and the patient's survival are correlated. It is therefore possible that screening causes a bigger reduction in incidence than in mortality rates. In Finland and Denmark the reduction in overall incidence was indeed somewhat bigger than that for mortality (Figure 6). The reverse was true for the rates among the age-groups with the most substantial reduction (Figure 7). The estimates for reduction depend somewhat on the reference year, but it seems fair to conclude that both incidence and mortality are equally valid in evaluating the effect of screening on risk of cervical cancer.

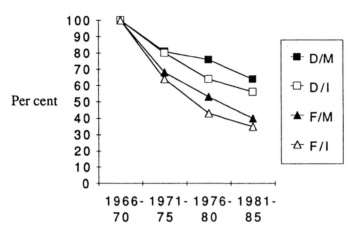

Figure 6 Percentage decrease in the age adjusted (world standard) incidence
(I) and mortality (M) rates of cervical cancer in Denmark (D) and
Finland (F) in 1966-1985.

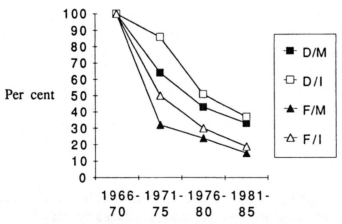

Figure 7 Percentage decrease in the incidence (I) and mortality (M) rates of
cervical cancer, age 40-44, in Denmark (D) and Finland (F) in
1966-1985

The differences in the reliability of death certificates between the countries and by time may have affected this conclusion, however. In Norway the official mortality statistics routinely utilize the information collected by the Cancer Registry of Norway. The time trends for Finland were also based on the total information accumulated at the Finnish Cancer Registry. The differences between the cancer registry-based and official statistics of cervical cancer mortality were small in Denmark in 1977 (Storm, 1984) and in Finland since the late 1960s (Hakama, 1978), and it is likely that the same applies to the other time periods covered in this review and to the other Nordic countries.

Data originating from different populations indicate an increase of preclinical lesions at young ages (Coppleson et al., 1987; Draper and Cook, 1983; Parkin et al., 1985). This increase was related to changes in sexual mores, allowing the spread of, e.g. human papilloma virus infections, rather than to an increase in smear-taking activity or changes in diagnostic criteria. The increase has led to proposals that screening at young ages be intensified.

Some increase has been reported in the invasive disease as well (Armstrong and Holman, 1981; Beral and Booth, 1986). In the Nordic countries there was some evidence for such an increase (Figure 3). At young ages the risk of cancer is low and the number of cases few. Comparing Figures 3 and 4, it appears that the increase at ages 20-24 was proportionally of the same magnitude as the decrease at ages 40-44. However, in absolute terms it appears that the increase at ages 20-24 is small indeed when compared with the decrease at ages 40-44, when the disease is much more common. Frankly invasive cervical cancer is rare under the age of 30, and deaths from cervical cancer occur infrequently at ages under 35. Thus the cost-effectiveness of screening remains low if rare occurrences of the disease are found by screening, and there is no good evidence, e.g., for screening those under 25 for cervical cancer. Viral infections which are thought to increase the risk of cervical cancer occur frequently among those younger than 25. If diagnosis and treatment of these infections prevents them from spreading, screening for papilloma virus and other infections should be done even if it is likely that the long-term adverse effects, such as invasive cancer, could be prevented later in life, when many of the original lesions have regressed spontaneously. Screening for viral infections should not be confused with screening for cancer, however. The purpose of screening for cervical cancer is to prevent invasive disease, and it is sufficient to start screening a few years before invasive disease appears.

Screening of women at high ages is problematic. In Denmark the recommendations have different frequency under 60 and at 60 years or more; in Finland there is a recent change to screen women at 60 also. The effect of screening at older ages is largely unknown, but the efficacy is probably smaller the higher the upper age limit. The person-years saved will ultimately become small, attendance seems to get lower and the biology of the disease may be more aggressive at older ages resulting in more cases in the target population not detected by screening. The change in the frequency and the variation in the upper age limit between time periods and countries reflects the uncertainty as to the effect.

5 CONCLUSION

It seems clear that opportunistic or spontaneous screening for cervical cancer covers a relatively limited and selected proportion of the target population, who undergo repeated screening at short intervals. Nonresponders to a spontaneous programme are likely to be those who would benefit most from regular screening for cervical cancer (Chamberlain, 1986; Miller, 1986). Organized screening with personal letters of invitation improves attendance and is a way to regulate the target age range and frequency of screening. This update on the Nordic countries confirms previous conclusions (Hakama, 1982; Läärä et al., 1987) that a population-based and well-organized screening programme with a valid target age range and the right frequency is more successful than opportunistic screening, and can thus be effective in reducing both the incidence of and the mortality from invasive cervical cancer.

Finland and Sweden probably have recorded the largest reduction in the incidence of cervical cancer as a result of screening. There has been also a substantial reduction in incidence in Denmark and Iceland. The reduction in risk closely correlates with the degree of organization. In many countries where there has been a substantial effect, the screening programme has been highly cost-effective. In Finland, for instance, the official recommendation that the screening programme be started at the age of 30 and that the smear be repeated every five years has resulted in one of the largest reductions in the risk of cervical cancer reported anywhere.

REFERENCES

Armstrong B, Holman D. Increasing mortality from cancer of the cervix in young Australian women. Med J Aust 1981; i:460-462.

Beral V, Booth M. Predictions of cervical cancer incidence and mortality in England and Wales. Lancet 1986; i:495.

Central Bureau of Statistics of Norway. Causes of death [1966-1985], Oslo (1967-1986).

Chamberlain J. Reasons that some screening programmes fail to control cervical cancer. In: Hakama M, Miller AB, Day NE (eds). Screening for Cancer of the Uterine Cervix, Lyon: IARC Scientific Publications No 76, 1986, pp.161-168.

Coppleson M, Elliott P, Reid B. Puzzling changes in cervical cancer in young women. Med J Aust 1987; 146:405-406.

Draper GJ, Cook GA. Changing patterns of cervical cancer rates. Br Med J 1983; 287:510.

Hakama M. Mass screening for cervical cancer in Finland. In: Miller AB (ed). Screening in Cancer. UICC Technical Report seires, Vol 40, UICC, Geneva 1978, pp.93-107.

Hakama M. Trends in the incidence of cervical cancer in the Nordic countries. In: Magnus K, ed. Trends in Cancer Incidence: Causes and Practical Implications. New York: Hemisphere, 1982, pp.279-292.

Hakama M, Chamberlain J, Day NE, Miller AB, Prorok PC. Evaluation of screening programmes for gynaecological cancer. Br J Cancer 1985; 52:669-673.

Hakama M, Louhivuori K. A screening programme for cervical cancer that worked. Cancer Surveys 1988; 7:403-416.

Hakulinen T, Andersen A, Malker B, Pukkala E, Schou G, Tulinius H. Trends in Cancer Incidence in the Nordic Countries. Acta Path Microbiol Immunol Scand Sect A 1986; 94:Suppl. 288:1-151.

IARC Working Group on Evaluation of Cervical Cancer Screening Programmes. Screening for squamous cervical cancer: the duration of low risk after negative result of cervical cytology and its implication for screening policies. Br Med J 1986a; 293:659-664.

IARC Working Group on Cervical Cancer Screening. Summary chapter. In: Hakama M, Miller AB, Day NE (eds). Screening for Cancer of the Uterine Cervix. Lyon: IARC Scientific Publications No 76, 1986b, pp.133-142.

Johannesson GE, Geirsson G, Day N, Tulinius H. Screening for cancer of the uterine cervix in Iceland 1965-1978. Acta Obstet Gynecol Scand 1982; Suppl 61:199-203.

Läärä E, Day NE, Hakama M. Trends in mortality from cervical cancer in the Nordic countries: association with organised screening programmes. Lancet 1987; i:1247-249.

Lynge E. Regional trends in incidence of cervical cancer in Denmark in relation to local smear-taking activity. Int J Epidemiol 1983; 12:405-413.

Lynge E, Madsen M, Engholm G. Effect of organized screening on incidence and mortality of cervical cancer in Denmark. Cancer Research 1989; 49:2157-2160.

Magnus K, Langmark F, Andersen A. Mass screening for cervical cancer in Ìstfold county of Norway 1959-1977. Int J Cancer 1987; 39:311-316.

Miller AB. Evaluation of the impact of screening for cancer of the cervix. In: Hakama M, Miller AB, Day NE, eds. Screening for Cancer of the Uteline Cervix, Lyon: IARC Scientific Publications No 76, 1986, pp.149-160.

National Board of Health. Causes of death in the Kingdom of Denmark [1966-1985], Copenhagen (1968-1987).

Parkin DM, Nguyen-Dinh X,Day NE. The impact of screening on the incidence of cervical cancer in England and Wales. Br J Obstet Gynaecol 1985; 92:150-157.

Pedersen E, Hoeg K,Kolstad P. Mass screening for cancer of the uterine cervix in Ostfold county, Norway: an experiment. Second report of the Norwegian Cancer Society. Acta Obstet Gynecol Scand 1971; Suppl 11:1-18.

Petterson F, Björkholm E, Näslund I. Evaluation of screening for cervical cancer in Sweden: trends in incidence and mortality 1958-1980. Int J Epidemiol 1985; 14:521-527.

Storm HH. Validity of death certificates for cancer patients in Denmark 1977. Cancerregisteret, Copenhagen, 1984.

17 The Organisation of Cervical Screening in England and Wales

J. CUZICK

Department of Mathematics, Statistics and Epidemiology
Imperial Cancer Research Fund, London

1 INTRODUCTION

A cervical screening service was introduced nationally into England and Wales in the mid 1960s. Few guidelines were provided for its use and no attempts were made to evaluate its effectiveness. This service has not led to any substantial reduction in the mortality rates from cervix cancer, despite notable successes in other countries (Hakama, 1982). Critics of the programme have pointed out that a major weakness of the system is its poor coverage of the population at risk and that successful programmes have actively invited women to participate and have monitored the performance of the system in terms of coverage, follow-up, and other indicators (ICRF Coordinating Committee on Cervical Screening, 1984). This has led the government to reorganise the programme and introduce a computerised call and recall system. More recently it has also introduced "targets" for general practitioners whereby they are paid a certain sum per women on their books who have been screened if they achieve an 80% overall coverage and a much smaller sum if they achieve 50% coverage but less than 80%. No fee is paid if less than 50% of eligible women have been screened in the last 5.5 years. The use of fixed cut-offs has received justifiable criticism, but some reward for a high coverage does seem to be a sensible approach.

Within England and Wales, responsibility for the cervical screening programme is delegated to each of the 211 district health authorities (DHAs). From a management and financial point of view these programmes are officially autonomous and completely independent of each other. However from a realistic and practical point of view this is infeasible and coordination and sharing of resources between districts is essential. In this paper, the groups involved and the organisational links within districts and between districts are described, the overall aims and objectives are recounted (ICRF Coordinating Committee on Cervical Screening, 1986), and the role of the programme coordinator at the district level is outlined (Pye, 1989).

2 PROGRAMME ORGANISATION WITHIN THE DISTRICT
Each district health authority is free to organise its programme as it chooses and local variations do exist. However the following model has been proposed and is used with some adaption in most districts. A schematic diagram of the main groups and their interactions is given in Figure 1.

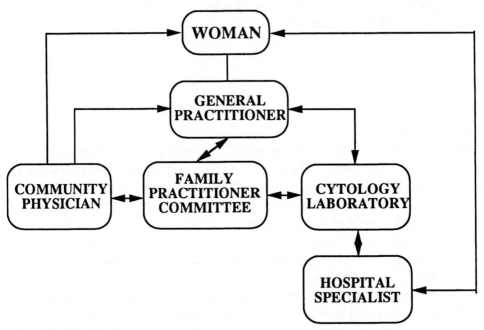

Figure 1 The main groups and their interactions

2.1 General Practitioners
General practitioners (GPs) now perform most cervical smears and are the direct link with the women who use the service. GPs need to be convinced of the efficacy of cervical screening and need help in implementing a call and recall system within their own practices. Each GP should receive data regularly in simple format to enable self assessment. Facilities should exist for patients of GPs who do not wish to offer the service and for women who prefer not to use their own GP for this purpose. Adequate completion of screening forms is of paramount importance and it is justifiable that item of service payments should depend on this.

2.2 Overall Responsibility at Local Level
The community physician (CP), who works within a DHA and whose remit is preventive medicine, is uniquely placed to undertake co-ordination of local screening services. His training should enable him to organise a screening programme according to District policy, oversee the implementation of that programme, and assess its efficacy. Each DHA should nominate one CP to take overall responsibility for its cervical screening service. The CP would not need to become directly involved in the day-to-day running of the service.

2.3 Routine Call and Recall

The generation of call and recall lists is undertaken by the Family Practitioner Committee (FPC) from their computerized register. A successful screening programme will require frequent contact between the CP and FPC. To facilitate this, one member of staff at the FPC should be identified to manage the database. Current policy is that this activity should be funded by the DHA involved. Screening histories are also held by the FPC and can be transferred to another FPC should women move out of the district.

A computerized system can only function well if provided with accurate data. Doctors should provide full name (including all Christian names and maiden name), date of birth and National Health Service (NHS) number when sending a smear to the laboratory. This information will be used by the laboratory when reporting to the FPC which will use it to identify a woman in their files. Addresses are not a reliable method for identification of a woman, but they should be checked at every opportunity. Regular use of the FPC database will help to improve the current inaccuracies in addresses and other relevant identifiers. FPCs will administer the computerized system, but they do not own the clinical information which the database contains. The system can be programmed to allow limited access to certain parts of the database. The CP should ensure that local policy states which members of staff or departments have access to confidential information. The system must also comply with the provisions of the Data Protection Act.

2.4 The Cytology Laboratory

The laboratory computer system will need to hold more information about each patient than the FPC computer, which will only need to keep a brief record of a woman's previous smears and her current recall interval. The non-routine follow-up of patients within the laboratory system should be divided into two categories - patients requiring another smear (for unsatisfactory smears, infections, most equivocal smears and some mild abnormalities) and patients who have been recommended for referral for specialist treatment (abnormal smears). If a further smear has been requested the system should check that it has been received. If so and if the result indicates that the patient does not require further active follow-up, the laboratory should inform the FPC that the women can rejoin the routine call and recall system. This may be at a shortened recall interval, and if so, this should be stated. If the result indicates the need for specialist referral, the system should note this fact. It is vitally important that a patient's GP (as well as the collector of the smear, if different) should be informed by the laboratory whenever a smear is abnormal, whatever the source of that smear. If the repeat smear has not been received a reminder should be issued to the collector of the original smear. If the reminder fails to elicit the repeat smear the CP should be informed. Under these circumstances CPs should approach the patient's GP or, if necessary, the patient herself.

2.5 Hospital Referrals

Gynaecologists will have short-term responsibility for patients referred to them. This will usually occur if a smear is abnormal. Their needs in terms of records and follow-up procedures should be accommodated within the laboratory computer system. Specialists must indicate to the system when a patient is discharged from their care and the recommended interval for the next smear, so that this information can be communicated to the FPC system and the recall status can be appropriately modified.

Laboratories also receive smears from (STD) clinics, where smears are almost always identified only by number and no other personal information is shown on the request form. These patients represent a high-risk group for malignant disease of the uterine cervix and their anonymity can lead to difficulty in ensuring that they receive appropriate follow-up. These patients, like all others, should always be informed that a cervical smear has been taken and should be told how they will be informed of its result. There is a strong case for obtaining names on smears from STD clinics. This should be done in a way to minimize any loss of confidentiality.

When names are not supplied, the staff of the STD clinic must assume full responsibility for further action when a smear is not negative. If the laboratory does not receive a repeat smear after one reminder has been issued, it should pass the number of the patient to the CP so that he can contact the clinic. When a smear is abnormal the case is even stronger for the patient to be identified by name.

2.6 Non-Coterminous Boundaries of Different Parts of the Service
DHAs, FPCs and the catchment areas of cytology laboratories are often not coterminous. As a result laboratories may receive smears from women in different FPCs. The laboratory must ensure that a result reaches the correct FPC. FPCs may contain more than one DHA and some DHAs are spread over more than one FPC so that the system must allow each district cervical screening committee to determine its own policy regarding screening interval, format of routine letters, etc. The system developed by the Exeter FPS Computer Unit has great flexibility in this regard.

3 PROGRAMME ORGANISATION ABOVE DISTRICT LEVEL
It has already been mentioned that many FPCs serve more than one district and this leads to a certain amount of inter-district co-operation. More organisation is needed however to coordinate policy and to share common resources. A first step has been to appoint a regional coordinator in each of the 14 regions and 3 celtic nations to act as a liaison person between districts within each region and to represent the region at a national level via a National Coordinating Network.

A National Coordinating Network has been set up by the NHS and is administered through the Faculty of Public Health Medicine within the Royal College of Physicians. It will bring together the five main groups involved in the development of Cervical Screening -

policy makers,

programme managers,
royal colleges and professional associations,
organisations representing women, and
the research workers.

The network will seek to create, develop, and co-ordinate national resources that will help people working at region and district level. Attention will be focussed on five main areas of work:

co-ordinating research,
evaluating the service and reviewing policy.
developing an information system,
improving programme management, and
education and training,

This group also publishes a newsletter "LINKS" which is sent to over 1000 people involved in providing this service.

A second major national resource is the Family Practitioner System Computer Unit (FPSCU) in Exeter. This group has been responsible for the development of software to computerise all the records of the local FPCs and has produced a module for administering the call and recall aspect of the cervical screening service and for keeping screening histories and transferring them between districts when a woman moves. They are also producing a statistical package for the monitoring and routine analysis of the performance of the programme. A Statistics Advisory Panel has been set up as well as a Cervical Cytology Computer System Users Group (CCCSUG) which coordinates and helps to prioritize requests for modifications to the system. The interaction of the FPSCU with these and other bodies is shown schematically in Figure 2.

A national cancer screening evaluation unit also exists. One of its activities is to perform a national evaluation of the screening programme. The interconnection of the activity of this group with that undertaken by the National Co-ordinating Network is not entirely clear yet, but there is an essential need to relate the occurrence of invasive disease with screening histories in order to see where the programme has failed, either due to lack of coverage, inadequate intervals between screens, failure to follow-up on abnormal smears, misreading of smears that were abnormal but passed as normal, or cancers occurring at such short intervals after screening that no feasible screening interval would have detected them. To do this a computer link between cancer registrations and screening histories must be established and this is not yet available.

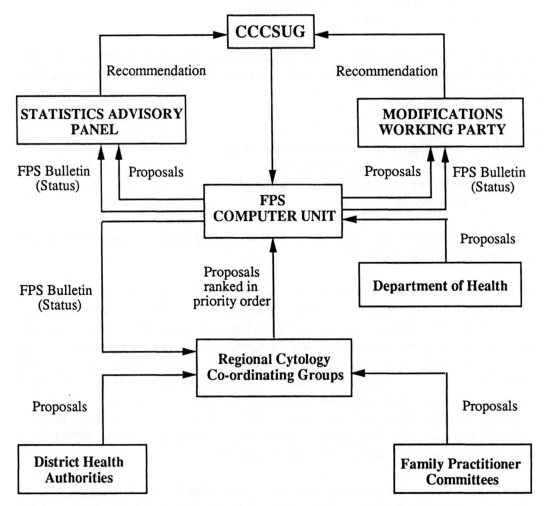

Figure 2 The interactions of the Family Practitioner System Computer Unit

4 MANAGEMENT GOALS:
Defining the job of the district programme co-ordinator

The aim of the screening programme is to reduce mortality and morbidity from cervix cancer by regularly screening all women at risk in order to detect and treat lesions at a pre-invasive stage. Responsibility for the organisation and effectiveness of each district health authority is placed in the hands of a named individual, usually the community physician. The lack of a specific budget and vagaries about the chain of command and individual responsibilities have hampered the ability of the person to properly coordinate a district's activities. However a number of specific goals and tasks have been identified in government circulars which further define the programme coordinator's role in taking action and delegating responsibility.   This list is by no means exhaustive.

Goal 1)   To provide a service which is acceptable to women and minimises the adverse effects of screening.

Tasks: a)   To communicate and consult with users of the service
       b)   To establish facilities for
             i) health education for all groups
             ii) counselling for women with non negative smears
       c)   Identify and monitor adverse effects of screening

Goal 2)   To provide a service as efficiently as possible making the best use of resources for the benefit of the whole population.

Tasks: a)   To identify the population to be screened
       b)   To define and promote an agreed policy for age and frequency
       c)   To identify the existing resources for the programme
       d)   To estimate resource requirements
       e)   To plan the service within the constraints identified

Goal 3)   To provide women who have normal smear tests with repeat tests at the recall interval determined by the programme.

Tasks: a)   To identify these women from FPC register
       b)   To ensure appropriate response from the FPC computer
       c)   To encourage GP's to help refine the call lists
       d)   To publicise the availability of alternative testing sites
       e)   To ensure the transfer of data between lab and FPC
       f)   To ensure the transfer of data on women who move
       g)   To monitor and respond to variations in the takeup rate

Goal 4)   To maximise the sensitivity and specificity of the programme

Tasks: a)   To minimise the number of inadequate smears
       b)   To provide a laboratory service capable of handling the workload generated by the defined population
       c)   To ensure that negative smears are correctly identified
       d)   To ensure that abnormal smears are correctly identified
       e)   To monitor all abnormal outcomes including the results of biopsy, cancer registration and deaths.

Goal 5)   To ensure that results are effectively communicated to women

  Tasks: a)   To provide results promptly to the sender of the smear
         b)   To ensure that the GP is always informed of the result
         c)   To clarify the responsibility for informing the woman
         d)   To ensure information is understandable and not alarming

Goal 6)   To ensure that all women with abnormal smears achieve appropriate follow up

  Tasks: a)   To reach agreement on referral and treatment protocols
         b)   To reach agreement on procedures to be followed for defaulters
         c)   To ensure that referral is made if necessary
         d)   To ensure that appropriate follow up is maintained
         e)   To provide a fail safe mechanism for women lost to follow up

Goal 7)   To provide effective treatment with minimal functional side effects

  Tasks: a)   To provide adequate, appropriate services for investigation, diagnosis and treatment.
         b)   To monitor medical and psycho social outcomes

Goal 8)   To evaluate the service and provide feedback to the users of the service

  Tasks: a)   To undertake the monitoring tasks above
         b)   To provide data for annual statutory returns
         c)   To provide data for the regional review
         d)   To report to the public in the DPH's annual report
         e)   To invite consultation with consumers and users of the service

The programme manager will also provide the necessary liaison between the DHA and the FPC computer system and will be responsible for ensuring that the laboratory computer system used is compatible with FPC requirements and can produce the statutory government returns. The main activities can also be grouped as follows:
  Information
  Planning
  Liaison
  Training
  Quality Assurance
  Evaluation

Responsibility for various areas can be shared or delegated according to the programme manager's professional background and prevailing local management arrangements.

5 CURRENT SCREENING POLICIES AND EVALUATION

The government's current recommendations are that all women age 20-65 who have ever been sexually active should be screened every 5 years. There is pressure to reduce the interval to 3 years and the government has indicated that it hopes to be able to recommend this in the future when more resources become available. Many districts appear to be operating a 3 year recall currently.

Returns have been made to the Department of Health by the district health authorities and the cytology laboratories providing details of coverage, utilisation, and positivity rates for the last two years. These data have not been made public and a report on this current functioning of the programme is eagerly awaited.

REFERENCES

Hakama M. Trends in incidence of cervical cancer in the Nordic countries. In Magnus K (ed). Trends in cancer incidence. New York, Hemisphere Publishing Corporation, 1982, pp 279-291.

ICRF Coordinating Committee on Cervical Screening. Organisation of a programme for cervical cancer screening. Br Med J, 1984, 289:894-895.

ICRF Coordinating Committee on Cervical Screening. The management of a cervical screening programme: a statement (October, 1985). Community Medicine, 1986; 8:179-184.

Pye M. Education and training needs of programme managers, NHS Cervical Screening Programme Document, 1989.

18 Indications for Colposcopy from a UK Viewpoint

R. ELLMAN

Cancer Screening Evaluation Unit, Institute of Cancer Research Section of Epidemiology, Sutton, Surrey, U.K.

1 INTRODUCTION

Colposcopy was first used in 1925, long before cervical smear screening. As a method of primary screening it was found inferior principally because it takes more time and because more equipment and more training are needed, but as a method of investigating women with an abnormal smear it is undoubtedly valuable. A punch biopsy can be taken from the most abnormal looking area so that if invasive cancer is detected an adequately extensive operation can be organized. If, on the other hand, a non-invasive lesion is found colposcopy enables the gynaecologist to see whether the whole area involved is visible and can be treated without a cone biopsy.

A dramatic increase in the use of colposcopy began in the mid-1970s accompanying innovations in treatment which enabled destruction of cervical lesions under local anaesthetic. Treatment, by diathermy, cold cautery, cryosurgery or laser was demonstrated to give satisfactory results, recurrence of CIN being only a little more likely than after cone biopsy. Women were subjected to less risk of haemorrhage or infection post-operatively, and cervical stenosis, with its possible effects on obstetric morbidity, was avoided. The introduction of colposcopy was advocated as a means of reducing the need for cone biopsy. Thus, in Winchester, Pill et al (1984) reported that the proportion of women with CIN3 who required cone biopsy fell from 100% to 39%. However the figures are deceptive as a measure of reduced costs. Colposcopically directed biopsy revealed more CIN3 lesions in patients with mild or moderate dyskaryosis. Consequently the number of women treated by cone biopsy or hysterectomy fell only moderately, to 73% of the number in the previous year, and when CIN1 and 2 cases are included the total number treated for CIN rose threefold.

The threshold for recommending investigation and treatment has fallen. In the early days of screening referral to a gynaecologist, usually without colposcopy, was reserved for patients with severe dyskaryosis whereas now some doctors consider that all patients with abnormal smears of whatever degree should be investigated immediately by colposcopy. The purpose of this paper is to examine what evidence there is that immediate referral of patients with mildly abnormal smears makes a significant contribution to health rather than an unnecessary addition to the costs of cervical screening programmes.

2   ESTIMATED NEED AND CURRENT PROVISION OF COLPOSCOPY

Little has been published on the cost of implementing a policy of liberal referral to colposcopy. Salfield and Sharp (1989) calculated the demand for colposcopy and for treatment under assumptions thought reasonable in Sheffield, that women with smears showing dyskaryosis or viral changes of any degree and women with a second inflammatory smear should also be referred; 5.6% were predicted to need colposcopic referral. This figure contrasts with the colposcopy referral rate in British Columbia in 1985 of 1.7% (Anderson et al, 1988). The criteria for referral in British Columbia were severe dyskaryosis, contributing 37% of referrals, or persistent mild or moderate dyskaryosis, which contributed 63% to the total.

The level of current provision in the UK is difficult to assess as colposcopy services are not covered in routine data gathering. Nearly all districts now provide colposcopy but the level of provision is variable.   An enquiry among 77 gynaecologists in West Midlands (Woodman & Jordan, 1989) found that few could provide quantitative information, services varied and there was no consensus on criteria for referral. In the South-East Thames Region we have found that the number of referrals in 1988 was between 1% and 3% of the number of smears examined in each district except for one Inner London teaching hospital district where it was 10%. Rates partly reflected the varied prevalence of abnormal smears but differences in referral policies and in the care taken to ensure that recommendations were followed also existed between districts. Colposcopic examination of 5% (Johnson & Rowland, 1989) and 16% (Chomet, 1987) of those screened have been reported from GP practices with colposcopy on their premises.

3   ROYAL COLLEGES' RECOMMENDATIONS

In 1987, a Working Party of the Royal Colleges of Pathology, General Practice, Community Medicine and Obstetrics and Gynaecology made these recommendations:

  1. No patient with CIN should be treated without prior colposcopy and biopsy.

  2. Ideally, where resources permit, all women with dyskaryotic smears are best investigated by colposcopy as soon as possible. In districts where this is not possible, in the interim, investigation of mild dyskaryotic smears may be deferred as follows:

  a) Mild dyskaryosis: Two normal smears required before going back into routine screening programme.

  If confirmed in second smear at say 3-6 months, refer for colposcopy.

  b) Moderate dyskaryosis: Refer for colposcopy/gynaecology

  c) Severe dyskaryosis: Refer for colposcopy/gynaecology

  3. Persisting doubtful or borderline abnormalities are an indication for colposcopy.

  4. Clinical suspicion of cervical malignancy requires urgent investigation regardless of the cytology.

Despite these recommendations the Intercollegiate Working Party observed that "The optimum management of women found to have a cytological diagnosis of mild or moderate dyskaryosis is not known".

4   EVIDENCE ON THE SAFETY OF A CONSERVATIVE POLICY FROM WELL-ORGANISED SCREENING PROGRAMMES

Well organized screening programmes have provided evidence on the long term risks of women with different screening histories, but the contribution of colposcopy to the programmes has not been evaluated. The British Columbia programme, with its restrictive policy on colposcopic referral has achieved a 78% reduction in cervical cancer incidence and found that 75% of recent cases were among women who had not been screened in the last 10 years indicating that full participation in screening rather than more thorough diagnostic follow-up remains the most important public health priority for cervical screening. Within the UK, Aberdeen is the only centre that has long experience of providing organized screening by invitation and has kept the person-based records which can provide detailed evidence on the long-term safety of a conservative policy. Further retrospective and prospective studies are currently in progress but it is clear from review of the screening histories of invasive cancer patients that inadequate follow-up of those with atypical smears made only a small contribution to the number of women suffering invasive cancer. The majority had simply not been screened. Out of 83 cases of invasive cancer occurring in 1960-1970 only four cases occurred in women who had had a previous atypical smear (MacGregor, 1976) despite the fact that gynaecological referral was reserved for severe dyskaryosis or three consecutive atypical smears.

Sweden is probably in the best position to provide the information needed. Not only have person-based records of screening on over a million women been kept since 1967 (Pettersson et al, 1986) but these can be linked with cancer registrations more reliably than in the UK. It would be interesting to know whether the risks of invasive cancer for women presenting at screening with mildly abnormal smears have diminished as the use of colposcopy has increased.

If we now focus on the management of mild dyskaryosis we find further evidence indicating that conservative management is reasonably safe. In Belfast (Robertson, 1988) the policy was to recommend six-monthly repeat smears for mildly dyskaryotic cases; only if severe dyskaryosis or clinical symptoms were found or if mild dyskaryosis continued for 18-24 months was referral recommended. Among 1781 cases of mild dyskaryosis detected between 1965-1984, 18% were biopsied for clinical reasons without waiting for smear progression and 24% were lost to follow-up. Table 1 shows the proportion who progressed or regressed among those who were followed up for two years. The study also found that with fourteen year follow-up 75% of those who regressed could be expected to remain relapse free.

A study of mild dyskaryosis in Stockholm produced similar results (Nasiell et al, 1986). The criterion for entry of one mildly dyskaryotic smear was modified by excluding a large number which were re-classified on review. In this study smears were taken under colposcopic view, thus reducing the possibility of missing invasive cases, had there been any, but biopsy was performed only if severe dyskaryosis developed, and the mean

Table 1 Outcome of smear follow-up for women with mild dyskaryosis

	Regression	Persistence	Progression	Duration of follow-up	Incomplete follow-up*
Robertson (1989) N = 1032 Recruited 1965-84	61%	25%	14%	2 years	(24%)
Nasiell (1986) N = 555 Recruited 1962-83	62%	22%	16%	2 years	(31%)
Armstrong (1980) N = 356 Recruited 1974-76	60%	27%	13%	4 years	(24%)

*Those with incomplete follow-up are classified by last follow-up smear. Those without any follow-up or with immediate biopsy are excluded completely.

---

follow-up period with close surveillance was two years. The slightly higher proportion reported to have regressed in the Stockholm study may result from the fact that in half of these regression was assumed to have taken place on the evidence of a single negative smear.

In another large series from London (Armstrong, 1980) where observation was over a four year period of follow-up, 420 women with a first mildly dyskaryotic smear were included. Again loss to follow-up was high, 16% having no repeat smear and a further 24% defaulting at a later stage. 13% progressed to more severe dyskaryosis, resulting in 9% showing CIN3 or worse on biopsy. 60% were normal on their last follow-up smear.

The proportion of cases progressing to CIN3 is not a measure of screening programme failure, since at this stage the disease is easily curable, but is used as an indicator of the danger of delaying referral on the assumption that if lesions are able to escape detection up to that stage a few may escape detection up to the stage of invasion. Cases detected by a mildly dyskaryotic smear which are already invasive by the time treatment is given are rare. In the three studies cited cancer registries were searched at the time of review for any cases additional to those discovered during follow-up. A total of thirteen cases of invasive cervical cancer who had suffered a delay of over three months from the first abnormal smear were identified but of these only one resulted from the false reassurance of two subsequent normal smears. Seven of the women had been lost to follow-up, two were falsely reassured by colposcopic findings, one suffered delay due to pregnancy, one suffered delay following a second abnormal smear and one had a recurrence after treatment for carcinoma-in-situ.   Thus, unless colposcopic referral reduces the likelihood of defaulting, among a total 1943 women with mild dyskaryosis, it could only have provided the benefit of earlier diagnosis for one or perhaps two invasive cancers.

Several smaller studies have reported on progression and regression and produced widely differing estimates; small numbers, varying terminology and selection criteria for entry, varying criteria for progression and varying follow-up periods make it difficult to provide a satisfactory overview of these studies. Some general observations, nevertheless, appear to hold good: the degree of dyskaryosis has some prognostic value; those with smear evidence of persistent dyskaryosis are more likely to show CIN on colposcopic biopsy than those who have been referred after a single abnormal smear; and, while the likelihood of one false negative smear is quite high, the likelihood of two in succession is small.

5   STUDIES RECOMMENDING RAPID REFERRAL TO COLPOSCOPY FOR WOMEN WITH MILDLY ABNORMAL SMEARS

In some reports, the recommendations drawn (as for example by Toon et al (1986) and Spitzer et al (1987)) that women with inflammatory smears should be referred for immediate colposcopy, are founded on the belief that treatment for any degree of CIN or human papilloma virus infection (HPV) is beneficial and that inflammatory changes may be masking evidence of CIN or HPV, though the benefit of such treatment has not been assessed.   It can be argued that ablative treatment for conditions which may regress spontaneously, and for which treatment can be safely deferred, should be counted a cost rather than a benefit of colposcopy.

Other studies recommending immediate referral are based on estimates that a high proportion will progress. Richart & Barron (1969) published a prediction, still often quoted, that 41% of women with smears showing 'very mild dysplasia' would progress to in-situ carcinoma with a median transit time of 86 months whilst only 6% would revert to normal. The prediction is based on Markov modelling for a series of nine follow-up examinations though only a single follow-up examination was carried out on the majority of the 557 women, with varying degrees of dyskaryosis, who were included in the study. At the first follow-up 1.5% of those with 'very mild dysplasia' had progressed to carcinoma-in-situ and a further 1.7% to 'severe dysplasia'. For reasons not specified, second and third examinations were only conducted on 41% and 13% of the cohort respectively. The authors reconciled their findings with those of studies giving a more optimistic prognosis on the assumption that their cases were more carefully selected, that punch biopsies which might promote regression were avoided, and that their diagnoses based on meticulous cytological assessment were more reliable than histological diagnoses. Conclusions based on such limited follow-up should not be given undue weight.

Confidence in the safety of following lesser degrees of dyskaryosis by smears has been further shaken by some recent studies. Campion and colleagues (1986) observed 100 consecutive women, under 30 years, referred to colposcopy from routine screening after three smears taken in the previous 16 weeks had shown persistent mild dyskaryosis. On follow-up without biopsy unless cytology and colposcopic appearance indicated CIN3, 26% progressed to CIN3, and only 7% regressed to normal and did not recur in a period of 19-30 months of observation. They concluded that these were real changes over time rather than cytological errors, because only one out of 30 women biopsied immediately showed CIN3.

A yet more alarming report from Campion et al (1987) described the cases of 14 young women all of whom presented with fully invasive cancer at one London hospital within a period of 12 months. It is not stated from how wide a field they were drawn, but 12 had had a mildly abnormal smear six months to 10 years before diagnosis. Though some of these women should have had smears examined more frequently or been referred earlier even with a conservative policy, it is argued that readier referral to colposcopy might have prevented these cases. This hospital perhaps attracted atypical patients, but the findings of the general practices referred to earlier are also disconcerting. In the Welsh practice (Johnson & Rowlands, 1989), two cases of invasive disease, one of microinvasive and 18 of CIN 2 or 3 were found among the 47 presenting with only mildly dyskaryotic smears. In the London practice (Chomet, 1987) 25% (15/60) of those with mild dyskaryosis and 18% of those with only inflammatory smears were found on biopsy to have CIN3.

6 CYTOLOGICAL AND HISTOLOGICAL CONSISTENCY

One explanation for varied estimates of rates of progression, or of the risk of missing severe dysplasia, lies in problems regarding the validity of pathological diagnoses. Two recent histopathology studies (Ismail et al, 1989; Robertson et al, 1989) indicate that problems in consistency still exist. In both studies a series of slides from 100 cervical biopsies were examined independently by 8-12 pathologists. Using Kappa statistics, both found agreement on CIN3 to be moderately good whilst agreement on CIN1 and CIN2 was poor. In Ismael et al's (1989) study the number of slides reported to show CIN3 varied from 7% to 32%.

Cytological diagnosis is equally liable to vary between observers. For example, Yobs et al (1987) compared the results when two well-reputed laboratories undertook to re-read 20,000 of each other's slides, using their routine screening procedures and in ignorance of the other laboratory's findings. The probability that the second laboratory would agree with the first that a smear showed mild dysplasia was only 9% with a further 6% reporting it as mild/moderate dysplasia. Observer variability could account for apparent regression to normal between two readings of 40%, and could account for apparent progression to severe dysplasia or worse in 4%.

Individuals may achieve much higher consistency than the inter-observer consistency found here, but in reporting research results of different management policies for mild dyskaryosis it is essential that smears and histopathological specimens are read blind and preferably re-read by an external observer. This was not reported in most of the studies reviewed.

7 SECULAR TRENDS

A recent change in the nature of the disease has been postulated as a reason for patients requiring more urgent follow-up (Elliot et al, 1989). In the United Kingdom the incidence of CIN is rising, particularly among younger women. This by itself increases demand for colposcopy, but epidemiological evidence does not indicate increasing aggressiveness of the disease. Silcocks and Moss (1988) have argued that an increase in the number of rapidly progressive cases of invasive cancer is explicable simply as a result of increasing disease incidence and of changes in the age structure of the population. Screening, by removal of the more readily detectable cases at a pre-invasive stage, leads to an increase in the proportion of endocervical and fast-developing cases. Robertson et al (1988) were unable to demonstrate a greater risk of relapse among women whose smears had reverted to normal in recent years compared with the risk in earlier cohorts, and Meanwell et al (1988) and Russell et al (1987) were unable to demonstrate any worsening of prognosis among younger or more recent cases of invasive cervical cancer after adjusting for stage at diagnosis. Thus there is no evidence that women with abnormal smears require more intensive investigation than in the past on grounds of increased risk of rapid progression.

8 SIZE OF LESIONS

A further recent explanation for the apparent contradiction between the success in preventing progression to invasive cancer of early screening programmes and the prevalence of CIN3 found when women with lesser degrees of dyskaryosis are now examined by colposcopy lies in observations on the size of lesions.

Toon et al (1986), in a study of women with non-specific inflammatory smears in which 12% were discovered by colposcopy to have CIN, commented on the small size of the lesions. Giles et al (1988), in a study of 200 women in one GP practice who were offered screening which combined colposcopy with cytology, found that colposcopy increased the apparent prevalence of CIN from 5% to 11% but that none of the cases missed by screening involved more than two quadrants of the transformation zone. Jarmulowicz et al (1989), in a series of cases which included several with a histological diagnosis more severe than suggested by the smear, found that the likelihood of smear underdiagnosis was inversely related to size, as measured microscopically. In 19 CIN cases, of which only two had shown severe dyskaryosis, the lesion could not be measured on the cone biopsy as it had disappeared after punch biopsy. Whether the punch biopsy removed a minute lesion or, as Nasiell et al (1983) have suggested, promoted regression, it is probable that patients with CIN and only mildly abnormal smears present a lower risk of progression than patients whose lesions are associated with severely abnormal cytology. Just as the risk of metastasis is related to the size of an invasive cancer, it is likely that the risk of invasion is related to the size of an in-situ lesion.

9   ADVERSE CONSEQUENCES OF REFERRAL FOR COLPOSCOPY OF WOMEN WITH MINOR CYTOLOGICAL ABNORMALITIES

Although the risk of invasive cancer among women with mildly abnormal smears is small, it is reasonable to suppose that colposcopy reduces it, at least to some extent.   However, before advocating colposcopy on these grounds, the disadvantages must be explored. The possible disadvantages of referring large numbers of women at low risk of invasive cervical cancer are the following:

From the Health Service viewpoint:
  Increased financial cost
  Crowded clinics and longer waiting lists
  Diversion of gynaecologists from other activities
  Employment of less experienced staff to do the job
  Increased histology workload
  Increased demand for treatment sessions
  Reduced benefit/cost ratio

From the patient's viewpoint:
  Increased time and travel cost
  Greater anxiety
  Risk of unnecessary treatment
  False reassurance from negative findings

The literature on economic evaluation of cervical screening has been recently reviewed (Brown, 1990), but there is little to be found on the costs of colposcopic investigation other than simple information on costs of equipment and outpatient sessions. The effect of increased workload on the quality of colposcopy should also be considered. Stafl (1976) suggested that 3-4 months of training for colposcopy was needed, and that full experience took at least a year to acquire, yet courses have only recently been organized and there is no system in Britain ensuring that those who perform colposcopy have had adequate training. Even experienced staff may perform less well when the volume of work is increased and the perceived probability of serious abnormality is reduced. The risk of false reassurance after a smear which failed to adequately sample cervical cells is well known but a misdirected colposcopic biopsy may also lead to false reassurance. If, however, staff are cautious and request further examinations, one of the main attractions of colposcopy, rapid resolution of uncertainty, is lost.

The extent of overtreatment as a result of early referral will vary with policy on treatment. Some consider that any sign of HPV infection or of CIN should lead to excision or destruction of the entire visible lesion and the entire transformation zone; others only treat CIN2 and CIN3. The type of treatment given for lesser degrees of dyskaryosis is not necessarily minor. If the margins of the transformation zone are not fully visible, cone biopsy or hysterectomy under general anaesthesia may be advocated. Cone biopsy causes post-operative haemorrhage or infection in up to 17% of cases (Coppleston, 1981) and causes cervical stenosis which can lead to obstetric problems.

Posner & Vessey (1988), who interviewed 153 women who had attended colposcopy, found that outpatient treatment was not trivial but very upsetting for many women. The profuse vaginal discharge for a month following cryocautery was particularly troublesome physically, and 52% had disturbed feelings about sexual relationships after colposcopy. Campion et al (1988), in a study comparing women under investigation for CIN, with women investigated as partners of men with sexually transmitted diseases, found that treatment of CIN had a strong negative effect on sexual feelings and behaviour six months later, whereas the psychosexuality of those who had not had CIN treatment did not change.

Early referral for colposcopy has been justified as a means of reducing the danger of patients being lost to follow-up. Much of the loss to follow-up, however, can be reduced by instituting 'fail-safe' mechanisms, by giving clearer cytology reports, and by seeking out and counselling non-attenders. The determined defaulter is often motivated by fear, which may be increased by hospital referral. Salfield & Sharp (1989) found that defaulting may be considerable even with colposcopy: 8% of women referred for colposcopy defaulted, 10% failed to attend for laser treatment and 21% defaulted from follow-up colposcopy. It is thus uncertain whether early colposcopic referral reduces the risk of non-compliance.

10 RESEARCH NEEDS
In order to make rational decisions on resource allocation research on the management of mild dyskaryosis is needed to determine the relative costs and benefits of smear follow-up by GPs and of colposcopic follow-up at hospital. The cheapness of the former policy may be illusory if most patients ultimately require hospital referral, and the safety of the latter may be reduced if avoidable treatment has side-effects of importance, or if it has little effect on the long term risk of recurrence. The greatest risk of invasive cancer, however, is among women who default, and hence the effect of different management strategies on risk of defaulting must be recorded.

Randomized controlled trials are ideal from the point of view of statistical analysis but may not be feasible. There is increased concern, especially following the unfortunate New Zealand experience (Paul, 1988), that patients should give informed consent before randomization, but discussion of alternatives and consent to randomization may increase the distress associated with follow-up and affect compliance.

Observational studies which compare districts with varied policies are easier to organize, and some are under way (Jenkins & Jones, 1988) but no study of a few hundred patients will be able to detect a significant difference in observed progression to invasive cancer, even with a follow-up of many years. It will therefore be necessary to make assumptions from the proportion who progress to CIN3. Yet, if progression does indeed depend on the size of the CIN3 lesion, assumptions derived from earlier studies on the progression of cases of carcinoma in-situ may not be valid. More detailed analysis of data from series in which treatment was unfortunately not given, such as the New Zealand experiment, and studies, under careful colposcopic surveillance, of changes in size as well as in smear grade of lesser CIN lesions are needed to provide further information on progression.

11 CONCLUSION

Referral for colposcopy is universally advocated for severe or persistent dyskaryosis but for lesser degrees of abnormality the policy adopted by a screening programme should be reached by discussion between all those involved, including GPs, pathologists and gynaecologists. It must reflect the resources available and the volume of work the policy would create. Confidential review of cases, to find the proportion of invasive cancers which might have been prevented by greater availability of colposcopy, provides the best indication of the priority which should be given to colposcopy, relative to other improvements such as increasing screening coverage, reducing defaulting on follow-up, and improving the quality of smear taking and reading. Hopefully current research, such as that on nuclear ploidy and human papilloma virus, will provide a means of determining with greater accuracy those who really need treatment. In the meantime health service managers should be aware that putting more resources into screening programmes in an attempt to eliminate completely the risk of invasive cervical cancer may produce very small marginal returns, and draw staff and funds away from other services where they might provide more benefit. Control of colposcopy provision may be less important as an economic issue in countries with larger health budgets, but in all countries the health consequences of management strategies for mild dyskaryosis merit review.

REFERENCES

Anderson GH, Boyes DA, Benedet JL et al. Organisation and results of the cervical cytology screening programme in British Columbia, 1955-85. BMJ, 1988; 296: 975-978.
Armstrong AE. Follow-up of women with dysplasia of the uterine cervix. Ph.D Thesis, University College Hospital Medical School, University of London, 1980
Brown J. An annotated bibliography of the economic literature concerning the evaluation of the screening for cervical cancer. In press, 1990.
Campion MJ, Cuzick J, McCance DJ et al. Progressive potential of mild cervical atypia:

prospective cytological, colposcopic, and virological study. Lancet, 1986; ii: 237-240.

Campion MJ, Singer A, Mitchell HS. Complacency in diagnosis of cervical cancer. BMJ,1987; 294: 1337-1339.

Campion MJ, Brown JR, McCance DJ et al. Psychosexual trauma of an abnormal cervical smear. Br J Obstet Gynaecol, 1988; 95: 175-181.

Chomet J. Screening for cervical cancer: a new scope for general practitioners? Results of the first year of colposcopy in general practice. BMJ, 1987; 294: 1326-1328.

Coppleson M. Gynaecological Oncology. Edinburgh, Churchill Livingstone, 1981; Vol 1, pg 420.

Elliott PM, Tattersall MHN, Coppleson M et al. Changing character of cervical cancer in young women. BMJ, 1989; 298: 288-290.

Giles JA, Hudson E, Crow J et al. Colposcopic assessment of the accuracy of cervical cytology screening. BMJ, 1988; 296: 1099-1102.

Ismail SM, Colclough AB, Dinnen JS et al. Observer variation in histopathological diagnosis and grading of cervical intraepithelial neoplasia. Journal? 1989; 298: 707-710.

Jarmulowicz MR, Jenkins D, Barton SE et al. Cytological status and lesion size: a further dimension in cervical intraepithelial neoplasia. Br J Obstet Gynaecol, 1989; 96: 1061-1066.

Jenkins D, Jones MH. Cervical intraepithelial neoplasia. Letter, BMJ, 1988; 297: 555.

Johnson DB, Rowland J. Diagnosis and treatment of cervical intra-epithelial neoplasia in general practice. BMJ, 1989; 299: 1083-1086.

MacGregor JE. Evaluation of mass screening programmes for cervical cancer in NE Scotland. Tumori, 1976; 62: 287-295.

Meanwell CA, Kelly KA, Wilson S et al. Young age as a prognostic factor in cervical cancer: analysis of population based data from 10,022 cases. BMJ, 1988; 296: 386-391.

Nasiell K, Nasiell M,Vaclavinkova V. Behavior of moderate cervical dysplasia during long-term follow-up. Obstet Gynecol, 1983; 61: 609-614.

Nasiell K. Roger V, Nasiell M. Behavior of mild cervical dysplasia during long-term follow-up. Obstet Gynecol, 1986; 67: 665-669.

Paul C. The New Zealand cervical cancer study: Could it happen again? BMJ, 1988; 297: 533-53

Pettersson F, Naslund I and Malker B. Evaluation of the effect of Papanicolaou screening in Sweden: Record linkage between a central screening registry and the National Cancer Registry. In: Screening for Cancer of the Uterine Cervix. (Eds: Hakama M, Miller AB, Day NE). IARC Scientific Publications No. 76, Lyon, International Agency for Research on Cancer, 1986; pp 91-105.

Pill CF, Letchworth AT, Noble AD. Effect of introduction of colposcopy into a district general hospital. Postgrad Med J, 1984; 60: 461-463.

Posner T, Vessey M. Prevention of Cervical Cancer. The Patient's View. King Edward's Hospital Fund for London. London, King's Fund Publishing Office, 1988.

Report of the Intercollegiate Working Party on Cervical Cytology Screening. Potters Bar, Herts, Progress Press Ltd., 1987.

Richart RM, Barron BA. A follow-up study of patients with cervical dysplasia. Am J Obstet Gynecol, 1969; 105: 386-393.

Robertson AJ, Anderson JM, Swanson Beck J et al. Observer variability in histopathological reporting of cervical biopsy specimens. J Clin Pathol, 1989; 42: 231-238.

Robertson JH, Woodend BE, Crozier EH et al. Risk of cervical cancer associated with mild dyskaryosis. BMJ, 1988; 297: 18-21.

Russell JM, Blair V, Hunter RD. Cervical carcinoma: prognosis in younger patients. BMJ, 1987; 295: 300-303.

Salfield NH, Sharp F. Planning colposcopy and gynaecological laser services. Community Med, 1989; 11: 140-147.

Silcocks PBS, Moss SM. Rapidly progressive cervical cancer: is it a real problem? Br J Obstet Gynaecol, 1988; 95: 1111-1116.

Singer A, Walker P, Tay SK et al. Impact of introduction of colposcopy to a district general hospital. BMJ, 1984; 289: 1049-1051.

Spitzer M, Krumholz BA, Chernys AE et al. Comparative utility of repeat Papanicolaou smears, cervicography, and colposcopy in the evaluation of atypical Papanicolaou smears. Obstet Gynecol, 1987; 69: 731-735.

Stafl A. New nomenclature for colposcopy. Report of the Committee on Terminology. Obstet Gynecol, 1976; 48: 123.

Toon PG, Arrand JR, Wilson LP et al. Human papillomavirus infection of the uterine cervix of women without cytological signs of neoplasia. BMJ, 1986; 293: 1261-1264.

Woodman CBJ, Jordan JA. Colposcopy services in the West Midlands region. BMJ, 1989; 299: 899-901

Yobs AR, Plott AE, Hicklin MD et al. Retrospective evaluation of gynecological diagnosis II interlaboratory reproducibility as shown in rescreening large consecutive samples of reported cases. Acta Cytol, 1987; 31: 900-910.

19 Screening for Cervix Cancer in Developing Countries

D. M. PARKIN

International Agency for Research on Cancer, Lyon

1 EPIDEMIOLOGY AND NATURAL HISTORY

In 1980, there were an estimated 465,000 new cases of cancer of the cervix in the world, 80% of which occurred in developing countries (Parkin et al., 1988). The regions of the world where the risk is highest are sub-Saharan Africa, Central & South America, and South-East Asia, where cancer of the cervix accounts for 20-30% of all cancers in women. The highest recorded incidence rates occur in South America and particularly in North Eastern Brazil (Table 1). In contrast, low incidence rates are found in middle-eastern populations: in Israel and Kuwait the age-standardized rate is below 4.0 per 10^5. A zone of relatively low risk, where cervical cancer accounts for less than 10% of female neoplasms, appears to extend from Pakistan to Egypt, but available evidence suggests considerably higher rates in Morocco, Algeria and Tunisia (Parkin, 1986).

In general, the form of the age-specific incidence curve is similar in all populations (Figure 1). Incidence rises rapidly from around age 20 to reach a plateau at about 40-50 years of age. The level of this plateau varies considerably, however, from about 10 per 100,000 in Kuwait and Israel, to 100-200 in Colombia and N.E. Brazil.

Aetiological hypotheses for cervix cancer tend to focus on the importance of a sexually transmitted agent (with HPV as the currently favoured candidate), a notion supported by consistent findings in epidemiological studies of the importance of sexual behaviour in affecting risk; cigarette smoking and possibly diet and use of oral contraceptives may also be of importance (Muñoz & Bosch, 1989). It is far from clear, however, how much of the very great inter-country differences in incidence are explicable in terms of exposure to these known risk factors. Certainly it seems hard, a priori, to believe that there are such enormous differences in the age at first intercourse and numbers of sexual partners, and the possible importance of males in the transmission of an infectious agent has been much discussed, and is now being investigated, particularly in Latin America (Brinton et al., 1989a).

It is clear that carcinoma of the cervix has a long pre-clinical phase identifiable by histological changes in the cervical epithelium. This stage of the disease process is conventionally described in terms of the histological degree of transition to malignancy

Table 1   Age standardized incidence of cervix cancer in developing countries

South & Central America		India	
Brazil, Fortaleza[1]	46.5	Bangalore[1]	40.2
Recife[1]	83.2	Bombay[1]	20.6
Porto Alegre[1]	23.7	Madras[1]	46.1
Sao Paulo[1]	35.1	Nagpur[1]	29.2
Colombia, Cali[1]	48.2		
Costa Rica[1]	36.9	**Western Asia**	
Martinique[1]	29.3	Israel: Jews[1]	4.0
Netherlands Antilles[1]	18.0	non Jews[1]	3.0
		Kuwait, Kuwaiti[1]	3.9
China			
Shanghai[1]	8.5	**Africa**	
Tianjin[1]	13.9	Algeria, Setif (1986-88)[8]	16.1
		Mali, Bamako (1987-88)[9]	20.8
South East Asia		Gambia (1986-88)[10]	11.0
Hong Kong[1]	23.7	Senegal, Dakar (1969-74)[2]	17.2
Philippines, Manila/Rizal	20.5	Nigeria, Ibadan (1960-69)[3]	21.6
(1980-82)[5]		Zimbabwe, Bulawayo	28.4
Singapore, Chinese[1]	17.0	(1968-72)[3]	
Malay[1]	9.9	Swaziland (1979-83)[4]	28.2
Indian[1]	28.0		
Thailand, Chiang Mai	29.2	**Oceania**	
(1983-87)[6]		New Caledonia, Melanesian	36.3
Khon Kaen (1985-88)[7]	24.1	(977-81)[4]	

Sources

[1] Muir et al. (1987)

[2] Waterhouse et al. (1982)

[3] Waterhouse et al. (1976)

[4] Parkin, (1986)

[5] Laudico et al. (1989)

[6] Martin et al. (1989)

[7] Vatanasapt et al. (1989)

[8] Hamdi-Cherif, H. (unpublished data)

[9] Bayo et al. (1990)

[10] Bah et al. (1990)

(CIN I-III, or dysplasia-carcinoma in situ), a categorization that has proved useful in conceptualizing the results of cytological screening, and deciding on therapeutic interventions, and which may even have some biological meaning. The rate of transition through this sequence, described most fully as the distribution of sojourn times in the different stages, and the rates of progression and regression between the different stages, have been estimated in western populations from longitudinal observations of women being

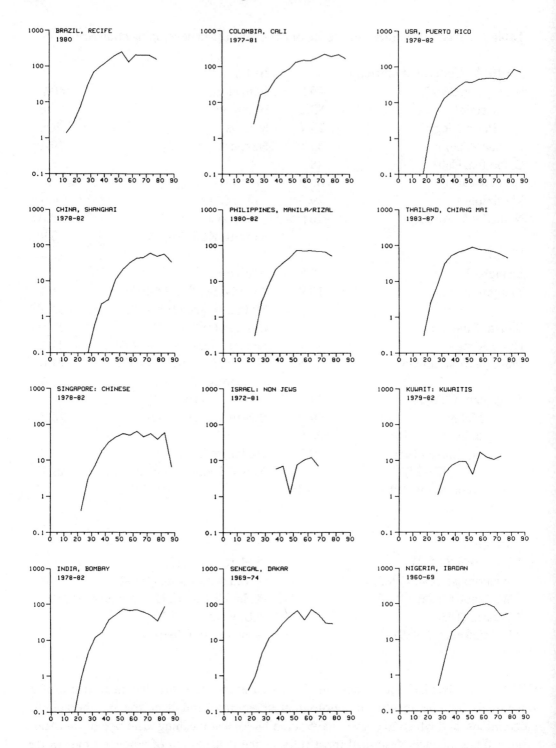

Figure 1 Age-specific incidence of cancer of the cervix in some developing countries.

repeatedly screened (e.g. Boyes et al., 1982), or from the analysis of screening histories of women developing invasive cancer (Day and Walter, 1984). It is not really clear where exactly in the natural history the different risk factors for cervix cancer identified in epidemiological studies act. An infectious agent might be responsible for initiating the sequence - indeed the histological features of papillomavirus infection seem to be those of CIN I or dysplasia (Campion, 1989). However, it is conceivable that some agents may act to enhance progression of pre-invasive disease or retard regression (e.g. dietary factors, or components of tobacco smoke). In any case, the possibility of different natural histories in different parts of the world should be considered, and this has important implications when the likely effectiveness of screening is deduced by extrapolating from the quantitative data derived from the study of screening programmes in Europe and North America.

2   SCREENING PROGRAMMES IN DEVELOPING COUNTRIES

It is probable that cytological examination of 'Pap' smears has been performed in almost all countries with access to histopathology services. Whether or not this is termed 'Screening' depends on the definition of the term. Thus, the most common circumstance - taking a Pap smear from women in gynaecological clinics - might be considered as selective screening of a very high risk group rather than a specific diagnostic investigation. Otherwise, there have been more or less extensive attempts to screen groups of asymptomatic women. Some of these have been reviewed by Lunt (1984). Mostly, the programmes are based in hospitals, and recruit women attending certain services (obstetric, gynaecology, family planning), or recruit volunteers for 'check-ups' from the surrounding population. These programmes are usually urban, and serve relatively selected populations. It was estimated (WHO, 1986) that less than 5% of women in developing countries had been screened within the previous 5 years, and that those who had been screened were mainly under 35 years of age. In addition, however, there have been several more extensive campaigns mounted in a variety of countries, the results of some of which are described in publications detailing numbers of tests, and prevalence of abnormalities detected.

Luthra and Rengachari (1986) provide results from some of the projects in India, including several rural programs using mobile cancer detection clinics, 'early cancer detection camps', or clinics in local dispensaries. The project carried out at the Cytology Research Centre, New Delhi recruited women attending gynaecology departments of six major hospitals. In 8 years, some 84.000 women were screened, the prevalence of dysplasia was 1.3% and of carcinoma 0.1%. Regular repeat smears allow the incidence of malignancy to be calculated in women with different degrees of dysplasia on the first smear.

Goes et al. (1981, 1987) report the results of the extensive screening program in Sao Paulo State, Brazil. Screening is carried out by paramedical personnel in state and municipal health centres. Between 1970 and 1985, some 981,000 women were examined, with the detection of 9,761 cases of dysplasia (1% of examinations) and 1460 cases of carcinoma in situ (0.15%). The quality of testing in these circumstances seemed to be good - values of about 70% for sensitivity and 99.6 for specificity can be calculated for a test result (and final diagnosis) of mild dysplasia or worse. Since 1980, some basic information on demographic and reproductive variables was collected, for comparison with the prevalence of abnormality. The prevalence of dysplasia appeared to vary little with age, but for carcinoma in situ it increased slowly to a maximum in the oldest age-group. The results for other variables are shown in Table 2. There is a clear relationship of prevalence of both dysplasia and carcinoma in situ to parity, age at first intercourse and educational level. Since only one-way frequencies are given, it is difficult to infer much about which relationships are likely to be the most important aetiologically, and which merely confounders, but the overall results are in keeping with what has been found in studies elsewhere.

Table 2   Screening programme in Sao Paulo (1980-85)
(from Goes et al., 1987)

	Prevalence (%)	
	Dysplasia	C.I.S.
No. of pregnancies:		
0	0.8	0.06
1-3	0.9	0.12
4-6	1.3	0.32
7+	1.4	0.52
Age at first intercourse:		
< 12	2.0	0.31
13-17	1.4	0.31
18-22	1.0	0.20
23+	0.8	0.12
Educational level:		
< Primary	1.2	0.25
Primary	0.8	0.11
Secondary ± University	0.6	0.07

Results from the long-established programme (since 1966) in Santiago, Chile, have been described by Dabancens (1989). Prevalence of mild dysplasia is highest at ages 25-29 (0.8%), and seems to be relatively little changed on subsequent annual examination; CIN grades II-III is most frequent at ages 40-44 (about 1% of smears), and prevalence is approximately halved after 2 or more previous negative smears. The results imply a rather insensitive test, or alternatively high incidence and regression rates of lower grade lesions.

Relatively few of the screening projects in developing countries permit any judgment as to their effectiveness. In four published case-control studies, however, the risk of invasive cancer has been reported in relation to screening history.

Aristizabal et al. (1984) presented data from Cali, Colombia where screening has been performed in pre-natal clinics since the early 1960's. A rise in the annual numbers of tests performed was accompanied by an increased detection of carcinoma in-situ and fall in incidence of invasive disease between 1964 and 1978. A case-control study of 204 cases of invasive disease, with two controls per case (one from the same health centre, one from the same neighbourhood) compared screening histories 12 months or more before diagnosis. The relative risks were 9.9 (neighbourhood) to 23.9 (health centre control) for never vs ever screened. In this study a positive history of screening was verified against clinic and hospital records, but not negative histories. The estimated annual screening frequency among the controls was lower for long intervals before diagnosis of their matched cases, which suggests failure to recall all previous tests. Any bias is likely, however, to result from better recall by cases, which in general would deflate estimates of relative protection.

Wangsuphachart (1987) report a hospital-based case-control study in Bangkok, Thailand, with 189 cases of invasive cancer and 1023 controls from other (non-gynaecological) hospital wards. Subjects were interviewed about their experience of Pap smears in the period up to 6 months before diagnosis. The results were presented as odds-ratios (adjusted for age, age at first intercourse, number of partners, number of episodes of vaginal discharge and years of education) (Table 3). 63% of controls reported never having had a test, but there were significantly reduced risks with more frequent screening.

Table 3   Relative risk in relation to frequency of Pap smears
             (Wangsuphachart et al., 1987)

Frequency	Cases*	Controls*	OR	95% C.I.
None	130	464	1.00	-
Only one	33	106	0.92	0.58-6.46
Once every 2-5 years	14	88	0.39	0.21-0.74
Once a year	7	63	0.25	0.12-0.59
> once a year	1	16	0.20	0.03-1.56

* Exclude subjects with no, or unknown, history of sexual intercourse

Zhang et al. (1989a) reported the results of an extensive screening project in a high risk rural community (Jingan County) in China. Screening began in 1974, with an invitation to all women aged 25 or more to attend, and 85% of those eligible did so. Subsequent invitations were sent to all women aged 30 or more, at 2 years intervals, until the 6th screening round in 1984-1985. During this 12 year period, over 22,000 women (95% of the eligible population) attended for screening at least once. A previous analysis (Zhang et al., 1989b) had demonstrated six variables which were independent risk factors for invasive cervix cancer. Two of these (number of sexual partners of the woman, and of her husband) were positively related to the number of screening tests, while for one (use of sanitary napkins), attendance was higher in the low risk category. Other risk factors related to genital washing and menstruation did not show a clear relation to screening history. A case-control analysis was carried out with 109 cases of invasive cancer and 5 controls per case (matched for age, area of residence, and attendance at the same screening round at which the case was diagnosed). The relative protection against cervix cancer in relation to the time since the last negative test (i.e. excluding the test at which the case was diagnosed, and the corresponding test in the matched controls) is shown in Table 4. Adjustment for the risk factors for cervix cancer, described above, made very little difference to the estimates of relative risk.

Table 4   Relative risk in relation to time since last negative test –
Jingan County, China   (Zhang et al., 1989a)

Years since last negative smear	Cases	Controls	Relative Risk*	95% C.I.
0 - 2	94	520	1.00	–
4 - 6	9	21	4.22	1.51-11.90
>8	6	4	11.41	2.38-63.66

* Stratified for number of previous tests

In a large case-control study in four Latin American countries (Panama, Costa Rica, Colombia and Mexico) 759 incident cervical cancer cases were compared with 1467 controls with respect to screening history, and a large number of other possible aetiological factors (Brinton et al., 1989b). Results relating to the history of Pap-smears have been presented in summary form (Herrero et al., 1990). 29% of controls and 50% of cases had never been screened, and screening was less common in older subjects, less educated women, non-users of oral contraceptives and women without histories of venereal diseases. There was no association with sexual behaviour. The relative risk of never vs ever screened was about 3, and varied little by the presence of other risk factors. Absence of screening was a stronger predictor of risk for advanced tumours - relative risk for Stage III and was about 5.

3 DIFFICULTIES IN THE ORGANIZATION OF SCREENING PROGRAMMES IN DEVELOPING COUNTRIES

Successful screening programmes demand a wide range of resources, human, material and organizational. The elements which appear to be essential components have been summarized by Hakama et al. (1985):
- the target population has been identified.
- the individual women are identifiable.

- measures are available to guarantee high coverage and attendance.
- there are adequate field facilities for taking the smears and adequate laboratory facilities to examine them.
- there is an organized quality control programme on taking of the smears and on interpreting them
- adequate facilities must exist for diagnosis and for appropriate treatment of confirmed neoplastic lesions.
- there is a carefully designed and agreed referral system, an agreed link between the woman, the laboratory and the clinical facility for diagnosis of an abnormal screening test, for management of any abnormalities found and for providing information about normal screening tests.
- evaluation and monitoring of the programme is organized ... at the level of the total target population.

It is usually very difficult to meet these criteria in developing countries. Thus, it is rarely possible to identify individually women in the target population, to take the appropriate measures to ensure that they will attend any screening service, to document which members of the population have or have not attended. Facilities for taking smears can usually be organized by training appropriate paramedical personnel, although poor technique in taking smears will reduce the validity of the test and the protection against cancer which is conferred by the screening (Husain, 1976). Interpretation of smears demands that trained cytotechnologists are available. These are usually in short supply, since there are rarely suitable facilities for training and employing such staff. One technologist is required for every 10-15,000 smears per year. Adequate facilities for the follow-up of suspicious or positive smears and for appropriate treatment of confirmed neoplastic lesions may not be available. Finally, the level of organization of services may be such that it is difficult to coordinate between the woman, the laboratory and the clinical facility so that abnormal screening tests are followed up according to an agreed protocol, and that information is provided about negative tests.

4 SCREENING STRATEGIES IN DEVELOPING COUNTRIES

As indicated above, it is generally implied that the natural history of cervix cancer is the same in all settings, and that variations in incidence reflect onset rates of precursor conditions rather than speed of progression or regression. If this is so, then the possible outcomes of different screening strategies can be evaluated using information on the duration of protection following a negative screening test, derived from the several studies which have been carried out in Europe or North America.

The relative protection provided by two or more negative tests, in relation to the duration of time elapsed since the last negative test, have been calculated from data from eight screening programmes in developed countries (IARC, 1986). The results are shown in Table 5.

Table 5 Geometric mean relative protection against cervical cancer in women
with two or more previously negative smears (IARC, 1986)

Months since last negative smear	Relative protection (95% C.I.)
0 - 11	15.3 (10.0 - 22..6)
12 - 23	11.9 (7.5 - 18.3)
24 - 35	8.0 (5.2 - 11.8)
36 - 47	5.3 (3.6 - 7.6)
48 - 59	2.8 (1.9 - 4.0)
60 - 71	3.6 (2.1 - 5.9)
72- 119	1.6 (0.6 - 3.5)
120+	0.8 (0.3 - 1.6)
Never screened	1.0 -

Using these data, the effects on cervical cancer incidence of different screening policies can
be estimated. Results for a population having the incidence rates observed in Cali,
Colombia in 1977-81 (as shown in Figure 1) are given in Table 6.

Table 6 Effects on cervical cancer incidence of different screening policies,
starting at age 20[a]

Screening schedule	Cumulative rate, 20-64, per 10^5	Reduction in rate (%)	No.of tests	No.of cases prevented per 10^5 tests
None	3311.5			
Every 10 years, 25-64	1298	61	4	503
Every 10 years, 35-64	1476	55	3	612
Every 10 years, 45-64	1895	43	2	708
Every 5 years, 20-64	544	84	9	308
Every 5 years, 30-64	630	81	7	383
Every 3 years, 20-64	303	91	15	201
Every year, 20-64	216	93	45	69

[a] From IARC Working Group (1986); assuming incidence rates from Cali, Colombia.
The first screening test is assumed to be 70% sensitive.

There are several interesting observations to be made from Table 6. Firstly, as noted on
many occasions, there is a diminishing return (in terms of number of cases prevented per

There are several interesting observations to be made from Table 6. Firstly, as noted on many occasions, there is a diminishing return (in terms of number of cases prevented per 100,000 tests) with increasing frequency of screening. Secondly, even very low intensity programmes - with 2-4 tests per lifetime spaced out at 10-year intervals - can reduce the incidence of cervix cancer by 40-60%. Thirdly, these results assume that all women will attend for screening - a programme of 5-yearly tests at ages 20-64 which was only attended by a third of the population at risk would reduce incidence by only about 28%, and yet would demand an average of 3 tests per lifetime for the entire population. The same number of tests (3 per lifetime) with 100% attendance can reduce incidence by 55%. This underlines the importance of securing good compliance with screening, rather than concentrating upon very frequent testing.

The estimation of the protective effects of screening using this simple model is rather critically dependent upon the assumed relative protection given in Table 5, and the constancy of these figures in different populations. They assume, for instance, that the duration of protection is independent of age, although it has been pointed out that it is rather unlikely that the duration of the preclinical phase of disease is independent of age, given the observed age-specific prevalence of c.i.n. and incidence of invasive cancer (Coppleson & Brown, 1975; Parkin, 1985). One case-control study (Klassen et al., 1989) has found that the duration of protection provided by a negative test declines with age, although a reduced effectiveness of screening in older age-groups was not observed in other studies (Clarke & Anderson, 1979; Aristizabal et al., 1984; Herrero et al., 1990).

The same study (Klassen et al., 1989) suggested that certain risk factors for cervix cancer (early age at first intercourse, non-use of barrier contraceptives) are associated with reduced duration of protection from a negative smear, which implies an effect on duration of the preclinical phase of disease (rather than on the rates of onset) and although in most case control studies of screening, adjustment for possible confounders (related to screening attendance and risk of invasive cancer) does not change the estimate of relative protection. This clearly requires further investigation. The need to incorporate assumptions about the effects of age and other risk factors on disease will usually require the use of rather more sophisticated simulation models to explore the relative benefits of different screening strategies (Eddy, 1980; van Oortmarssen et al., 1981; Parkin, 1985).

5   APPROACHES TO THE ORGANIZATION OF SCREENING SERVICES

5.1 Organized Programmes
It is not possible to do more than generalize, since specific patterns of service must clearly be adapted to particular countries. Fairly detailed principles were described in a WHO meeting report (WHO, 1986). In summary, an organized programme of screening must have identifiable control and co-ordinating mechanism, responsible for planning the screening policy, and ensuring that the various services involved (in taking and interpreting smears, and in clinical management of the women) work in a defined, co-ordinated

manner. The level of screening activity should <u>never</u> exceed the facilities for clinical management of women with abnormal findings. Services for cytology, and histopathology must be organized to permit adequate training, supervision, and quality control. Smear taking should be fitted into the existing health care infrastructure (ideally in primary health care facilities), whilst ensuring that staff are well trained and follow agreed procedures.

While all of these prescriptive recommendations are eminently sensible, and probably indispensable for efficient screening programmes, it has to be admitted that there are relatively few model programmes which demonstrate how they may all be put into effect. An optimal programme would require that women in specific age-groups in the target population are identified, and called for screening (with follow-up of non-attenders). Screening more than once (inevitable in all but the most basic service) implies that information on the previous screening history of women in the population is available. An organized programme must avoid taking smears from individuals more frequently than the prescribed interval. The presence of several organizations taking and reading smears - frequently charitable bodies operating mobile or open-access clinics - greatly complicates the process of record keeping. Almost inevitably, any sort of control at the population level requires some complex form of data storage and record linkage - a feat which has proved beyond the organizational skills of quite sophisticated health services. There is clearly scope for pilot schemes of simplified call/recall schemes.

The choice of policy (ages and frequency of screening) is necessarily the result of cost-effectiveness considerations. The number of screening examinations which can be carried out is dictated by the availability of facilities for taking and interpreting the smears, and following up women found to be positive. Their optimal spacing is determined by the type of calculation in Table 6, plus information on the size of the female population. Because of the young age structures of many developing countries, concentrating tests at older ages will permit a higher coverage for the same number of examinations - thus in a typical country of sub-Saharan Africa, there may be rather more than two women aged 25-29 for every one aged 45-49.

5.2 Opportunistic or Incidental Screening
The opportunity should be taken to use existing health-care contacts in the most efficient way possible. Thus, many of the smears taken in developing countries are obtained by family planning or maternal and child health (MCH) clinic staff. Generally, relatively young age of women attending these services means that the efficiency of such examinations is very low (see Parkin, 1985). However, in many developing countries, childbearing is prolonged for much longer than in the developed world (Table 7), and there is also evidence that high parity is associated with an increased risk of disease (Brinton et al., 1989b). Examinations taken at the time of such contacts could, for example, be limited to a single examination in each decade of life (30-39; 40-49). Women attending clinics for gynaecological disorders (and especially for s.t.d.) are known to be a particularly high risk group, with observed high prevalences of preclinical disease (Parkin et al., 1982).

Examination of all such women should be a priority for cytology services, since although only a relatively small percentage of the population is covered, the efficiency of such testing, in terms of disease prevented per 1000 tests, is particularly high (Parkin, 1985).

Table 7   Average number of births per woman. Calculated for 10 year age groups, with rates specific to year shown *

Country	Year	Age-group 30-39	40-49
Malawi	1977	2.2	1.2
Rwanda	1978	3.4	1.6
Tunisia	1980	2.1	0.6
Jamaica	1982	0.9	0.14
Mexico	1980	1.0	0.2
Brazil	1984	0.7	0.13
Venezuela	1984	1.1	0.2
Bangladesh	1981	1.5	0.3
Kuwait	1984	1.9	0.3
Philippines	1980	1.5	0.3
Malaysia	1984	1.5	0.2
Pacific Islands	1979	1.8	0.3
Fed. Rep. of Germany	1985	0.4	0.02
USA	1984	0.4	0.02

*Source: United Nations. 1986 Demographic Yearbook (Table 24) New York, 1986

6 ALTERNATIVES TO SCREENING BY CERVICAL CYTOLOGY

Because of the logistic difficulties of cytological screening for pre-invasive disease, an alternative strategy has recently been advocated for developing countries - so-called 'down-stage' screening (Stjernswärd et al., 1987). This advocates the systematic search for early stage disease by visual inspection of the cervix by non-medical health workers, with the objective of reducing mortality. It is not clear how effective this would prove to be, experience in screening for early stage disease in other cancers (e.g. breast and colon) indicates that the reduction in mortality is likely to be very small in comparison to cytological screening. The logistics would also seem to be quite formidable, given the probably very low prevalence of unknown invasive cancers in the population.

Detection and treatment of cancers at early stage would, however, provide a benefit to the patient in terms of quality of life, even if mortality were not reduced. However, this would seem to be better achieved by programmes of population education which alert women with suspicious symptoms to consult health care personnel, rather than by active case-finding.

7   CONCLUSIONS

Some of the conclusions reached by the IARC/UICC working group (Hakama et al., 1986) remain particularly pertinent.

(1) Applied research is required to develop appropriate screening strategies for developing countries.

(2) Research is needed to clarify the natural history of pre-cancerous lesions in developing countries, and to clarify the long term effects of screening at all ages.

(3) Research on the aetiology of cervical cancer to provide useful markers of women at very high risk - although screening only of high risk groups defined on the basis of epidemiological risk indicators other than age, is likely to be inappropriate.

(4) Research on the effectiveness and long term effects of different methods of treatment of pre-cancerous lesions.

REFERENCES

Aristizabal N, Cuello C, Correa P, Collazos T and Haenszel W. The impact of vaginal cytology on cervical cancer risks in Cali, Colombia. Int J Cancer 1984; 34: 5-9.

Bah E, Hall AJ and Inskip HM. The first two years of the Gambian National Cancer Registry. Brit J Cancer 1990; in press.

Bayo S, Parkin DM, Koumaré AK, Diallo AN, Ba T, Soumaré S and Sangaré S. Cancer in Mali, 1987-1988. Int J Cancer 1990; 45 (in press).

Boyes DA, Morrison B, Knox EG, Draper GJ and Miller AB. A cohort study of cervical cancer screening in British Columbia. Clin Invest Med 1982; 5: 1-29.

Brinton LA, Reeves WC, Brenes MM, Herrero R, Gaitan E, Tenorio F, de Britton RC, Garcia M and Rawls WE. The male factor in the etiology of cervical cancer among sexually monogamous women. Int J Cancer 1989a; 44: 199-203.

Brinton LA, Reeves WC, Brenes MM, Herrero R, de Britton RC, Gaitan E, Tenorio F, Garcia M and Rawls WE. Parity as a risk factor for cervical cancer. Am J Epidemiol 1989b; 130: 486-496.

Campion MJ. Human cervical papillomavirus infection: a clinical perspective. In: Muñoz N, Bosch FX and Jensen OM (eds). Human Papillomavirus and Cervical Cancer. IARC Scientific Publications No. 94, Lyon, International Agency for Research on Cancer,1989; pp 41-65.

Clarke EA and Anderson TW. Does screening by 'Pap' smears help to prevent cervical cancer? Lancet 1979; ii, 1-4.

Coppleson LW and Brown B. Observations on a model of the biology of carcinoma of the cervix: a poor fit between observation and theory. Am J Obstet Gynecol 1975; 122:127-136.

Dabancens A. Tasas estandarizadas de patologia cervical preclinica obtenidas por el programe de control precoz de cancer cervico-uterino, en el area metropolitana de Santiago. Rev Chil Obstet Ginecol 1989; 54: 217-224.

Day NE and Walter SD. Simplified models for screening: estimation procedures from mass-screening programmes. Biometrics 1984; 40: 1-14.

Eddy DM. Screening for Cancer: Theory, Analysis and Design. Prentice Hall Inc., Englewood Cliffs, N.J., USA ,1980.

Goes JS, Goes JCS, Zyngier SB, Dias JCS, Lemos LB, Donoso NF, Sampaio Tosello JR, de Oliveira Filho W, Mesquita L, Pereira Cortez A, Miniccelli CA and Pinheiro LR. Cervical cancer prevention and control in developing countries: A model program. Bull Pan Am Health Organ 1981; 15: 216-225.

Goes JS, Lemos LB, Donoso NF, Pinheiro LR, Goes JCS, Dias JCS and Zyngier SB. Practical Approaches to Screening for Cervical Cancer. Cancer Detection and Prevention 1987; 10:265-277.

Hakama M, Chamberlain J, Day NE, Miller AB and Prorok PC. Evaluation of screening programmes for gynaecological cancer. Br J Cancer 1985; 52:669-673.

Hakama M, Miller AB and Day NE (eds). Screening for cancer of the uterine cervix. IARC Scientific Publications No. 76, Lyon, International Agency for Research on Cancer 1986.

Herrero R, Brinton LA, Reeves WC and Brenes MM. Screening for cervical cancer in Latin America: A case-control study. Abstract for presentation at Society for Epidemiological Research, 1990.

Husain OAN. Quality control in cytological screening for cervical cancer. Tumori 1976; 62:303-314.

IARC Working Group on Evaluation of Cervical Cancer Screening Programmes. Screening for squamous cervical cancer: duration of low risk after negative results of cervical cytology and its implication for screening policies. Br Med J 1986; 293:659-664.

Klassen AC, Celentano DD and Brookmeyer R. Variation in the duration of protection given by screening using the Pap test for cervical cancer. J Clin Epidemiol 1989; 42:1003-1011.

Laudico AV, Esteban D and Parkin DM. Cancer in the Philippines (IARC Technical Report No. 5). Lyon, International Agency for Research on Cancer, 1989.

Lunt R. Worldwide Early Detection of Cervical Cancer. Obstet Gynecol 1984: 63:707-713.

Luthra UK and Rengachari R. Organization of screening programmes in developing countries with reference to screening for cancer of the uterine cervix in India. In: Hakama M, Miller AB and Day NE (eds). Screening for cancer of the uterine cervix. IARC Scientific Publications No. 76, 1986; pp 273-285.

Martin NC, Lorvidahya V, Changwaiwith W, et al. Cancer incidence and mortality 1983-1987 in Chiang Mai Province. Faculty of Medicine, Chiang Mai University, Thailand, 1989.

Muir CS, Waterhouse J, Mack T, Powell J and Whelan S (eds). Cancer Incidence in Five Continents, Vol. V. IARC Scientific Publications No. 88. Lyon, International Agency for Research on Cancer, 1987.

Muñoz N and Bosch FX. Epidemiology of cervical cancer. In: Muñoz N, Bosch FX and Jensen OM (eds). Human Papillomavirus and Cervical Cancer. IARC Scientific Publications No. 94. Lyon, International Agency for Research on Cancer, 1989; pp 9-39.

Parkin DM, Leach K, Cobb P and Clayden AD. Cervical cyology screening in two Yorkshire areas: Results of testing. Public Health (London) 1982; 96: 3-14.

Parkin DM. A computer simulation model for the practical planning of cervical cancer screening programmes. Br J Cancer 1985; 51:551-568.

Parkin DM (ed). Cancer Occurrence in Developing Countries. IARC Scientific Publications No. 75. Lyon, International Agency for Research on Cancer, 1986.

Parkin DM, Läärä E and Muir CS. Estimates of the worldwide frequency of sixteen major cancers in 1980. Int J Cancer 1988; 41:184-187.

Stjernswärd J, Eddy D, Luthra U and Stanley K. Plotting a new course for cervical cancer screening in developing countries. World Hlth Forum 1987; 8:42-45.

Van Oortmarssen GJ, Habbema JDF, Lubbe JTN, de Jong GA and van der Maas PJ. Predicting the effects of mass screening for disease - a simulation approach. Evr J Operational Res 1981; 6:399-409.

Vatanasapt V, Titapant V, Tangvoraphonkchai V & Pengsaa P. Cancer Incidence in Khon Kaen, Thailand, 1985-1989. Khon Kaen University, Thailand, 1989.

Wangsuphachart V, Thomas DB, Koetsawang A and Riotton G. Risk factors for invasive cervical cancer and reduction of risk by 'Pap' smears in Thai women. Int J Epidemiol 1987; 16:362-366.

Waterhouse J, Muir CS, Correa P and Powell J (eds). Cancer Incidence in Five Continents, Vol. III. IARC Scientific Publications No. 15. Lyon, International Agency for Research on Cancer, 1976.

Waterhouse J, Muir CS, Shanmugaratnam K and Powell J, eds. Cancer Incidence in Five Continents, Vol. IV. IARC Scientific Publications No. 42. Lyon, International Agency for Research on Cancer, 1982.

WHO. Control of cancer of the cervix uteri. Bull. WHO, 1986; 64:607-618.

Zhang ZF, Yu SZ, Estève J and Yang XZ. Risk factors for cancer of the cervix in a rural Chinese population. Int J Cancer 1989; 43:762-767 .

Zhang ZF, Parkin DM, Yu SZ, Estève J, Yang XZ and Day NE. Cervical screening attendance and its effectiveness in a rural population in China. Cancer Detection and Prevention 1989; 13:337-342.

20 Summary of Discussion on Screening for Cancer of the Cervix

It was emphasised that there were many aspects of quality control on which attention should be focussed in an organized programme. These include taking the smear, interpreting the smear, the subsequent diagnostic work-up and evaluation of the impact of the programme. In the Nordic countries personal invitations appear to be the best mechanisms for ensuring high compliance with screening. The invitations are complete, that is they indicate the place and time assigned for attendance, they are however easy to change if necessary. All women are informed independently of the result. They are told to go to a gynaecologist if they have problems.

Organized programmes have so far resulted in a larger reduction in the risk of invasive cervical cancer than opportunistic screening, because they achieve higher compliance by the at risk groups and can ensure a higher quality of the screening examination in taking the smear and in the laboratory interpretation of the smear. There is also a potential for major cost saving from organized programmes because they could prevent the overuse of services as compared to unorganized programmes. However, for this to be achieved in countries such as Canada and the United States, it will be necessary to persuade the governments to provide the necessary up-front resources to introduce the appropriate organisational framework (including the mechanisms to identify women in the population and invite them for screening) and persuade the medical profession to accept less frequent screening for many women not at increased risk so that resources can be released to ensure that higher risk women are brought into the programme. It has yet to be demonstrated that this is possible.

In England there has been an increase in the incidence of invasive cancer at all ages up to 35, with a large increase in those aged 20-29. There has also been some increase at ages 20-29 in Finland. These increases suggest that there may be important increases at older ages in another 10 years if there is a cohort effect. In Canada there has been a small increase at age 20-24, and there is no longer a decline in incidence at ages 25-34. It is not felt that these changes dictate a change in the frequency of rescreening, rather efforts are required in order to ensure that all at risk women attend for screening. It is important to note that the increase at younger ages is still small in absolute terms. Money will be better used in most countries to improve coverage of screening at older ages, rather than making heroic efforts to improve coverage at younger ages. Indeed, many programmes are failing because they do not ensure good coverage at older ages.

In all countries screening more frequently than every three years provides only marginally improved protection. Even five-year intervals between the screening rounds has resulted in equally good protection in Finland and Aberdeen at the population level as more frequent screening in other countries and at far less cost. In addition, screening at ages younger than age 25 provides marginal extra benefit at the population level because of the infrequency of invasive cancer at young ages, while the costs are substantial because of the high prevalence of preclinical lesions, the majority of which will not progress within the next few years after detection, while many will regress. Nevertheless, in many countries decisions have been taken to start screening at younger ages because of the substantial weight given to cases of invasive cancer of the cervix at young ages. The age-specific incidence of cancer of the cervix, and the trends in recent years, should be considered in each country therefore to guide such decisions. For maximal cost-effectiveness screening should commence at an age only a few years before invasive disease appears at a level that is high enough to justify screening. Because the protective effect is known it is possible to estimate the marginal benefit corresponding to any change in the age to start screening and make recommendations that are specific to the age-specific rates in the population.

The protective effect at ages older than 65 is largely unknown in women who have been previously screened. Because of problems in taking smears, attendance for screening and possibly a lesser protection at older ages (because of more rapid progression of preclinical lesions at older than younger ages) it may be appropriate not to extend screening beyond the age of 65 for women who have had a number of negative smears in the last 10 years and no positive smears. Women older than 65 who have not had a number of negative smears should continue to be screened until they have achieved such a record (at least two negative smears).

It should be recognised that decisions on the age to start and stop screening, and the frequency of rescreening are dependent on an assessment of the marginal benefits and disadvantages of such changes and the resources that are available in the country concerned. Apart from the age to stop screening, which can still be considered to be a research issue, quantitative data are available to facilitate such decisions. Not all lesions that are diagnosed as neoplastic and treated would have progressed to invasive cancer. Estimates of rates of progression are strongly related to local diagnostic practices and age. The problem of over-diagnosis is particularly great if viral abnormalities on cytology or viral lesions on colposcopy are considered preneoplastic in the absence of moderate or severe dysplasia.

There are many difficulties in the way of introducing screening programmes in developing countries, in spite of the urgency of the task because of the high incidence of the disease. The resources are limited, there are other health problems with higher priority and there may be little opportunity for diagnostic work-up and treatment. Without such facilities screening should not be undertaken. Nevertheless even low level activities, appropriately directed, could be quite valuable. An appropriately timed smear, once in a woman's lifetime, could have a major effect. This should be taken at a sufficiently old age (at least 40 or 45). Because of the age structure of developing countries costs would be much less if tests are concentrated on older women; there are far fewer of them. There are some programmes in developing countries where women are receiving smears every 6 months. Resources are being overused on a small segment of the population, with very little benefit. Much more effect would be achieved with high coverage of the population and limited numbers of smears in a lifetime, than with low coverage and intensive screening of a few. When programmes are introduced in developing countries careful consideration should be given to starting screening no earlier than age 35. This will largely eliminate the dysplasia problem in younger women, as evidence increasingly shows that the large majority of these lesions regress spontaneously. With the extended families in many developing countries use could be made of maternal and child health services, not to screen the young mothers, but to ensure through the young mothers that the grandmothers and aunts are screened. In addition, every opportunity should be taken through primary health care in the community to ensure that contacts with older women for other health reasons are utilised to ensure that appropriately timed smears are taken.

It has been suggested that in the absence of laboratory facilities a programme of clinical examination with a speculum should be introduced in developing countries to find invasive cancers and result in "down-staging". It has to be emphasised that there is no evidence available on the effectiveness of such an approach. Given the costs associated with locating and examining women, a more cost-effective approach may be to combine a cervical smear with the speculum examination of all women included in such programmes. This would seem to be a high priority research issue for any country that considers adopting such a programme.

State of the Art on Screening for Ovarian Cancer

At the present time there are no data on the effect of screening on ovarian cancer mortality, and screening for ovarian cancer cannot be recommended as public health policy.

Recommendations for Research
Data on intermediate outcomes (eg, on the sensitivity and specificity of a combination of tests, the extent to which early cancers are diagnosed and the effect of screening on advanced cancer) should be obtained.

When satisfactory data on intermediate outcomes are available well-planned randomized studies of screening for ovarian cancer with mortality as an endpoint should be supported. However, such trials, either individually or in combination, will have to be large; involving at least 150,000 postmenopausal women.

21 Tumour Markers in Screening for Ovarian Cancer

A. P. DAVIES, D. ORAM, and I. JACOBS

Academic Department of Obstetrics and Gynaecology, The London Hospital, London, UK

1 INTRODUCTION

Of all the gynaecological cancers, ovarian cancer has the poorest prognosis. In the United Kingdom over 4,000 women die from the disease each year (OPCS, 1983). As a result of the anatomical position of the ovaries, and the lack of early symptoms, at diagnosis the cancer is already at an advanced stage in 60% of cases. The 5 year survival figure for FIGO Stage III and IV disease combined is currently 10.4% (Kottmeier, 1982) (Table 1).

Table 1 Five year survival rates by stage at presentation for epithelial ovarian cancer (after Kottmeier, 1982).

Stage	% incidence	5 year survival (%)
Ia	17.9	69.7
Ib	4.3	63.9
Ic	3.0	50.3
Total stage I	25.2	67.1
IIa	4.8	51.8
IIb+c	12.8	42.4
III	39.5	13.3
IV	17.7	4.1
Total stages III+IV	59.2	10.4
Total all stages:	100.0	30.6

However, 5 year survival greater than 95%, with complete cure possible after surgery alone, may be achieved for the minority of women diagnosed with disease still confined to the ovary (Dembo et al, 1990). Recent research has therefore been directed towards finding a method of diagnosing ovarian cancer at a pre-clinical stage, in the hope that this will improve the outlook for women with the disease (Jacobs and Oram, 1988; Smith and Ol, 1984a and 1984b).

The ideal screening test would detect pre-invasive disease and hence provide a method for prevention of ovarian cancer. However, unlike cervical dysplasia or atypical endometrial hyperplasia, a pre-invasive ovarian lesion has not been recognised. The duration of the pre-clinical but screen positive phase of the disease is also unclear. If this phase is short and there is rapid progression to advanced disease, the window in which screening and treatment could be effective would be too narrow for screening to be practicable.

2 REQUIREMENTS OF A SCREENING TEST

Although approximately 1 in 70 women in the USA will develop ovarian cancer in their lifetime, the overall incidence of the disease is quite low. This places limitations on the performance of prospective screening tests. Employing a test with 100% sensitivity and 99% specificity for ovarian cancer in the general female population would result in 1 case of cancer being diagnosed per 10,000 women tested - and 100 women with a false positive result (Smith and Ol 1984a). As a false positive may lead to an operation under general anaesthesia, the positive predictive value of an abnormal test has to be high for a screening programme to be acceptable. The positive predictive value of a test can be improved, without altering the test, by targeting the screening programme to a higher risk population, eg by screening women of 45 years and above. Even with an incidence of 40/100,000 per year (which is the United Kingdom incidence of ovarian cancer in women in this age group), a test with 100% sensitivity would require 99.6% specificity in order to detect 1 case of ovarian cancer for every 10 operations performed (a positive predictive value of 10%). To date, no single screening test for ovarian cancer has combined such levels of specificity or sensitivity.

Methods currently under evaluation for screening for asymptomatic ovarian cancer include:

a) The detection of morphological changes in the ovary using ultrasound (Andolf et al, 1986; Campbell et al, 1982; Campbell et al, 1989; Bourne et al, 1989).

b) The detection of changes in circulating substances reflecting either an alteration in ovarian function or surface molecular structure, or a "general" response to malignancy (Smith and Ol, 1984a, 1984b; Bast and Knapp, 1987).

3 TUMOUR MARKERS

Over the years numerous substances have been associated with ovarian cancer. They have included qualitative and/or quantitative changes in circulating enzymes (van Kley et al, 1982; Awais, 1978; Gauduchon et al, 1983; Barlow et al, 1981; Cramer et al, 1989), hormones (Heinonen et al,1982; Backstrom et al, 1983), non-specific inflammatory proteins (Lukomska et al 1981; Astedt et al, 1971), and placental and fetal antigens (Donaldson et al, 1980; Stone et al, 1977; Nouwen et al, 1985; Doellgast and Homesley, 1984; Sunderland et al, 1984) (Table 2). Apart from the association of alpha-feto protein (AFP) with germ cell ovarian cancer (especially endodermal sinus and embryonal tumours) (Gallion et al 1983; Talerman et al, 1977; Talerman et al, 1980) and human chorionic gonadotrophin (ßHCG) in monitoring choriocarcinoma (Bagshaw, 1976), these other markers have not shown sufficient sensitivity or specificity, even for advanced disease, to be used as single screening agents for asymptomatic epithelial ovarian cancer (Sarjadi et al, 1980; Kikuchi et al, 1984; van Nagell et al, 1981).

Table 2 Serum markers for ovarian cancer

ENZYMES	FETO-PLACENTAL MARKERS
galactosyl transferase	alpha-feto protein
alpha l-fucosidase	human chorionic gonadotrophin
amylase	placental alkaline phosphatase
lactic dehydrogenase	carcinoembryonic antigen
cystine aminopeptidase	
HORMONES	MISCELLANEOUS
progesterone	circulating immune complexes
oestrogen	d-dimer of fibrin

4 MONOCLONAL ANTIBODIES

More recent advances in monoclonal antibody techniques have resulted in the improved definition of antigens expressed on the malignant cell surface (Old, 1981; Taylor-Papadimitiou and Griffiths, 1985; Boyer et al, 1988). The anatomical site of the ovaries may make ovarian cancer particularly suitable for detection by serum markers. An antigen expressed on malignant ovarian cells may reach the peripheral circulation by two routes; either via the diaphragmatic lymphatics and thoracic duct having been shed into the peritoneal cavity, or through the lymphatics or vessels supplying the ovarian stroma (Bast et al, 1990). The ideal tumour antigen would be expressed by all individuals with a tumour of a certain histotype, and only by tumours of that histotype. To date however, the antigens defined on epithelial ovarian cancer cells have been tumour-associated rather than tumour-specific and are therefore also expressed by other cells, both diseased and healthy.

The first ovarian cancer antigens to be detected in serum were OCC and OCA, which were defined by rabbit polyclonal hetero-antiserum (Bhattacharya and Barlow, 1973, 1978; Bhattacharya et al, 1982; Knauf and Urbach, 1980). 70% of patients with Stage I and II ovarian cancer had raised serum OCA levels, but as 10% of healthy women also had elevated serum OCA levels, the positive predictive value of an abnormal result precludes its use as a screening test in healthy women.

Later attempts at improving antigen sensitivity and specificity using monoclonal antibodies resulted in the identification of a fragment of the OCC antigen, designated NB/70K (Knauf and Urbach, 1981; Dembo et al, 1985; Knauf et al, 1985). Preliminary work using radioimmunoassay showed serum NB/70K levels to be elevated (> 11 KU/ml) in all women in whom ovarian cancer was diagnosed, while none of the healthy controls and only 5% of "gynaecology controls" (women in the first trimester of pregnancy or presenting with fertility problems etc.) showed such an elevation. However 90% of women with benign ovarian pathology (endometriosis, dermoid cysts, fibroids etc.) also had serum NB/70K levels > 11 KU/ml, limiting its value as a potential screening test for ovarian cancer in apparently healthy women.

5 CA 125

Numerous ovarian tumour-associated antigens have been defined (Table 3), the most extensively studied being CA 125, an antigen which is recognised by a murine monoclonal antibody OC 125 (Bast et al, 1981;1983). The distribution of CA 125 in immuno-histochemical studies suggest that cells expressing CA 125 are derived from the embryonal Mullerian duct and coelomic epithelium (Kabawat et al, 1983). Serum CA 125 levels are elevated in 82% of women with epithelial ovarian cancer, more frequently in serous, clear cell, and endometrioid than mucinous histological types (Bast et al, 1983, 1987; Hawkins et al, 1989a; Jacobs and Bast, 1989). Serum CA 125 levels may also be raised in association with other conditions, both benign and malignant, including benign ovarian cysts, endometriosis, pregnancy and during menstruation, and colon, breast and pancreatic cancers (Niloff et al, 1984a, 1984b; Halila et al, 1986). These observations potentially decrease the specificity of an elevated serum CA 125 level as a screening test for epithelial ovarian cancer. However the benign conditions associated with an elevated serum CA 125 are not common in the high risk population for ovarian cancer.

Table 3   Antigens associated with ovarian cancer.

OVARIAN CANCER
    OOCA
    OCA

    CA 125
    ID3
    NB/70K
    OC 133
    MOV-2

COLONIC CANCER
    CA 19-9

BREAST CANCER
    DF3
    CA 15-3
    F36/22

MILK FAT GLOBULE
    HMFG1/2
    AUA1

PLAC.ALK.PHOS.
    NDOG2

PANCREATIC CANCER
    DUPAN-2

A radioimmunoassay has been developed for measuring serum CA 125 concentrations (Klug et al, 1984). An upper limit of 35 µ/ml, which is associated with over 80% of ovarian cancers, will exclude 99% of apparently healthy female blood donors. A higher cut-off of 65 µ/ml excludes 99.7% of the normal population, but at the expense of decreased sensitivity for ovarian cancer. Tumour grade and differentiation do not appear to have an effect on serum CA 125 expression.

A large number of studies have investigated the role of serum CA 125 in the pre-operative differential diagnosis of an adnexal mass and in monitoring the treatment of ovarian cancer post-operatively or during and after chemotherapy (Schwartz, 1988; Malkasian et al, 1988; Mogenson et al, 1989; Bast et al, 1984; Hawkins et al, 1989b; Sevelda et al, 1989; Schilthuis et al, 1987). These studies indicate:

1). In the preoperative differential diagnosis of benign and malignant disease in patients with a pelvic mass:
- CA 125 measurement alone has a diagnostic accuracy of approximately 80%.
- Diagnostic accuracy can be improved by combined consideration of CA 125, ultrasound and menopausal status.

2). In monitoring disease status in patients receiving treatment for ovarian cancer:
- A rising or persistently elevated serum CA 125 is a reliable indicator of poor response to therapy and may provide a basis for discontinuing or altering the therapeutic regime.
- A falling serum CA 125 indicates response to treatment but a fall to < 35 µ/ml is not a reliable indicator of complete pathological response.
- The rate of fall of CA 125 during treatment (CA 125 half-life) is a strong prognostic indicator of survival.

Although the reports of serum CA 125 in women with ovarian cancer are numerous, only a few studies have investigated serum CA 125 in the general population. The largest such study is a population based retrospective study using stored serum (Zurawski et al, 1988a). Cases comprised 105 women who developed ovarian cancer at varying intervals following venepuncture. Stored serum samples from these cases were assayed for CA 125 and compared with levels in 323 apparently healthy matched controls. Cases had a higher median serum CA 125 concentration than controls (18 µ/ml cf 10 µ/ml). However this is of little practical value as 18 µ/ml results in poor specificity. Serum CA 125 levels of >35 µ/ml were measured in 50% of cases within 18 months of ovarian cancer being diagnosed, and a third had serum CA 125 levels > 65 µ/ml within 18 months of diagnosis.

This study suggested that it may be possible to detect ovarian cancer prior to the development of symptoms in a proportion of women by measurement of serum CA 125 levels. Subsequent prospective studies have been performed to determine the limitations of sensitivity and specificity of CA 125 measurement for early asymptomatic ovarian cancer. Means of improving the detection rate and positive predictive value of an abnormal test are currently under investigation.

6 IMPROVING SPECIFICITY

6.1 CA 125 and Ultrasound
The specificity of serum CA 125 may be improved by using a combination of screening methods. At The London Hospital, a research programme incorporating a multimodal, stepwise screening programme for ovarian cancer using CA 125, ultrasound and vaginal examination was initiated in 1985 (Jacobs et al, 1988). The study population consists of post-menopausal women of 45 years and above. In the original, phase I, protocol both venepuncture and a vaginal examination were performed on recruitment. If either of these tests proved abnormal (ie a serum CA 125 level of > 30 μ/ml or a palpable pelvic mass neither colonic or uterine in origin) a trans-abdominal ultrasound scan was performed (recently trans-vaginal ultrasound scanning has been introduced). Women found to have a pelvic abnormality on ultrasound scanning underwent surgical investigation by laparoscopy or laparotomy. The results of the first 4,000 women to have undergone screening show that a combination of a raised serum CA 125 and an abnormal ultrasound scan give an acceptable specificity (>99.6%) and hence positive predictive value for an abnormal screening test (Table 4) (Jacobs & Oram, 1990).

Table 4   Specificity for ovarian cancer of vaginal exam, CA 125 and ultrasound.

TEST	SPECIFICITY (%)
CA 125	97.0
Vaginal examination	87.3
Vaginal examination & ultrasound	99.0
CA 125 & ultrasound	99.8
CA 125 & vaginal examination	100.0
CA 125, vaginal examination & ultrasound	100.0

The London Hospital ovarian cancer screening project in post menopausal women.
n = 4,000

Subsequently a phase II study has been initiated using CA 125 as a single first line test, and ultrasound and vaginal examination as secondary tests (Figure 1). The sensitivity of this screening method is currently being assessed. Preliminary results of 20,000 women indicate a detection rate for ovarian cancer of 78%, with 11 of the 14 diagnosed ovarian cancers having been detected by the programme (Table 5).

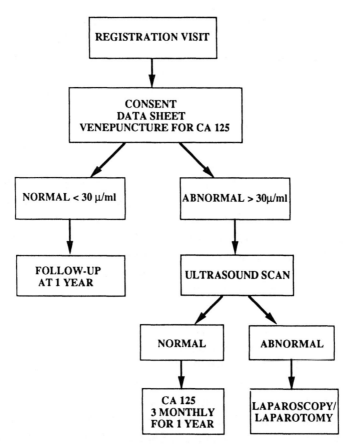

Figure 1   Study design.

Table 5   Study results (incomplete 1 year follow up).

	SCREEN NEGATIVE			SCREEN POSITIVE
CA 125 < 30μ/L	CA 125 > 30μ/L Normal ultrasound			CA 125 > 30μ/L Abnormal ultrasound
n = 19,719	n = 259			n = 22
	3 false negatives:			11 true positives

				11 false positives
stage	histology	CA 125	interval	
III	granulosa	10	8/12	
III	serous	22	13/12	
III	clear cell	85	6/12	

Of the three cases not detected, in 1 case, histological examination showed the cancer to be of granulosa cell type. One of the other 2 women classified as a "false negative" had in fact refused an ultrasound examination despite having an elevated serum CA 125 level. Long term follow up will undoubtedly alter the sensitivity of the screening programme as further cases of ovarian cancer in women with negative screening tests are documented.

6.2 CA 125 - Other Tumour Markers

The specificity of serum CA 125 as a screening test for ovarian cancer may also be improved by using a combination of monoclonal antibodies directed against a spectrum of different ovarian tumour-associated antigens. These determinants may be different epitopes on the same complex (eg, HMFG1 and HMFG2 which recognise different epitopes on a mucin glycoprotein molecule present on some epithelial cell membranes) (Xing et al, 1989; Ward et al, 1987b) or may be distinct antigens. At Duke University Medical Centre, Bast et al (1990) studied serum from patients with known ovarian cancer and from women with a "false positive" elevation of CA 125 using radioimmunoassays for a number of other antigens including CA 15-3, TAG 72, PLAP, HMFG1, HMFG2, NB/70K. CA 125 and NB/70K rose in tandem, and in combination showed an increased sensitivity rather than specificity for ovarian cancer. CA 15-3 and TAG 72 seemed to be the more useful antigens in differentiating ovarian cancer from benign disease. Seventy seven percent of women with ovarian cancer had elevated serum levels of all 3 serum antigens compared with only 5% of women with benign disease. The improved specificity for ovarian cancer using this combination of markers has been confirmed in a subsequent study (Einhorn et al, 1989). The specificity for malignancy when all 3 antigens were raised was 98% compared with 83% for CA 125 alone. Other combinations of antigens have also been assessed, eg DF3 (Sekine et al, 1985) and PLAP (Eerdekens et al, 1985).

These studies suggest that it may be possible to provide a screening programme for pre-clinical ovarian cancer using a sequence of monoclonal antibodies. The serum of women with elevated CA 125 levels would be tested against a panel of other monoclonal antibodies, eg CA 15-3, TAG 72. Women with multiple positive antigens would undergo an ultrasound scan, a CAT-scan or immunoscintigraphy to identify the source of the shed antigen. However, the increase in specificity obtained by using a panel of antigens is likely to be at the expense of sensitivity. Ultimately the overall sensitivity of the screening test will be dependent upon the sensitivity of the least sensitive marker. A fall in sensitivity for ovarian cancer to 53% has been documented using a combination of serum CA 125, CA 15-3 and TAG 72 (Jacobs and Bast, in preparation).

7 IMPROVING SENSITIVITY

A highly specific ovarian cancer screening programme incorporating serum CA 125 with other methods is therefore possible. The programme may, however, prove unacceptable because it would lack sufficient sensitivity for early stage disease. Although overall over 80% of women with clinically apparent ovarian cancer have elevated serum CA 125 levels, there is a correlation with stage. Ninety percent of women with stage III and IV disease have serum CA 125 levels greater than 35 µ/ml, while only 50% of women with Stage I disease have circulating levels of this value (Table 6). With a disease as fatal as ovarian cancer, an overall improvement in mortality may be seen should only 50% of cases be diagnosed at Stage I. However this degree of sensitivity may not be acceptable for women with false negative results feeling that they have been falsely reassured.

Table 6   The proportion of women with ovarian cancer with an elevated pre-operative serum CA 125 level in relation to FIGO Stage (after Jacobs and Oram, 1990).

FIGO Stage

Author:	I	II	III	IV	TOTAL
Bast et al (1983)	1/1	2/2	15/16	3/3	21/22
Brioschi et al (1987)	4/13	3/3	29/30	22/23	58/69
Canney et al (1984)	–	–	–	–	48/58
Crombach & Wurtz (1984)	3/5	5/6	13/19	10/10	31/40
Cruickshank et al (1987)	3/12	2/3	15/16	10/10	31/42
Fuith et al (1987)	4/6	4/5	16/18	8/10	32/39
Heinonen et al (1985)	0/3	– 9/9 stages II-IV –			9/12
Kaesemann et al (1986)	– 31/46 –		– 135/153 –		166/199
Kivinen et al (1986)	3/3	10/10	15/15	1/1	29/29
Krebs et al (1986)	3/4	8/8	25/25	7/8	43/45
Li-juan et al (1986)	1/2	3/3	22/23	–	26/28
Ricolleau et al (1985)	–	–	–	–	35/38
Schilthuis et al (1987)	6/8	5/5	20/20	13/13	44/46
Zanaboni et al (1987)	8/15	3/4	29/34	3/4	43/57
Zurawaski et al (1988b)	12/24	10/12	–	–	#
TOTAL	48/96	55/61	199/216	77/82	615/723
%	50.0%	90.0%	92.1%	93.9%	85.1%

= not included in total as this was a study of stage I and II disease

Methods of improving the detection rate - whilst retaining specificity - are therefore being investigated. One such method involves serial measurements of serum CA 125. Progressively elevating levels, with rapid increases in the serum CA 125 concentration, have been associated with the subsequent diagnosis of ovarian cancer. Zurawski has reported 1 such case, when ovarian cancer was diagnosed 21 months following a normal ultrasound scan performed in order to investigate a serum CA 125 of >35 µ/ml (Zurawski et al, 1990). In the interim, the serum CA 125 level had markedly increased. Similarly, the ovarian cancer screening programme at The London Hospital has documented 3 cases of ovarian cancer diagnosed at intervals of 3, 6 and 9 months following an apparently normal ultrasound scan performed on women with serum CA 125 levels >30 μ/ml. All 3 women had progressively and rapidly elevating serum CA 125 levels.

In addition to using temporal changes in serum CA 125 levels to increase the detection rate, improvements may be gained by using a combination of markers directed at different epitopes. CA 125 and NB/70K (Knauf et al, 1985) together achieve a sensitivity for ovarian cancer greater than that of either when used as single tests. Other antigens which have been shown to improve the detection rate in conjunction with CA 125 include MOV 2 (Miotti et al, 1985), DF 3 (Sekine et al, 1985), PLAP (Ward et al, 1987a), and HMFG2 (Dhokia et al, 1986; Ward et al 1987a & 1987b) (Table 7).

Table 7   Improving sensitivity using a panel of tumour-associated antigens.

Elevated Serum CA 125, HMFG1, HMFG2 and PLAP in 85 Women with Epithelial Ovarian Cancer (Dhokia et al, 1986)

CA 125	HMFG1	HMFG2	Any of 3	Any of 3 or PLAP
85%	56%	65%	95%	98.8%

Elevated Serum CA 125, PLAP and HMFG2 in 41 Women with Ovarian Cancer by Stage (Ward et al, 1987)

	CA 125	+ HMFG2 or PLAP
Stage I + II	2/11 (18%)	7/11 (64%)
Stage III + IV	25/26 (96%)	26/26 (100%)

8 FUTURE ADVANCES IN IMMUNOLOGICAL DETECTION

The search for structurally altered molecules on cancer cells may lead to the identification of cancer specific antigens that are present in most tumours of a particular histotype. Monoclonal antibodies may then be raised against the mutated protein. It has been suggested that molecules of small molecular weight, eg AFP or HCG, which are able to traverse basement membranes and enter the circulation easily - may be more appropriate as markers for early disease, than proteins of a higher molecular weight (Duffy, 1989).

9 ONCOGENES AND GROWTH FACTORS IN THE DETECTION OF OVARIAN CANCER

The uncontrolled growth of cancer cells is believed to be due to aberrant expression of cell growth regulatory genes, or cell growth suppressor genes, which usually keep cell division in check. This may occur as a result of transduction by viruses, chromosome translocations, gene amplification, mutation or deletion (Willman and Fenoglio-Preiser, 1987). Molecular studies of many solid tumours have confirmed oncogene or altered proto-oncogene expression. For example, the ras oncogene has been found in up to 40% of colo-rectal cancers (Bos et al, 1987; Forrester et al, 1987). A few studies have been conducted on oncogene expression in ovarian cancer (Tyson et al, 1988). These have shown variable expression of c-fos, c-myc, v-fms, c-Ha-ras and c-erb B2, but not 1 myc, c-myb, c-erb B, or c-mos by ovarian cancers. Oncogenes (or proto-oncogenes) cannot be detected in serum. However, in the future it may be possible to detect circulating oncogene products - oncoproteins - which may be a means of screening for ovarian cancer.

Macrophage-colony stimulating factor (M-CSF) (Ramakrishnan et al, 1989), which is similar to c-fms proto-oncogene, is produced by both fibroblasts and endothelial cells. Elevated serum levels have been detected in women with ovarian cancer. In vitro, M-CSF stimulates both the proliferation and functional activity of macrophages and granulocytes. Although the role of M-CSF in regulating the proliferation of ovarian cancer and its relationship to any oncogene of proto-oncogene is still unclear, serum M-CSF levels may be a useful tumour marker for epithelial ovarian cancer either alone or in combination with serum CA 125 (Bast et al, 1990) or other markers.

10 CONCLUSION

The ideal humoral marker for ovarian cancer is yet to be defined. Monoclonal antibodies have provided a means of monitoring disease, and may also be of value in the differential diagnosis of an adnexal mass. To date, the most sensitive and specific monoclonal antibody for ovarian cancer is CA 125, yet, as a single test, CA 125 does not have sufficient validity to be used for screening for asymptomatic disease. A combination of markers or screening methods may provide an adequate screening programme. If, or when a screening protocol for ovarian cancer combining satisfactory sensitivity and specificity is available, demonstration that it results in a reduction in mortality in the screened population will be required. This will only be obtained by performing a large (and expensive) population based, randomised controlled study.

REFERENCES

Andolf E, Svalenin SE, Astedt, B. Ultrasonography for early detection of ovarian carcinoma. Br J Obstet Gynaecol 1986; 93:1286-1289.

Astedt B, Svanberg L, Nilsson IM. Fibrin degradation products in ovarian tumours. Br Med J 1971: 458-459.

Awais GM. Carcinoma of the ovary and serum lactic dehydrogenase levels. Surg Gynecol Obstet 1978; 146:893-895.

Backstrom T, Mahlck C-G, Kjellgren O. Progesterone as a possible tumour marker for 'nonendocrine' ovarian malignant tumours. Gynecol Oncol 1983; 16:129-138.

Bagshaw KD. Risk and prognostic factors in trophoblastic neoplasia. Cancer 1976; 38:1373-1385.

Barlow JJ, DiCioccio RA, Dillard PH et al. Frequency of an allele for low activity of ã-L-fucosidase in sera: possible increase in epithelial ovarian cancer patients. JNCI 1981; 67:1005-1009.

Bast RC, Boyer CM, Olt GJ et al. Identification of markers for early detection of epithelial ovarian cancer. In: Sharp F, Mason WP, Leake RE (eds). Ovarian cancer biological and therapeutic challenges. London: Chapman & Hall Medical, 1990, p.265.

Bast RC, Freeney M, Lazarus, H et al. Reactivity of a monoclonal antibody with human ovarian carcinoma. J Clin Invest 1981; 68:1331-1337.

Bast RC, Hunter V, Knapp RC. Pros and cons of gynecologic tumour markers. Cancer 1987; 60:1984-1992.

Bast RC, Klug TL, St John E et al. A radioimmunoassay using a monoclonal antibody to monitor the course of epithelial ovarian cancer. N Engl J Med 1983; 309: 883-887.

Bast RC, Klug TL, Schaetzl E et al. Monitoring human ovarian carcinoma with a combination of CA 125, CA 19-9 and CEA. Am J Obstet Gynecol 1984; 149: 553-559.

Bast RC, Knapp R C. Humoral markers for epithelial ovarian carcinoma. In: Piver MS (ed). Ovarian Malignancies. Diagnostic and Therapeutic advances. London: Churchill Livingstone, 1987, pp. 11-25.

Bhattacharya M, Barlow JJ. Immunologic studies of human serous cystadenocarcnoma of ovary. Demonstration of tumor-associated antigens. Cancer 1973; 31:588-595.

Bhattacharya M, Barlow JJ. Ovarian tumour antigens. Cancer 1978; 42:1616-1620.

Bhattacharya M, Chatterjee SK, Barlow JJ et al. Monoclonal antibodies recognising tumor-associated antigen of human ovarian mucinous cystadenocarcinomas. Cancer Res 1982; 42:1650-1654.

Bos JF, Fearson ER, Hamilton SR. Prevalence of ras gene mutations in human cancers. Nature 1987; 327:293-297.

Bourne T, Campbell S, Steer C et al. Transvaginal colour flow imaging: a possible new screening technique for ovarian cancer. Br Med J 1989; 299:1367-1370.

Boyer CM, Lidor Y, Lottich C et al. Antigenic cell surface markers in human solid tumours. Antibody, Immunoconjugates and Radiopharmaceuticals 1988; 1:105-162.

Brioschi PA, Irion O, Bischoff P et al. Serum CA 125 in epithelial ovarian cancer. A longitudinal study. Br J Obstet Gynaecol 1987; 94:196-201.

Campbell S, Bhan V, Royston P et al. Transabdominal ultrasound screening for early ovarian cancer. Br Med J 1989; 299:1363-1367.

Campbell S, Gressens L, Goswamy R et al. Real-time ultrasonography for determination of ovarian morphology and volume. Lancet 1982; i:425-426.

Canney PA, Moore M, Wilkinson PM et al. Ovarian cancer antigen CA 125: a prospective clinical assessment of its role as a tumour marker. Br J Cancer 1984; 50:765-769.

Cramer DW, Harlow BL, Willet WC et al. Galactose consumption and metabolism in relation to the risk of ovarian cancer. Lancet 1989; ii:66-71.

Crombach G, Wurz H. CA 125, PA, and CEA in ovarian cancer -a critical evaluation of single and contained determinations of serum markers. In: Geten H, Klapdor R (eds). New Tumour-associated antigens. Stuttgart-New York: George Viene Verland, 1984, p. 134.

Cruickshank DJ, Fullerton WT, Klopper A. The clinical significance of pre-opertive serum CA 125 in ovarian cancer. Br J Obstet Gynaecol 1987; 94:692-695.

Dembo AJ, Chang P-L, Urbach GI. Clinical correlations of ovarian cancer antigen NB/70K: a preliminary report. Obstet.Gynecol 1985; 65:710-714.

Dembo AJ, Davy M, Stenwig AE et al. Prognostic factors in patients with stage I epithelial ovarian cancer. Obstet.Gynecol 1990; 75:263-273.

Dhokia B, Canney PA, Pectasides D et al. A new immunoassay using monoclonal antibodies HMFG1 and HMFG2 together with an existing marker CA 125 for the serological detection and management of epthelial ovarian cancer. Br J Cancer 1986; 54:891-895.

Doellgast GJ, Homesley HD. Placental-Type alkaline phosphatase in ovarian cancer fluids and tissues. Obstet Gynecol 1984; 63:324-329.

Donaldson ES, van Nagell JR, Pursell S et al. Multiple biochemical markers in patients with gynecologic malignancies. Cancer 1980; 45:948-953.

Duffy MJ. New cancer markers. Ann Clin Biochem 1989; 26:379-387.

Eerdekens MW, Nouwen EJ, Pollet DE et al. Placental alkaline phosphatase and cancer antigen 125 in sera of patients with benign and malignant diseases. Clin Chemistry 1985; 31:687-690.

Einhorn N, Knapp RC, Bast RC et al. CA 125 assay used in conjunction with CA 15-3 and TAG-72 assays for discrimination between malignant and non-malignant diseases of the ovary. Acta Oncologica 1989; 28:655-657.

Forrester K, Almoguera C, Han K, et al. Detection of high incidence of C-ras oncogenes during human colon tumor genesis. Nature 1987; 327:298-303.

Fuith LC, Daxenbichler G, Dapunt O. CA 125 in the serum and tissue of patients with gynecological disease. Arch Gynecol Obstet 1987; 241:157-164.

Gallion H, van Nagell JR, Donaldson ES. Immature teratoma of the ovary. Am J Obstet Gynecol 1983; 146:361-365.

Gauduchon C, Tillier C, Guyonnet C et al. Clinical value of serum glycoprotein galactosyltransferase levels in different histological types of ovarian carcinoma. Cancer Res 1983; 43:4491-4496.

Halila H, Stenman U-H, Seppala M. Ovarian cancer antigen CA 125 levels in pelvic inflammatory disease and pregnancy. Cancer 1986; 57:1327-1329.

Hawkins RE, Roberts K, Wiltshaw E et al. The clinical correlates of serum CA125 in 169 patients with epithelial ovarian carcinoma. Br J Cancer 1989a; 60:634-637.

Hawkins RE, Roberts K, Wiltshaw E et al. The prognostic significance of the half-like of serum CA 125 in patients responding to chemotherapy for epithelial ovarian carcinoma. Br J Obstet Gynecol 1989b; 96:1395-1399.

Heinonen PK, Tontti K, Koivula T et al. Tumour associated antigen CA 125 in patients with ovarian cancer. Br J Obstet Gynaecol 1985; 92:528-531.

Heinonen PK, Tuimala R, Pyykko K et al. Peripheral venous concentrations of oestrogens in postmenopausal women with ovarian cancer. Br J Obstet Gynaecol 1982; 89:84-86.

Jacobs I, Bast RC. The CA 125 tumour-associated antigen: a review of the literature. Human Reprod 1989; 4:1-12.

Jacobs I, Oram DH. Screening for ovarian cancer. Biomed & Pharmacother 1988; 42:589-596.

Jacobs I, Oram DH. Potential screening tests for ovarian cancer. In: Sharp F, Mason WP, Leake RE (eds). Ovarian cancer. Biological and therapeutic challenges. London: Chapman and Hall Medical, 1990, pp.197-205.

Jacobs I, Oram DH, Bast RC. Approaches to improve the specificity for ovarian cancer with tumour-associated antigens CA 125 , CA 15-3, TAG-72. (in preparation).

Jacobs I, Stabile I, Bridges J et al. Multimodal approach to screening for ovarian cancer. Lancet, 1988; i:268-271.

Kabawat SE, Bast RC, Welch, WR et al. Immunopathologic characterization of a monoclonal antibody that recognizes common surface antigens of humanr ovarian tumours of serous, endometrioid, and clear cell types. Am J Clin Pathol 1983; 79:98-104.

Kaesemann H, Caffier H, Hoffman F J et al. Monoklonale Antikorper in diagnostik und verlaufskontrolle de ovarial karzinomas. CA 125 als tumormarker. Klin Wochenshr 1986; 64:781-785.

Kikuchi Y, Kizawa I, Koyama E et al. Significance of serum tumour markers in patients with carcinoma of the ovary. Obstet Gynecol 1984; 63:561-566.

Kivinen S, Kuoppala T, Leppilampi M et al. Tumor-associated antigen CA 125 before and during the treatment of ovarian carcinoma. Obstet Gynecol 1986; 67:468-472.

Klug TL, Bast RC, Niloff JM et al. Monoclonal antibody immunoradiometric assay for an antigenic determinant (CA 125) associated with human epithelial ovarian carcinomas. Cancer Res 1984; 44:1048-1053.

Knauf S, Anderson DJ, Knapp RC et al. A study of the NB/70K and CA 125 monoclonal antibody radioimmunoassays for measuring serum antigen levels in ovarian cancer patients. Am J Obstet Gynecol 1985; 152:911-913.

Knauf S, Urbach GI. A study of ovarian cancer patients using a radioimmunoassay for human ovarian tumor-associated antigen OCA. Am J Obstet Gynecol 1980; 138:1222-1223.

Knauf S, Urbach GI. Identification, purification and radioimmunoassay of NB/70K, a human ovarian tumor-associated antigen. Cancer Res 1981; 41:1351-1357.

Kottmeier H (ed). Annual report in the results of treatment in gynaecological cancer, 1982; 18, FIGO, Stockholm.

Krebs H-B, Goplerud DR, Kilpatrick SJ et al. Role of CA 125 as tumour marker in ovarian carcinoma. Obstet Gynecol 1986; 67:473-477.

Li-juan L, Xiu-feng H, Wen-shu L et al. A monoclonal antibody radioimmunoassay for an antigenic determinant CA 125 in ovarian cancer patients. Chin Med J 1986; 99:721-726.

Lukomska B, Olszewski WL, Engeset A. Acute phase reactive proteins and complement components and inhibitors in patients with ovarian cancer. Gynecol Oncol 1981; 11:288-298.

Malkasian GD, Knapp RC, Lavin PT et al. Preoperative evaluation of serum CA 125 levels in premenopausal and postmenopausal patients with pelvic masses: Discimination of benign from malignant disease. Am J Obstet Gynecol 1988; 159:341-346.

Miotti S, Aguanno S, Canevari S et al. Biochemical analysis of human ovarian cancer-associated antigens defined by murine monoclonal antibodies. Cancer Res 1985; 45:826-832.

Mogenson O, Mogensen B, Jakobsen A et al. Preoperative measurement of cancer antigen 125 (CA 125) in the differential diagnosis of ovarian tumors. Acta Oncologica 1989; 28:471-473.

Niloff JM, Klug TL, Schaetzl E et al. Elevation of serum CA 125 in carcinomas of the fallopian tube, endometrium, and endocervix. Am J Obstet Gynecol 1984a; 148:1057-1058.

Niloff JM, Knapp RC, Schaetzl E et al. CA125 Antigen levels in obstetric and gynecologic patients. Obstet Gynecol 1984b; 64:703-707.

Nouwen EJ, Pollet DE, Schelstraete JB et al. Human placental alkaline phosphatase in benign and malignant ovarian neoplasia. Cancer Res 1985; 45:892-902.

Old LJ. Cancer immunology: The search for specificity. Cancer Res 1981; 41:361-375.

OPCS Cancer Statistics, Registrations. Cases of diagnosed cancer registered in England and Wales. HM Stationery Office, London. 1983.

Ramakrishnan J, Xu FJ, Branat SJ. Constitutive production of macrophage colony stimulating factor by human ovarian and breast cancer cell lines. J Clin Invest 1989; 3: 921-926.

Ricolleau G, Chatal JF, Fumoleau P et al. Radioimmunoassay of the CA 125 antigen in ovarian carcinomas: advantages compared with CA 19-9 and CEA. Tumour Biol 1985; 5:151-159.

Sarjadi S, Daunter B, Mackay E et al. A multiparametric approach to tumor markers detectable in serum in patients with carcinoma of the ovary or uterine cervix. Gynecol Oncol 1980; 10:113-124.

Schilthuis MS, Aalders JG, Bouma J et al. Serum CA 125 levels in epithelial ovarian cancer: relation with findings at second-look operations and their role in the detection of tumour recurrence. Br J Obstet Gynaecol 1987; 94:202-207.

Schwartz PE. The role of CA 125 in the evaluation of palpable or enlarged postmenopausal ovaries. Am J Obstet Gyneco 1988; 158:1072-1073.

Sekine H, Hayes DF, Ohno T et al. Circulating DF3 and CA 125 antigen levels in serum from patients with epithelial ovarian carcinoma. J Clin Oncol 1985; 3:1355-1363.

Sevelda P, Schemper M, Spona J. CA 125 as an independent prognostic factor for survival in patients with epithelial ovarian cancer. Am J Obstet Gynecol 1989; 161: 1213-1216.

Smith LH, Ol RH. Detection of malignant ovarian neoplasms: A review of the literature. II. Laboratory detection. Obstet Gynecol Survey 1984a; 39:329-345.

Smith LH, Ol RH. Detection of malignant ovarian neoplasms: A review of the literature. III. Immunological detection and ovarian cancer-associated antigens. Obstet Gynecol Survey 1984b; 39:346-360.

Stone M, Bagshaw KD, Kardona A et al. ß human chorionic gonadotrophin and carcino-embryonic antigen in the management of ovarian carcinoma. Br J Obstet Gynaecol 1977; 84:375-379.

Sunderland CA, Davies JO, Stirrat GM. Immunohistology of normal and ovarian cancer tissue with a monoclonal antibody to placental alkaline phosphatase. Cancer Res 1984; 44:4496-4502.

Talerman A, Haije WG, Baggerman L. Serum alpha fetoprotein (AFP) in patients with germ cell tumurs of the gonads and extragonadal sites. Cancer 1980; 46:380-385.

Talerman A, Haije WG, Baggerman L. Alpha-1 antitrypsin and alpha fetoprotein in sera of patients with germ cell neoplasia. Int J Cancer 1977; 19:741-746.

Taylor-Papadimitiou J, Griffiths AB. Development of monoclonal antibodies with specificity for human epithelial cells. In: Receptor-mediated targeting of drugs, 1985, p 201-234. Ed: Gregoiadis G, Poste G, Senio, J, Trouet A. Plenum Publishing Corporation.

Tyson FL, Soper JT, Daly L, et al. Overexpression and amplication of the C-erb B-Z (HER Z/neu) proto-oncogene in epithelial ovarian tumours and cell lines. Proc Am Assoc Cancer Res 1988; 29:471.

van Nagell JR, Donaldson ES, Hanson MB et al. Biochemical markers in the plasma and tumours of patients with gynaecological malignancies. Cancer 1981; 48:495-503.

van Kley H, Cramer S, Burns DE. Serous ovarian neoplastic amylase (SONA). Cancer 1981; 48:1444-1449.

Ward BG, Cruickshank DJ, Tucker DF et al. Independent expression in serum of three tumour-associated antigens: CA 125, placental alkaline phosphatase and HMFG2 in ovarian carcinoma. Br J Obstet Gynecol 1987a; 94:696-698.

Ward BG, Lowe DG, Shepherd JH. Patterns of expression of a tumor associated antigen, defined by the monoclonal antibody HMFG2, in human epithelial ovarian carcinoma. Cancer 1987b; 60:787-793.

Willman CL, Fenoglio-Preiser CM. Oncogenes, suppressor genes and carcinogenesis. Hum.Pathol 1987; 18:895-902.

Xing PE, Tjandra JJ, Reynolds K et al. Reactivity of anti-human milk fat globule antibodies with synthetic peptides. J Immunol 1989; 142:3503-3509.

Zanaboni F, Vergadoro F, Presti M et al. Tumor antigen CA 125 as a marker of ovarian epithelial carcinoma. Gynecol Oncol 1987; 28:61-67.

Zurawski VR, Orjaseter H. Andersen A et al. Elevated serum CA 125 levels prior to diagnosis of ovarian neoplasia: relevance for early detection of ovarian cancer. Int J Cancer 1988a; 42:677-680.

Zurawski VR, Knapp RC, Einhorn N et al. An initial analysis of preoperative serum CA 125 levels in patients with early stage ovarian carcinoma. Gynecol Oncol 1988b; 30:7-14.

Zurawski VR, Sjovall K, Schoenfeld DA et al. Prospective evaluation of serum CA 125 levels in a normal population, Phase I. The specificities of single and serial determinations in testing for ovarian cancer. Gynecol Oncol 1990; 36:299-305.

22 Phase I Investigation for Early Diagnosis of Ovarian Carcinoma; What Problems are to be Expected in a Larger Screening Programme?

K. SJÖVALL [1], R. C. BAST JR [2], G. EKLUND [1], P. HALL [2], R. C. KNAPP [2], D. A. SCHOENFELD [3], V. R. ZURAWSKI JR [2], and N. EINHORN [1]

[1] Karolinska Institutet, Stockholm Sweden
[2] Duke University Medical Center, Durham (NC), USA
[3] Harvard Medical School, Boston (MA), USA

1 INTRODUCTION

An important issue in the diagnosis of ovarian cancer, is whether the CA 125 ratio immunoassay (RIA) might provide a means for early detection of this disease. As a first step towards evaluating this issue, both the sensitivity of elevated serum CA 125 levels associated with early stage disease and the specificity of the test have been investigated. CA 125 levels have been determined in patients with pelvic masses (Einhorn, Bast, Knapp et al. 1986; Malkasian, Knapp, Lavin et al, 1988; O'Connell, Ryan, Murphy et al. 1987), in a group of Roman Catholic nuns in the Philadelphia area (Zurawski, Broderick, Pickens et al. 1987) and in a multicentre study of early stage ovarian cancer (Zurawski, Knapp, Einhorn et al. 1988). These studies made it evident that it would be worthwhile to investigate whether it would be feasible to use the CA 125 RIA as a screening method.

A Phase I investigation was initiated in 1985 in Sweden, where very well functioning regional cancer and in-patient registries provide the possibility for satisfactory follow-up. The first results of 1082 women screened with CA 125 have recently been analyzed. The results of this analysis included evaluation of single and serial CA 125 levels and the specificity of the RIA in different age groups (Zurawski, Sjövall, Schoenfeld et al. 1990).

The aim of the present study was to evaluate the results of a four-year follow-up of these 1082 women in the cancer registry and the in-patient registry, and to analyse the consequences of detecting other pathological and pseudopathologial conditions during the screening procedure.

2 MATERIALS AND METHODS

From a population registry in the Stockholm region, 1082 women 40 years of age or older were enrolled in this study between May 1985 and January 1986. Each woman completed a questionnaire in order to define her current status. Blood samples from the study group were collected annually for each of two years. Sera were frozen and thawed once. Then CA 125 levels were determined as described (Zurawski, Sjövall, Schoenfeld et al. 1990). Women with elevated values - ≥35 µ/ml - and an equal number of age-matched controls with CA 125 levels less than 35 µ/ml underwent gynaecological examinations semiannually. Additional CA 125 levels were then determined quarterly for a period of two years. The gynecological examination was performed by one of the two participating gynaecologists blinded to CA 125 levels. In cases of suspected pathological changes in the ovaries transabdominal sonograms were also obtained. Patients with gynaecological symptoms were referred for further investigations, e.g. curettage, needle biopsy or radiologic investigation. Laparotomy was performed when, based on clinical and sonographic evidence, surgery was indicated.

In February 1987 the code was broken for the first time and information from the cancer registry and the in-patient registry could be correlated to the study population. Additional registry follow-up was completed in November 1988 and in February 1989.

3 RESULTS

The distribution of CA 125 levels according to age groups and analysis of single and serial levels during the first year of examination has been described (Zurawski, Sjövall, Schoenfeld et al. 1990). In this report 1082 women, among them 36 women with levels ≥ 35 µ/ml and the same number of matched controls with CA 125 levels < 35 µ/ml, were followed for at least three years. During this period two of the negative matched controls had occasional elevated values. At the second screen of the entire study population another six women, previously negative, were determined to have elevated CA 125 levels. A total of 44 women with elevated CA 125 levels were found during the 2-year study (Table 1).

Table 1 Women with positive values

One-year observation	36
Changes in controls	2
Two-year observation	6
Total	44

Among them the cancer registry revealed one ovarian carcinoma patient whose first blood sample with increased CA 125 level had been obtained 20 months before clinical diagnosis and one malignant lymphoma patient with a pleural efusion whose elevated CA 125 level had been noted 27 months before clinical diagnosis. There were no other malignancies among the patients with increased CA 125 levels. In the in-patient registry 17 nonmalignant diagnoses were discovered in the group of women with elevated CA 125 levels (Table 2).

Table 2 Diagnoses for women (n=44) with elevated CA 125 values.
Follow-up through In-patient Registry and Cancer Registry

Malignant	Benign
1 ovarian carcinoma	4 endometriosis
	4 fibromata
1 malignant lymphoma	5 irregular bleedings
	1 Crohns disease
	1 liver cirrhosis
	1 pneumonia
	1 abdominal pain

No diagnosis was found in either registry for the remaining 25 women with elevated CA 125 levels. In 22 of these 25 the CA 125 levels decreased to normal during the observation period, while three continued with moderately increased levels. An additional 12 nonovarian cancers were detected in the cancer registry among the 1038 women with nonelevated C 125 levels (Table 3).

Table 3 Nonovarian malignancies found in the screened
population (n=1038) with CA 125 values < 35 µ/ml

Diagnosis	Intervals between test and diagnosis in months
1 skin cancer	8
2 colon carcinomas	9, 10
5 breast cancer	0, 5, 8, 11, 21
1 brain tumor	15
1 cancer of ampulla Vater	4
2 cervical cancer	4, 9
2 malignant melanoma	13, 16

At the second follow-up in the cancer and in-patient registries, two additional patients were detected with ovarian cancer; 24 months and 20 months respectively after their CA 125 levels had been recorded as negative (Table 4).

Table 4 Ovarian malignancy in the screened population with CA 125 values < 35 µ/ml

Diagnosis	Interval between test and diagnosis	Values
Stage I C	41 m	2.8 µ/ml
endometrioid	24 m	10.2 µ/ml
Stage III C	32 m	29.6 µ/ml
seropapillary	20 m	28.1 µ/ml

Among the 44 women with elevated levels and their age-matched controls, gynaecological examination was supplemented with ultrasound in 10 cases. Among these 88 women, nine laparotomies and three curettages were performed (Table 5).

Table 5 Surgical interventions

	< 35 µ/ml	≥ 35 µ/ml
Laparotomies	3	6
Curettages	2	1

Surgical intervention was recommended in an additional two cases but was not carried out. The three patients undergoing curettage had benign histopathology; two of them had non-elevated CA 125 levels and the third had an increased level. Of the three patients undergoing laparotomy with non-elevated CA 125 levels; two of them were diagnosed with uterine leiomyomas and one with chronic salpingitis. Among the six laparotomy patients with elevated CA 125 levels, three were diagnosed with endometriosis, two with uterine leiomyomas, and one with ovarian cancer (Table 6). Only the patient with ovarian cancer had continuously increasing CA 125 levels.

Table 6 Findings on laparotomy

Diagnosis	< 35 μ/ml	≥ 35 μ/ml
Endometriosis	-	3
Fibromata	2	2
Chronic salpingitis	1	-
Ovarian carcinoma	-	1

The CA 125 levels of the 1082 women were also correlated with age. There were 483 women under 50 years of age and 599 were 50 years of age or older. In the younger group, 24 patients (4.96%) had CA 126 levels above 35 μ/ml. Among the older women, 12 (2%) had levels above 35 μ/ml. In the whole study population of 1082 women there were 11, equally divided between the the age groups, who had levels above 65 μ/ml. When the levels were correlated not to age but to menopausal status, only 0.6% of the postmenopausal study population had levels above 35 μ/ml.

4 DISCUSSION

Development of a screening programme for ovarian carcinoma is a more complex issue than for those tumours which are already subject to screening procedures, i.e. carcinomas of the cervix and breast. Much less is known about the natural history of carcinoma of the ovary. Consequently we are still quite ignorant about the actual prevalence of the disease in an asymptomatic population. Even supposing the prevalence were high and that a test were very sensitive, the specificity of the screening method also must be very high because of the consequences - laparotomy - for women with false positive tests. In well organized screening programmes for cervical cancer decreased mortality has been observed in several countries. In Sweden the annual number of new cases of invasive carcinoma of the cervix has decreased from 958 in 1958 to 593 in 1986 and the mortality has decreased by 45%. This has been achieved at the cost of about 8000 conizations a year. The screening programme for carcinoma of the breast has led to a 30% decrease in mortality among the screened population. It is impossible to determine whether it has also led to many unnecessary operations in cases where spontaneous regression would have occurred. Nevertheless, we are satisfied with the results of the screening programmes for carcinomas of the cervix and breast because a decrease in mortality is regarded as an indication of efficacy of a screening programme.

The questions and considerations associated with screening for carcinoma of the cervix and the breast may also be considered in a discussion of screening for ovarian carcinoma. The mortality in these three tumour types differs considerably. Case fatality due to carcinoma of the ovary is 64-68%. Case fatality due to carcinoma of the cervix and breast is 35% and 40% respectively.

Analysis of our own study with regard to pathologic findings and consequences, hospitalization and surgical intervention, indicated that the Phase I screening programme resulted in only a modest number of interventions. In the study population with clinical follow-up there were as many women with normal as with elevated CA 125 levels. Among 44 women with elevated levels only six underwent laparotomy. Three of those were over 50 years of age representing only 0.5% of the total screened study population in this age group. Totally, 2% of the women over 50 years of age had elevated CA 125 levels. Based on this experience and on the results presented here the following conclusion can be drawn: A screening programme for early detection of ovarian carcinoma utilizing the CA 125 RIA should only include women 50 years of age or older. Many fewer elevated CA 125 levels are detected in postmenopausal women, but for practical reasons the population probably has to be chosen by age and not by menopausal status.

Additionally, it is noteworthy that, with one exception, other nonovarian malignancies were not associated with elevated CA 125 levels in the present study. This finding suggests that false positive results in a screen using the CA 125 RIA should not pose an overwhelming problem. Our findings are in agreement with the reports indicating that benign gynecological conditions such as endometriosis and leiomyoma are sometimes associated with elevated CA 125 values (Barbieri et al. 1986).

One purpose of the present analysis was to estimate the amount of invasive procedures to be expected in the population of women screened with CA 125. Although the gynaecological examinations were blind and all invasive procedures were done on strict clinical findings, it should be noted that after breaking the code for CA 125 levels, twice as many laparotomies had been performed in the group with elevated CA 125 levels as in the group with non-elevated levels.

A summary of the experience of the Phase I investigation indicates that in a large population of women 50 years of age or older, one would expect to find 2% with elevated CA 125 levels. A pelvic mass indicating laparotomy might be found in one in four of these women.

A Phase II study including 5500 women has also been completed. Among 175 women with elevated CA 125 levels six ovarian cancer patients were detected clinically or sonographically with 2 in surgical stage IA, 2 in stage IIB , and 2 in Stage III, all on women above 50 years of age (Einhorn et al. 1990).

In conclusion, we believe that a large screening trial for ovarian cancer using the CA 125 RIA is warranted provided that only women 50 years of age or older are screened in a well-designed randomized 2-arm study and that mortality be used as the final endpoint demonstrating utility of the screen.

REFERENCES

Barbieri RL, Niloff JM, Bast RC et al.: Elevated serum concentrations of CA 125 in patients with advanced endometriosis. Fertil Steril 45:630-634, 1986.

Einhorn N, Bast RC, Knapp RC et al.: Preoperative evaluation of serum CA 125 levels in patients with primary epithelial ovarian cancer. Obstet Gynecol 67:414-417, 1986.

Einhorn N, Sjövall K, Schoenfeld DA et al. Early detection of ovarian cancer using the CA 125 radioimmunoassay (RIA). ASCO abstract, 1990.

Malkasian GD, Knapp RC, Lavin PT et al.: Preoperative evaluation of serum CA 125 levels in premenopausal and postmenopausal patients with pelvic masses: Discrimination of benign from malign disease. Am J Obstet Gynecol 159:341-146, 1988.

O'Connell GJ, Ryan, Murphy J et Al.: Predictive value of CA 125 for ovarian carcinoma in patients presenting with pelvic masses. Obstet Gynecol 70:930-932, 1987.

Zurawski VR, Broderick SF, Pickens P et al.: Serum CA 125 levels in a Group of Nonhospitalized Women. Relevance for the Early Detection of Ovarian Cancer. Obstet Gynecol 69:606-611, 1987

Zurawski VR, Knapp RC, Einhorn N et al.: An Initial Analysis of Serum CA 125 Levels in Patients with Early Ovarian Carcinoma. Gynecol Oncol 30:7-14, 1988.

Zurawski VR, Sjövall K, Schoenfeld DA et al.: Prospective evaluation of serum CA 125 levels in a normal population Phase I: The specificities of single and serial determinations in testing for ovarian cancer. Obstet Gynecol 36:299-305, 1990.

23 Screening for Ovarian Cancer

H. CUCKLE and N. WALD

Department of Environmental and Preventive Medicine, Medical College of
St Bartholomew's Hospital, Charterhouse Square, London, UK.

1 INTRODUCTION

Ovarian cancer is the most common gynaecological malignancy in the UK, with about
twice as many new cases each year than cervical cancer. Two features of the disease which
are relevant to screening are the much longer survival when the disease is confined to the
ovary compared to when the disease is more advanced and the fact that most cases present
clinically with abdominal symptoms when there is already spread into the peritoneum and
beyond (Table 1).

Table 1 Relative survival from ovarian cancer in two countries according to stage.

Stage		No. women	Relative survival (%)		
			1 year	5 years	15 years
Localised	USA	975 (29%)	89	69	60
	Norway	1292 (33%)	86	63	54
Regional	USA	515 (16%)	68	30	24
	Norway	284 (7%)	60	32	27
Distant	USA	1822 (55%)	35	7	4
	Norway	2352 (60%)	31	11	9
Total	USA	3312 (100%)	57	29	25
	Norway	3928 (100%)	51	30	26

Sources: USA = The SEER Program (Axtell et al, 1976)
Norway = Cancer Registry of Norway (1975)

Screening therefore has every opportunity to improve prognosis unless the observed differences in survival are entirely due to lead time and length bias. The issue can only be resolved by a trial with mortality as the endpoint. Since older women who agree to be screened may have, for reasons that are not understood, a different risk of the disease, this would be a randomised trial and it would need to be large (more than 100,000 women randomised). Before considering such an undertaking it is, of course, necessary to find a screening test with a reasonably high sensitivity and specificity.

Table 2 CA-125 perioperative detection rate and false-positive rate in 27 studies*

Study	Detection rate	False-positive rate
Australia (Dodd et al, 1985)	78% (14/18)	-
Austria (Fuith et al, 1987)	82% (32/39)	-
Canada (Atack et al, 1986)	33% (3/9)	-
China (Li-juan et al, 1986)	93% (26/28)	-
Finland (Heinonen et al, 1985)	69% (9/13)	0% (0/16)
Finland (Halila et al, 1986)	69% (9/13)	-
Finland (Kivinen et al, 1986)	86% (25/29)	-
France (Ricolleau et al, 1985)	92% (35/38)	4% (3/67)
Germany (Crombach et al, 1985)	78% (31/40)	5% (3/58)
Germany (Kaesemann et al, 1986)	83% (166/199)	14% (34/251)
Holland (Rodenburg et al, 1985)	67% (16/24)	-
Holland (Schilthuis et al, 1987)	96% (44/46)	-
International (Zurawski et al, 1988a)	61% (22/36)	-
Italy (Pansini et al, 1986)	100% (16/16)	-
Italy (Zanaboni et al, 1986)	75% (43/57)	-
Japan (Haga et al, 1986)	-	5% (13/258)
Norway (Vergote et al, 1987)	92% (34/37)	-
Norway (Zurawski et al, 1988b)	-	5% (15/323)
Spain (Ruibal et al, 1984)	-	2% (4/226)
Sweden (Einhorn et al, 1986)	78% (14/18)	-
Switzerland (Brioschi et al, 1987)	84% (58/69)	-
UK (Canney et al, 1984)	83% (48/58)	-
UK (Cruickshank et al, 1987)	73% (30/41)	-
UK (Jacobs et al, 1989)	-	1% (13/1009)
USA (Bast et al, 1983)	95% (21/22)	1% (5/351)
USA (Malkasian et al, 1988)	82% (49/60)	-
USA (Patsner and Mann, 1988)	63% (29/46)	-
Total	81% (774/956)	4% (90/2559)

    * using a 35 µ/ml cut-off

2 SCREENING TECHNIQUES

Three general categories of screening modality are available, namely, the use of a tumour marker in blood or urine, the use of an imaging technique such as ultrasound, and physical examination.

2.1 Tumour Markers

Ovarian tumours are associated with the increased production of various substances, many of which reach the peripheral circulation. Some of them are strong enough determinants of the presence of tumour cells to be used in clinical practice, primarily to monitor relapse after the surgical removal of the tumour and associated tissues. The most effective marker described so far is CA-125, and this is the main candidate for use as a potential screening test.

2.2 CA-125

In women who present clinically with ovarian cancer serum CA-125 levels are raised before or soon after initial surgery. Table 2 shows that on the basis of data from 956 women with ovarian cancer from 27 studies CA-125 levels exceeded 35 μ/ml in 81% of affected women and 4% of unaffected women.

Table 3 CA-125 perioperative detection rate according to stage*

Study	Stage I	Stage II	Stage III	Stage IV
Austria (Fuith et al, 1987)	67% (4/6)	80% (4/5)	89% (16/18)	80% (8/10)
China (Li-juan et al, 1986)	50% (1/2)	100% (3/3)	96% (22/23)	-
Finland (Heinonen et al, 1985)	0% (0/3)	100% (2/2)	100% (4/4)	75% (3/4)
Finland (Halila et al, 1986)	-	0% (0/1)	57% (4/7)	100% (5/5)
Finland (Kivinen et al, 1986)	25% (1/4)	100% (5/5)	90% (9/10)	100%(10/10)
Germany (Crombach et al, '85)	60% (3/5)	83% (5/6)	68% (13/19)	100%(10/10)
Holland (Schilthuis et al, 1987)	75% (6/8)	100% (5/5)	100% (20/20)	100%(13/13)
Internatl. (Zurawski et al,'88a)	50% (12/24)	83% (10/12)	-	-
Italy (Zanaboni et al, 1986)	53% (8/15)	75% (3/4)	85% (29/34)	75% (3/4)
Norway (Vergote et al, 1987)	100% (1/1)	-	89% (24/27)	100% (9/9)
Switzerland (Brioschi et al,'87)	31% (4/13)	100% (3/3)	97% (29/30)	96%(22/23)
UK (Cruickshank et al, 1987)	25% (3/12)	67% (2/3)	94% (15/16)	100%(10/10)
USA (Bast et al, 1983)	100% (1/1)	100% (2/2)	94% (15/16)	100% (3/3)
USA (Malkasian et al, 1988)	29% (4/14)	100% (6/6)	100% (37/37)	67% (2/3)
USA (Patsner and Mann,'88)	40% (8/20)	100% (2/2)	93% (13/14)	100% (2/2)
Total	44%(56/128)	88%(52/59)	91%(250/275)	94%(100/106

* using a 35/μ ml cut-off

Some of the reports of the studies allow detection rates to be estimated according to the clinical stage of the disease (using the FIGO scheme): 44%, 88%, 91% and 94% at stages I, II, III, and IV respectively (Table 3). This suggests that the test is likely to have a detection rate much less than 81% when applied to asymptomatic women.

The principal source of published information on the detection rate of CA-125 in an apparently healthy population is the report of the JANUS study based on prospectively collected and stored serum samples (Zurawski et al, 1988b). In addition there is the report of the London Hospital Study in which a single case of ovarian cancer was detected with a CA-125 level of 32 μ/ml - no others presented after a minimum follow up period of 2 years (Jacobs et al, 1988). In the JANUS study serum samples from healthy women were stored and later retrieved and tested for CA-125 after ovarian cancer had presented clinically in 105 women. Table 4 shows that a cut-off level of 35 μ/ml would be expected to yield a detection rate of about one-third for cancers that presented within 18 months. The detection rate would have been one-fifth for those that presented within 5 years. In general the odds of being affected given a positive result is low (eg. 1:200 for a 55 year old using a 25 μ/ml

Table 4   CA-125 in the JANUS study: detection rate according to level and time to clinical presentation after blood sampling together with the corresponding false-positive rate and odds of being affected given a positive result.*

CA-125 (μ/ml)	Detection rate (%) Time to presentation (years)				False positive rate (%)	Odds of being affected given a positive result Time to presentation (years)			
	≤1.5	≤3	≤5	≤12		≤1.5	≤3	≤5	≤12
≥25	50	43	33	30	13	1:500	1:300	1:200	1:90
≥30	50	32	24	24	7	1:300	1:200	1:150	1:60
≥35	33	25	20	17	5	1:250	1:150	1:100	1:60
≥65	33	14	9	6	1	1:50	1:60	1:60	1:30
≥100	25	11	6	5	0.5	1:50	1:50	1:50	1:30

* for a 55 year old woman in UK.
(derived from Zurawski et al, 1988b)

cut-off level and considering only those presenting within 5 years). Only if an extreme cut-off level were adopted and a long presentation time considered (eg 1:30 using a 100 μ/ml cut-off and a 12 year period) would the odds be high enough to warrant the further investigations. CA-125 levels tend to be raised in the presence of benign disease of the reproductive and digestive tracts, as well as with cancers at various sites (Jacobs & Bast, 1989). Screening for ovarian cancer will therefore lead to the incidental diagnosis of some of these disorders, possibly leading to over-treatment.

2.3 Combining Markers

If other tumour markers were used with CA-125 that were, at least, to some extent independent indicators of the risk of ovarian cancer, a greater screening efficiency could be achieved, combining the information in much the same way as is being done in antenatal screening for Down's syndrome (Wald et al, 1988). For example human milk fat globule antigen and placental alkaline phosphatase showed little correlation in 198 serum samples from women with ovarian cancer (Ward et al, 1987). However, so far no combination of markers has been investigated in sufficient detail to derive reliable information on screening performance.

2.4 Ultrasound

The ovary can be visualised using ultrasound, computer tomography, magnetic resonance and immunoscintography. Only the first is suitable as a population screening technique, although the others may have a role in the subsequent investigation of women with positive ultrasound results. The ultrasound examination is used to determine whether the ovary is enlarged (judged either by the maximum diameter or the volume estimated from the product of 3 orthogonal diameters times $\pi/6$) or whether the outline and internal structure is indicative of malignancy (abnormal 'morphology').

As with CA-125 most experience to date is with women who present clinically with ovarian cancer. In seven studies the scan was done prior to surgery to investigate a pelvic mass, hence the main criteria for judging abnormality was morphology rather than ovarian volume. Table 5 summarises the results of these studies including 339 women who were later shown to have ovarian cancer; the detection rate was 77% and the false positive rate was 6%. The detection rate may be higher than it would be in asymptomatic women because the ultrasonographers may have been influenced in reaching their judgement by the clinical history and any physical findings.

Routine ultrasound performed on women attending gynaecological out-patients clinics is of more relevance to screening than the examiniation of patients with specific symptoms or signs suggestive of ovarian cancer. Two such series have been reported from Lund, Sweden based on women aged 40-70 years. The first series included 795 women with a variety of symptoms (Andolf et al, 1986) the second series included 801 women selected because of epidemiological risk factors such as nulliparity, and previous family or personal history of cancer or with abdominal symptoms which could not be obviously explained

Table 5   Preoperative ultrasound: detection rate and false positive rate in seven studies.

Study	Detection rate	False-positive rate
Japan (Kobayashi, 1976)	70% (43/61)	4% (14/345)
Japan (Takeuchi et al, 1978)	74% (76/103)	7% (29/399)
UK (Meire et al, 1978)	83% (15/18)	6% (3/51)
USA (Requard et al, 1981)	88% (28/32)	-
China (Ling et al, 1983)	92% (35/38)	8% (9/119)
Switzerland (Herrmann et al, 1987)	82% (41/50)	6% (14/254)*
USA (Finkler et al, 1988)	62% (23/37)	5% (3/65)
Total	77% (261/339)	6% (72/1233)

* including those thought on ultrasound to be malignant at sites other than the ovary

(Andolf et al, 1990). Out of the total of 1596 women, 97 (6%) had a surgical operation following a positive ultrasound results; 10 were later shown to have ovarian cancer, 2 endometrial cancer and 1 cancer of the caecum. Formal follow up of women with negative ultrasound examinations was not undertaken but no ovarian cancers were known to the authors between the study and the time of publication despite the hospital being the gynaecological referral centre for the area. A similar study from Gottingen, Germany found 2 ovarian cancers in 27 "positives" from 212 women (Osmers et al, 1989).

Routine ultrasound examination of the ovaries is sometimes carried out in pregnancy. In three published studies a total of 85,130 women were examined, 101 ovarian cysts were operated on and 4 ovarian malignancies were found (Booth, 1963; White, 1973; Hogston & Lilford, 1986). The only available information on screening asymptomatic women specifically for ovarian cancer comes from a study at King's College Hospital, London and another in Lexington, Kentucky. In the King's Study 5479 volunteers mostly aged 40 or more recruited from all over the country in response to wide media publicity, had at least one scan (90% had 2 and 77% had 3, at an average interval of about 18 months) (Campbell et al, 1989). Over the three scans an average of 2.3% were referred to a surgeon and eight women were found to have ovarian cancer, of whom five had primary cancer (all stage I including one bilateral cancer) and three had metastatic disease (one bilateral) from the breast or colon and one other patient presented clinically two years after the third ultrasound screening examination. The odds of being affected given a positive result was 1:70, not dissimilar to the position with CA-125. In the Kentucky study 506 women aged 40 or more were scanned and 10 (2%) had surgery including one found to have ovarian cancer which was a metastatis from a primary cancer of the colon (Higgins et al, 1989).

2.5 Physical Examination
This is a less sensitive method of screening than ultrasound. In the two Swedish ultrasound studies 4 of the 10 ovarian cancers detected by ultrasound had negative findings on vaginal examination. In the King's study only one of the 5 primary cancers was detected by physical examination.

3 DIAGNOSTIC PROCEDURES
A difficulty with both CA-125 and ultrasound is the low odds of being affected given a positive screening result. This is largely the result of positives due to benign ovarian disease. In the King's College Hospital Study one-third of the false-positives had benign tumours and one-half had tumour-like conditions such as teratoma and endometrioma.

The usual way of distinguishing benign from malignant masses in the ovary is by laparotomy, although some might use laparoscopy first to select those suitable for surgery. Other less invasive approaches have been proposed. Firstly there is immunoscintography, in which radiolabelled markers (usually human milk fat globule antigen and placental alkaline phosphatase) are injected and after a period the abdomen is scanned. In one study all 15 primary ovarian malignancies had positive scanning results preoperatively (Shepherd et al, 1987). Secondly there is fine needle aspiration but this seems to be an inadequate method: in a series of 59 cysts aspirated prior to laparotomy, only two of the seven cancers were identified and one of the 52 benign cysts was wrongly classified (Diernaes et al, 1987). Thirdly there is Doppler ultrasound colour flow imaging. This can identify new blood vessel formation which is a common result of cancer. In three published studies of ovarian masses prior to surgery a total of 184 women have been scanned: there was prominent blood flow indicating new blood vessel formation in 97% (36/37) of those found to have malignant tumours compared with 2% (3/147) when a benign condition was found (Hata et al, 1989; Bourne et al, 1989; Kurjak & Zalud, 1990). Computer tomography (Sanders et al, 1983) and magnetic resonance imaging (Hricak et al, 1985) have also been studied but on insufficient numbers.

It may therefore be possible to avoid carrying out a laparotomy in many women with positive screening results with little loss in detection. Whether or not this is the case is unknown and depends on the natural history of benign ovarian lesions. Some take the view that many benign lesions will inevitably lead to medical problems (eg torsion) and so benefit from early non-emergency removal. Pathologists are divided on the malignant potential of some of the benign tumours (Fox, 1990; Anderson, 1990). If benign tumours were precursors of malignant tumours with a high rate of progression then the removal of benign tumours may be useful. But we do not know, and it may be that only a randomised trial of screening in which benign tumours were removed could resolve the question.

4 RANDOMISED TRIAL

Of the screening methods currently available ultrasound appears to be the most sensitive. A trial would need to be carried out in women with a high enough risk of ovarian cancer to yield a large number of cases and who are likely to accept screening and subsequent investigation. Women with a family history of ovarian cancer could be studied but they present two problems. Firstly if the familial risk were great enough such women may not accept randomisation to a group that was not routinely screened and second there is no simple means of identifying a large number of women in this category. Another approach in the UK would be to study women already attending for breast cancer screening, as part of the National Health Service Breast Cancer Screening Programme, which is targeted at women aged 50-64 years. The national programme is population based with a recall interval of three years, though more frequent screening may be needed with ovarian cancer.

If we assume that (i) screening transfers two-thirds of those who would have presented with distant disease to the localised stage, (ii) the mortality rate in the additional women with an early diagnosis is similar to that in those presenting clinically at that stage, and (iii) 75% of those offered randomisation agree, then 150,000 women would be needed and, if followed up for 7 years, would yield an expected 66 deaths in the arm offered screening compared with 99 in the control arm. Such a trial would have 80% power to establish the benefit at the 5% level of significance and could be carried out in just six breast screening centres. We have started a pilot study for such a trial in the Reading Screening Centre, one of the screening centres participating in the National Breast Cancer Screening Programme.

The aim of the pilot study is to determine the acceptance rate, to explore ways of minimising the proportion of women referred for a laporotomy and to evaluate the practical problems involved. Women attending the screening centre for their mammographic examination are if eligible invited to join the ultrasound trial. Women aged 62-64 are ineligible since there is insufficient time for two 3-yearly screens and a small number of women are ineligible on account of having had bilateral oophorectomy. In the first 1160 eligible women invited to join the trial 1002 (86%) agreed to randomisation. Initially both vaginal and abdominal screening is being performed, in order to obtain comparable normal ranges for both methods. Because abdominal scanning requires a full bladder an appointment is made for screening to be performed on another day. It is planned that in the full study vaginal scanning will be used on the same day as the breast screening examination and abdominal scanning restricted to women who do not want a vaginal examination.

The practical problems we have encountered so far relate to the definition of a large ovarian volume (ie. the cut-off level). Our early results reveal that there can be considerable variation in determining the ovarian size from centre to centre. The King's College Hospital group have published data on the median volume for the larger of the two ovaries according to age and menopausal status (Campbell et al, 1990). On average we found results that were about one-third of those published. Most of these centre-to-centre differences can be overcome by expressing all results as multiples of the appropriate median. When this is done the proportion of positive results is similar in the two centres, so that, for example, the 90th centile for postmenopausal women is 1.68 times the median at King's College Hospital and 1.72 at the Reading Screening Centre.

A second problem relates to establishing menopausal status. Ovarian volume in post-menopausal women is about two-thirds of that in premenopausal women of the same age, when menopause is defined in terms of the time since the last menstrual period. Separate ovarian volume cut-off levels are therefore needed for pre- and post-menopausal women. However women who have had a hysterectomy before the time of their natural menopause have intermediate volumes with a wide variability. This is presumably because they are a mixed group including both post-menopausal women and those who would have been menstruating had they not have had a hysterectomy. Also difficulty of distinguishing adhesions from ovarian tumours may contribute to the wide variability. Screening will therefore be less discriminatory in this group and since they have a low risk of ovarian cancer one solution might be not to include them in a trial.

It is too early to estimate the surgical intervention rate from the pilot study; there is, as yet, virtually no information upon which to judge the appropriate use of the diagnostic options other than surgery.

5 CONCLUSION
There are sufficient grounds for carrying out a randomised trial of ovarian cancer screening by ultrasound. If such a trial is not started soon screening is likely to be introduced into clinical practice without proper evaluation and it will then be difficult to examine its efficacy in an unbiased way.

REFERENCES
Anderson MC. Malignant potential of benign ovarian cysts: the case "for". In: Sharp F, Mason WP, Leake RE (eds). Ovarian Cancer. Chapman and Hall Medical, London, 1990; 187-190.
Andolf E, Svalenius E, Astedt B. Ultrasonography for early detection of ovarian carcinoma. Br J Obstet Gynaecol 1986; 93:1286-1289.
Andolf E, Jorgensen C, Astedt B. Ultrasound examination for detection of ovarian carcinoma in risk groups. Obstet Gynecol 1990; 75:106-109.
Atack DB, Nisker JA, Allen HH et al. CA 125 surveillance and second-look laparotomy in ovarian carcinoma. Am J Obstet Gynecol 1986; 154:287-289.
Axtell IM, Asire AJ, Myers MH (eds). Cancer Patient Survival, Cancer Surveillance, Epidemiology and End Results (SEER) Program, Report Number 5. US Department of Health Education and Welfare, Washington, 1976.
Bast RC, Klug TL, St John E et al. A radioimmunoassay using a monoclonal antibody to monitor the course of epithelial cancer. N Eng J Med 1983; 309:883-887.
Booth RT. Ovarian tumours in pregnancy. Obstet Gynecol 1963; 21:189-193.

Bourne T, Campbell S, Steer C et al. Transvaginal colour flow imaging: a possible new screening technique for ovarian cancer. Br Med J 1989; 299:1367-1370.

Brioschi PA, Irion O, Bischof P et al. Serum CA 125 in epithelial ovarian cancer: a longitudinal study. Br J Obstet Gynaecol 1987; 94:196-201.

Campbell S, Collins WP, Royston P et al. Developments in ultrasound screening for early ovarian cancer. In: Sharp F, Mason WP, Leake RE (eds). Ovarian Cancer. Chapman. pp 217-227.

Campbell S, Bhan V, Royston P et al. Transabdominal ultrasound screening for early ovarian cancer. Br Med J 1989; 299:1363-1367.

Cancer Registry of Norway. Survival of Cancer Patients. Cases diagnosed in Norway 1953-1967. The Norwegian Cancer Society, Oslo, 1975.

Canney PA, Moore M, Wilkinson PM et al. Ovarian cancer antigen CA 125: A prospective clinical assessment of its role as a tumour marker. Br J Cancer 1984; 50:765-769.

Crombach G, Zippel HH, Wurz H. Erfahrungen mit CA 125, einem Tumormarker fur maligne epitheliale Ovarialetumuren. Geburtsh Frauenhildkd 1985; 45:205-212.

Cruickshank DJ, Fullerton WT, Klopper A. The clinical significance of pre-operative serum CA 125 in ovarian cancer. Br J Obstet Gynaecol 1987; 94:692-695.

Diernaes E, Rasmussen J, Soerensen T et al. Ovarian cysts: management by puncture? Lancet 1987; i:1084.

Dodd J, Tyler JPP, Crandon AJ et al. The value of the monoclonal antibody (cancer antigen 125) in serial monitoring of ovarian cancer: a comparison with circulating immune complexes. Br J Obstet Gynaecol 1985; 92:1054-1060.

Einhorn N, Bast RC, Knapp RC et al. Preoperative evaluation of serum CA 125 levels in patients with primary epithelial ovarian cancer. Obstet Gynecol 1986; 67:414-416.

Finkler NJ, Benacerraf B, Lavin PT, et al. Comparison of Serum CA 125, Clinical Impression, and Ultrasound in the Preoperative Evaluation of Ovarian masses. Obstet Gynecol 1988; 72: 659.

Fox H. Malignant potential of benign ovarian cysts: the case "against". In: Sharp F, Mason WP, Leake RE (eds). Ovarian Cancer. Chapman and Hall Medical, London, 1990; 185-186.

Fuith LC, Dazenbickler G, Dapunt O. CA 125 in the serum and tissue of patients with gynecological disease. Arch Gynecol Obstet 1987; 241:157-164.

Haga Y, Sakamoto K, Egami H et al. Evaluation of serum CA 125 values in healthy individuals and pregnant women. Am J Med Sci 1986; 292:25-29.

Halila H, Stenman UH, Seppala M. Ovarian cancer antigen CA 125 levels in pelvic inflammatory disease and pregnancy. Cancer 1986; 57:1327-1329.

Hata T, Hata K, Senoh D et al. Doppler Ultrasound Assessment of Tumor Vascularity in Gynecologic Disorders. J Ultrasound Med 1989; 8:309-314.

Heinonen PK, Tontti K, Koivula T et al. Tumour- associated antigen CA 125 in patients with ovarian cancer. Br J Obstet Gynaecol 1985; 92:528-531.

Herrmann UJ, Locher GW, Goldhirsch A. Sonographic patterns of ovarian tumors: prediction of malignancy. Obstet Gynecol 1987; 69:777-781.

Higgins RV, van Nagell JR, Donaldson ES. Transvaginal Sonography as a Screening Method for Ovarian Cancer. Gynecol Oncol 1989; 34:402-406.

Hogston P, Lilford RJ. Ultrasound study of ovarian cysts in pregnancy: prevalence and significance. Br J Obstet Gynaecol 1986; 93:625-628.

Hricak H, Lacey C, Schriock E et al. Gynecologic masses: value of magnetic resonance imaging. Am J Obstet Gynecol 1985; 153:31-37.

Jacobs IJ, Stabile I, Bridges J et al. Multimodal approach to screening for ovarian cancer. Lancet 1988; i:268-271.

Jacobs I, Bast RC. The CA 125 tumour-associated antigen: a review of the literature. Hum Rep 1989; 4:1-12.

Kaesemann H, Caffier H, Hoffman FJ et al. Monoklonale Antikorper in diagnostik und verlaufskontrolle de ovarialkarzinomas. CA 125 als tumormarker. Klin Wochenshr 1986; 64:781-785.

Kivinen S, Kuoppala T, Leppilampi M et al. Tumour- associated antigen CA 125 before and during the treatment of ovarian carcinoma. Obstet Gynecol 1986; 67:468-472.

Kobayashi M. Use of diagnositc ultrasound in trophoblastic neoplasms and ovarian tumors. Cancer 1976; 38:441-452.

Kurjak A, Zalud I. Transvaginal colour imaging and ovarian cancer. Br Med J 1990; 300:330.

Li-juan L, Xui-feng, H, Wen-shu L et al. A monoclonal antibody radioimmunoassay for an antigenic determinant CA 125 in ovarian cancer patients. Clin Med J 1986; 99:721-726.

Ling X, Mei-ling H, Yu-fang C et al. Grey scale ultrasonography in diagnosis of pelvic mass and early ovarian carcinoma. Chinese Med J 1983; 96 (11):829-834.

Malkasian GD, Knapp RC, Lavin PT et al. Preoperative evaluation of serum CA 125 levels in premenopausal and postmenopausal patients with pelvic masses: Discrimination of benign from malignant disease. Am J Obstet Gynecol 1988; 159:341-346.

Meire HB, Farrant P, Guha T. Distinction of benign from malignant ovarian cysts by ultrasound. Br J Obstet Gynaecol 1978; 85:893-899.

Osmers R, Völksen M, Rath W et al. Die Vaginalsonographie: eine Screeningmethode zur Früherkennung von Ovarialtumoren und Endometriumkarzinomen? Arch Gynecol Obs 1988; 245 (1-4):602-606.

Pansini F, Bellinazzi A, Rainaldi V et al. Serum CA 125 in ovarian pathology and its variation in ovarian carcinoma after integrated therapy. Gynecol Obstet Invest 1986; 21:47-51.

Patsner B, Mann WJ. The value of preoperative serum CA 125 levels in patients with a pelvic mass. Am J Obstet Gynecol 1988; 159:873-876.

Requard CK, Mettler FA, Wicks JD. Preoperative sonography of malignant ovarian neoplasms. Am J Roentgen 1981; 137:79-82.

Ricolleau G, Chatal JF, Fumoleau P et al. Radioimmunoassay of the CA 125 antigen of ovarian carcinomas: advantages compared with CA 19-9 and CEA. Tumour Biol 1985; 151-159.

Rodenburg CJ, de Maaker GA, Trimbos JBMZ. Moolenaar AJ, van Oosterom AT. CA 15 and TPA as markers in ovarian carcinoma. Neth J Med 1985; 28:536-539.

Ruibal A, Encabo G, Martinez-Miralles E et al. CA 125 seric levels in non malignant pathologies. Bull Cancer 1984; 71:145-148.

Sanders RC, McNeil BJ, Finberg HJ et al. A prospective study of computer tomography and ultrasound in the detection and staging of pelvic masses. Radiology 1983; 146:439-442.

Schilthuis MS, Aalders JG, Bouma J et al. Serum CA 125 levels in epithelial ovarian cancer: relation with findings at second-look operations and their role in the detection of tumour recurrence. Br J Obstet Gynaecol 1987; 94:202-207.

Shepherd JH, Granowska M, Britton KE et al. Tumour-associated monoclonal antibodies for the diagnosis and assessment of ovarian cancer. Br J Obstet Gynaecol 1987; 94:160-167.

Takeuchi H, Kawamata C, Sugie T et al. Grey scale ultrasonic diagnosis of ovarian carcinoma. Excerpta Medica International Congress Series 1978; 436:113-121.

Vergote IB, Bormer OP, Abeler VM. Evaluation of serum CA 125 levels in the monitoring of ovarian cancer. Am J Obstet Gynecol 1987; 157:88-92.

Wald NJ, Cuckle HS, Densem JW et al. Maternal serum screening for Down's syndrome in early pregnancy. Br Med J 1988; 297:883-887.

Ward BG, Cruickshank DJ, Tucker DF et al. Independent expression in serum of three tumour-associated antigens: CA 125, placental alkaline phosphatase and HMFG2 in ovarian carcinoma. Br J Obstet Gynaecol 1987; 94:696-698.

White KC. Ovarian tumours in pregnancy. Am J Obstet Gynecol 1973; 116:544-548

Zanaboni F, Vergadoro F, Presti M et al. Tumor antigen CA 125 as a marker of ovarian epithelial carcinoma. Gynecol Oncol 1987; 28:61-67.

Zurawski VR, Knapp RC, Einhorn N et al. An initial analysis of preoperative serum CA 125 levels in patients with early stage ovarian carcinoma. Gynecol Oncol 1988a; 30:7-14.

Zurawski VR, Orjaseter H, Andersen A et al. Elevated serum CA 125 levels prior to diagnosis of ovarian neoplasia: relevance for early detection of ovarian cancer. Int J Cancer 1988b; 42: 677-680.

24 Summary of Discussion on Screening for Ovarian Cancer

The incidence of ovarian cancer in Western populations is relatively high and in many the mortality from ovarian cancer exceeds all other gynaecological cancers combined, in large part because of the inaccessibility of the ovaries and the late stage at diagnosis of many cancers. The screening tests so far available are based on tumour markers, especially Ca 125, and ultrasound. High specificity of the tests is a prerequisite because diagnostic confirmation is invasive. In premenopausal women low specificity of the tests and a relatively low incidence make screening inapplicable. In postmenopausal women acceptable levels of specificity appear to be obtained by optimally combining several tests or by applying the same test twice within a given interval. However, it seems likely that the sensitivity of the screens has been reduced in such combinations, though the extent of this reduction is not known. Further evaluation of the specificity and sensitivity of such combinations should be obtained. One approach that has been applied is to follow a positive test with repeats after an interval. A rising titre is indicative of ovarian cancer. One risk of such an approach is that delay in diagnosis caused by the necessity to wait for a rise in titre may result in a poorer outcome.

There are some grounds for question as to whether screening for ovarian cancer with the present tests will be cost-effective, because of the low incidence of the disease, as well as the specificity problem, even if testing is restricted to post-menopausal women. It must also be bourne in mind that studies to investigate ovarian cancer screening will have to be large. Studies based on samples of 10,000 or so will only be able to assess the validity of the screening test used. The studies that have been done so far are in the nature of pilot studies. It may be necessary to pool the results from a number of studies to detect an effect on mortality.

The studies that have been performed on ultrasound do not yet suffice to determine whether the test will pick up early stage disease to the same extent as Ca 125. However, in the UK pilot study the 5 cancers detected so far were all impalpable and early stage. Whether or not the UK ultrasound study will be expanded nation-wide will depend on whether or not at least twice the expected annual incidence is detected in the prevalent screen, with a high proportion of early stage cancers.

State of the Art on Screening for Melanoma

Screening for malignant melanoma is in an early stage of development. No evaluation studies have been completed to determine the impact of screening on mortality. Until such data are available, screening for malignant melanoma is not recommended as public health policy. Health promotion programmes advocating enhanced individual awareness may be beneficial but data are not available to confirm this.

Recommendations for Research
Monitor trends in the distribution of lesion depth at diagnosis.
Determine the value of using the early signs of melanoma in population programmes.
Determine the value of high risk markers, including their frequency in the population and their reproducibility.
Conduct a randomized controlled trial to determine the value of screening for melanoma in reducing the mortality from the disease, if a suitable opportunity occurs.
Ongoing programmes of public education and self-examination as well as of physician examination should be evaluated for reduction in mortality.

25 Screening and Early Diagnosis for Melanoma in Australia and New Zealand

J. MARK ELWOOD

Hugh Adam Cancer Epidemiology Unit, Department of Preventive & Social Medicine
University of Otago Medical School, Dunedin, New Zealand

1 SCREENING FOR MELANOMA

There are no major programmes which come under the true definition of "screening", for melanoma in Australia or New Zealand, if we reserve the term "screening" for an organised programme in which unsuspected lesions in asymptomatic subjects are found, either through self-screening stimulated by an appropriate campaign, or through screening by health professionals.

However, the use of self-assessment for lesions which may be early melanoma or suspicious moles is being encouraged by public education campaigns which have usually mixed and unclear objectives. They tend to aim simultaneously to: (a) prevent melanoma by giving advice about sun exposure and its reduction; (b) encourage a rapid response to suspicious lesions which the subject has already noticed by emphasising the importance of seeking medical advice for skin lesions which have certain "danger" signs; and (c) encourage the recognition of the early signs of melanoma by giving advice about these signs, and by encouraging people to inspect their own bodies and perhaps those of families and close friends. These education campaigns are often related not only to melanoma but to other skin cancers. It is often difficult to correctly assess even the objectives of some of these programmes, never mind attempting to evaluate whether these objectives are met.

1.1 Screening for Melanoma in Australia

The lifetime risk of developing melanoma is estimated as 1 in 55 in Australia, compared to 1 in 1.5 for non-melanoma skin cancer (MacLennan, 1987). There is a "National Skin Cancer Awareness" programme with activities being conducted in each state, mainly in early summer. Such programmes have been running since at least 1985, and are based mainly on screening caravans, referred to as "battle stations", which are placed at beaches, in city squares, and at other sites. The screening procedures offered have differed. Some, such as those in Victoria and South Australia, have offered only to examine a particular lesion about which the person is concerned. Others, for example in New South Wales and Western Australia, have offered to perform a fuller body examination of a person who has not presented with any particular lesion. Queensland has used a combination of these techniques.Usually no specific diagnoses are made, but patients with suspicious lesions are encouraged to visit their own doctor (R. Marks, personal communication).

There have been many other free screening clinics offered throughout the various states at different times of the year. The state cancer councils have advised on how these should be run, being in general along the lines of the screening caravans. The evaluation of outcome of these screening caravans has been relatively crude. Total numbers of subjects presenting, and the number of potential skin cancers diagnosed, have been the most widely used methods. There have also been a number of programmes based on workplaces, using videos relating to behaviour in the sun, the early recognition of suspicious lesions, and self-screening. The evaluation of the effect of professional education programmes has also been relatively limited. In most cases the number of booklets sent to doctors, whether or not they received them, and their opinions of them have been all that has been assessed.

The Anti-Cancer Council of Victoria is undertaking research on the feasibility and value of self-examination for melanoma, testing whether words, photographs, or a combination are better for various subgroups of the community. This research project still has several years to go before the investigators will be confident enough on the issue of whether a specific self-examination programme should be proposed to the public.

In 1990 the National Skin Cancer Awareness Programme is again focussing on the early detection of skin cancer. Material is being prepared on the management of skin cancer as a way of improving the professional's ability in early detection and management of melanoma and other skin cancers. The possibility of screening selected high-risk populations, for example subjects with dysplastic naevi, has been put on the agenda for discussion as part of the cancer control plan in Australia. Preliminary plans for the identification of high risk subjects and setting up registers have been made. For example in Queensland subjects with a family history of melanoma or evidence of the dysplastic naevus syndrome are entered onto a register, and their own doctors kept advised of the need for regular checking with the aim of early detection of changing lesions (McLeod,1988; R.McLeod, personal communication).

Anecdotally, many physicians feel that the greatest impact has been made by specific television programmes rather than media campaigns with a health education message. Professor McCarthy, of the Sydney Melanoma Programme, produced a television documentary based on a young patient who was dying from melanoma, which was shown on a peak time current affairs programme, and produced a major reaction with great increases in referrals for melanoma in the subsequent weeks. The programme was shown for the second time in the summer of 1989 with similar results. Professor McCarthy states that some 750 melanomas were diagnosed as a direct result of the television programme. In 1990 the Sydney melanoma group is conducting a further television, radio, and print media campaign entitled the "Mole Patrol", designed specifically to encourage people to look at their moles. It uses a 30 second television cartoon backed up by brochures (W. McCarthy, personal communication).

Consideration has been given to the need to set up more systematic screening programmes, either for high risk individuals, self-referred individuals, or whole populations. The suggestion has been made that technicians could be specially trained for such screening analagous to the professional input required for cervical or breast screening.

1.2 Screening for Melanoma in New Zealand

The problem of melanoma in New Zealand was reviewed in 1988 by an academic group (Elwood et al, 1988) who recommended a national policy including (1) an assessment of the current situation with regard to melanoma diagnosis; (2) a programme to improve early diagnosis by improving biopsy and referral facilities, refreshing the knowledge of medical practitioners, and by public education; (3) developmental work in health education aimed at primary prevention, and the development of evaluable public education projects; (4) an assessment of the potential value of the identification and surveillance of high risk subjects; and (5) monitoring the melanoma problem by assessing incidence, mortality, depth distribution, and treatment results.

In New Zealand, the main focus of activity has been the educational campaigns run for the public by the Cancer Society of New Zealand. These have been directed primarily to melanoma over the last two summers, and have used television, radio and magazine advertising, and publicity material sent to doctors, pharmacies, and schools primarily on the dangers of excessive sun exposure and suggestions on how it can be moderated. This is linked to messages on the danger signs for melanoma and the importance of rapid referral to a medical practitioner.

In addition, the Cancer Society has sponsored skin check days in most major urban centres and towns. These are sessions usually held on a Saturday, in which doctors, (general practitioners, dermatologists, and surgeons) operate a free very informal clinic to which people can come with skin lesions about which they are concerned. These patients are either reassured or advised to go back to their own doctors with a brief note about the lesion. The programmes have been given extensive local publicity. For the programme in the summer of 1988-89, a limited evaluation is in progress. From September 1988 to April 1989, the Cancer Society supported 22 skin spot check assessment days attended by 12,811 people (0.4 percent of the whole population). Results for the follow-up of the 746 patients attending one clinic are available; histologically confirmed tumours comprised 3 melanomas, 2 squamous cell carcinomas, and 8 basal cell carcinomas (K Cooke, personal communication).

A recent development (December 1989) has been that the Minister of Health of New Zealand has specified ten health targets to be the focus of the actions of area health boards over the next few years (New Zealand Department of Health, 1989). One of these is the early diagnosis of melanoma, the target being that the proportion of invasive melanomas diagnosed and treated at a thickness of less than 0.76mm should increase to at least 60 percent by 1995 and to 80 percent by 2000. These targets were set in the absence of good data on the current depth distribution of melanomas over the whole country. The setting of targets of depth distribution is of limited value because the ability to detect shifts is fairly limited. For example, data from the areas which have been surveyed suggest that currently about 56 percent of invasive melanomas are less than 0.76mm in thickness. This is very close to the first target of 60 percent recently set. To detect a shift in depth distribution from 50 to 60 percent, at 80 percent power using a one-sided test, would require the survey of some 300 melanomas in each time period, that is almost half the total number in New Zealand in a year. Thus surveillance over most of the country for a year would be required to adequately monitor a shift in depth distribution which may be of significant public health importance. Such surveillance requires a great improvement in current data sources. A larger shift, such as from 60 to 80 percent in the thinner category, could be ascertained on approximately 60 subjects, which is a much more reasonable number as it would be typical of the annual number of new cases in one of New Zealand's 15 health board areas.

The methods suggested to achieve this include the education of medical practitioners and the public about early diagnosis and treatment, and the extension and improvement of referral services to ensure reduction in delays for consultations for suspected malignant lesions (Elwood et al, 1988; New Zealand Department of Health, 1989). A committee is being set up to advise Area Health Boards about appropriate steps to take, which are likely to be based on the recommendations of Elwood et al (1988).

1.3. Monitoring for the Effect of Education Campaigns
To examine some of the effects of the New Zealand educational campaigns, a system has been set up to register and record the depth of melanomas in a number of areas in New Zealand. Preliminary data for two areas show that before the campaign, 55 percent of invasive melanomas were under 0.76mm in depth, with no change seen after the campaign; but more areas will be studied before conclusions are reached (K Cooke, personal communication). This pre-campaign depth distribution is favourable in comparison to that in Glasgow after successful programmes, suggesting an already high level of awareness.

It is not yet clear whether pre-invasive melanoma should be regarded as a separate entity or in continuum with thin, invasive melanoma. If it is a separate state which is a precursor of invasive melanoma, the progression rate to invasive melanoma may be much below 100 percent. The prime objective of screening can be seen as being to reduce the total frequency of invasive melanoma, an increased rate of diagnosis of pre-invasive melanoma being seen as a necessary nuisance; the analogy is with the detection of pre-invasive carcinoma of the cervix. The effect of screening on the depth distribution of invasive melanoma could be paradoxical; if for example, screening caused earlier detection primarily of the slower growing lesions, the proportion of invasive tumours detected while thin could decrease despite a partially effective screening programme. If pre-invasive melanoma is seen as a continuum with thin, invasive melanoma, screening could be assessed by a downward shift in depth distribution of total melanoma. However, in either scenario, the absolute rates of deep melanoma on a population basis, and in the longer term the death rates, are a better guide.

2.0 THE OPTIONS FOR SCREENING

2.1 General Population Screening by Professionals

Consideration of melanoma in comparison with the classic guidelines for the applicability of general population screening (Burr and Elwood, 1985) does not produce an unequivocal response. In terms of frequency, melanoma is currently the most common invasive cancer (that is, excluding in situ carcinoma of the cervix) in adults aged 20-40 in New Zealand, and probably in all areas of Australia (Elwood et al, 1988; Giles et al, 1982). Its relative frequency is lower at older ages, but in total it is a frequent cancer, causing more deaths than for example uterine cervical cancer, although it is still relatively small in comparison with breast or colo-rectal cancer.

Melanoma is a serious disease, although current survival rates are relatively high, with five year survival rates of around 85 percent being reported from the South Australian Registry (South Australia Cancer Registry, 1986). To some extent of course these good survival rates may reflect the impact of past programmes of public and professional awareness, even in the absence of organised screening.

In terms of natural history, there is a very rapid change in post-diagnosis survival rates in terms of the depth of invasion of the initial tumour. While this does not necessarily mean that chronologically earlier diagnosis will result in a truly better survival, beyond the effects of lead time, it certainly carries an implication that earlier diagnosis may produce better survival. The variation in survival with total tumour burden at diagnosis, as assessed by depth of invasion in these relatively small area tumours on a visible surface, seems very considerable and is likely to be greater than that of other cancers. Thus in terms of the prevalence of the disease, its seriousness, and its natural history, there does appear to be a reasonable prima facie case for the consideration of screening.

The great difficulty arises with the definition of a suitable test. We can consider three issues; the early warning signs of an in situ or invasive melanoma; the existence of specific precursor lesions; and the existence of markers of high risk which are not necessarily precursor lesions.

Early signs of melanoma   Screening procedures can be orientated towards the recognition of early signs of invasive disease, either before these are known to the patient, or even (by a moderate extension of the definition of screening) before the patient has had sufficient motivation to take action.

Clinical experience of melanoma has resulted in a number of lists of early signs and symptoms of melanoma, such as the A,B,C,D,E list used by Fitzpatrick et al (1988) in the United States, and the seven point check list suggested by MacKie in Glasgow (MacKie and Doherty, 1988) (Table 1).

Table 1 Warning signs of melanoma (from Elwood et al, 1988)

First indication of a melanoma*	Percent	Signs of melanoma: the ABCDE list **	Signs of melanoma: the Glasgow 7 point checklist ***
(a) classic presentation	65	Asymmetry - in shape	1. mild itch
changes in a mole one or more of: enlargement, colour change, pain or bleeding		Border is irregular - edges scalloped Colour - haphazard display of shades of brown, blue gray, white	2. over 1cm diameter 3. recent growth 4. irregular edge 5. irregular pigmentation
(b) suspicious lesion, not noted by patient	24	Diameter is large - greater than a pencil: 6.0 mm	6. inflammation 7. oozing and crusting
(c) new mole	8	Elevation is almost always present - assessed by side lighting if subtle	

* First event noticed by the patient or other person which led to the diagnosis of melanoma; percentages refer to first sign in 651 patients from a defined population, 3 percent had other or unrecorded first signs (Elwood and Gallagher, 1988)

** Suspicious signs in a pigmented skin lesion (Fitzpatrick et al, 1988)

*** Suspicious signs and symptoms in a pigmented skin lesion, referral recommended if 3 or more are present (MacKie and Doherty, 1988)

These are put forward as clinical guides, but their usefulness is limited. For example the A,B,C,D,E list consists of five factors which are given as suspicious signs in a pigmented skin lesion, given that the patient has already taken the initiative of coming to a physician. Decision criteria related to the presence of one, several, or all of these signs have not been specifically suggested. The Glasgow checklist, although still based on clinical experience rather than empiric testing, is a little more specific in that Professor MacKie intends its use primarily for general practitioners, stating that patients who have lesions in which three of more of the seven signs or symptoms are present should be referred for a specialist opinion. In a recent study in Nottingham (England), we were able to demonstrate some validity of this technique, in that of 23 melanomas detected in a specific population over a given time period, 21 had at least three of the seven signs, whereas in all patients referred for a hospital opinion 326 out of 861 patients without melanoma had these signs (Whitehead et al, 1989). Thus, the 'sensitivity' is 91 percent, 'specificity' is 62 percent - clearly very low, and 'predictive value positive' is 6.4 percent. But these figures relate only to patients referred by the general practitioner and will be over-optimistic if applied to all patients visiting a general practitioner. We do not know the frequency of these signs in all patients coming for a general practitioner's opinion, or indeed in the general population.

Lists based on clinical experience can be supplemented by studies in which a systematic assessment has been made in a representative series of patients. In the Western Canadian study, subjects were asked in an unprompted question what were the first indications of the melanoma which was ultimately diagnosed (Elwood and Gallagher, 1988). This showed that four changes were most commonly present, that a substantial proportion of lesions were not noted by the patient but were regarded as suspicious by a health professional or a lay person, and that a small proportion of melanomas arose from what the patient regarded as new moles. In a similar although less detailed study in Queensland, 23 percent of melanomas were recognised by a doctor before the patient had noticed anything wrong and a further 20 percent were noticed by a lay person other than the patient, usually a family member (Green, 1982). The corresponding proportions in Western Canada were 14 percent and 25 percent (Elwood and Gallagher, 1988). These high proportions indicate the potential value of simple screening, that is inspection of skin, by health professionals or by relatives or friends of the subject.

2.2 Screening in the General Population

It may be useful to consider specific screening interventions which could be applied for melanoma in a general population, and see how they relate to the criteria for a suitable screening test (Burr and Elwood, 1985). A suitable test should be simple and capable of rapid application; acceptable in terms of inconvenience, discomfort, and risks; reproducible in its results; and with known validity and performance characteristics. The first is a regular examination of the skin by the patient's general practitioner. This can hardly be regarded as a simple technique capable of rapid application; it involves a patient visit to a general practitioner, taking some 15-30 minutes if done thoroughly, and complete undressing. It is quite expensive, as at least the normal consultation fee for a general practitioner, (around $30 in New Zealand) would be necessary, and perhaps a further charge given the length of time involved.

In regard to the second criterion, that it should be acceptable to the subject, this may well be true at least in high risk areas such as Australia, but has not really been tested, and would probably in practice depend considerably on the costs involved. The procedure can certainly be regarded as free of major discomfort or side effects, although not free of inconvenience. In terms of reproducibility and validity, there is little information available. Efforts in research studies to achieve high reproducibility in counting naevi, or assessing dysplastic versus normal naevi, have not been very encouraging, showing that inter-observer variation in the assessment of pigmented lesions is very considerable. The greatest difficulty at present is that there is no research which assesses what measures should be emphasised during a general skin examination, and the frequencies in a general population of the early signs given by various authorities (Table 1), are unknown. The effects of general skin examinations done regularly on the number and cost of further follow-up visits, hospital referrals, and biopsy rates, are unknown.

Thus the use of a general skin examination by a health professional on a general population basis cannot be recommended as a screening test on current evidence, mainly because the performance of the test procedure is unknown. "A complete annual examination of the skin by a physician" has been recommended by many US authorities (e.g.Friedman et al, 1985). Such a recommendation is unjustified without information on its validity, reproducibility, and ill effects such as unnecessary biopsies or anxiety, and the costs involved make it unrealistic as part of a comprehensive health care service for whole populations, as distinct from a private practice situation.

In the US, the main impetus for such screening is from dermatologists. In New Zealand, there are about one million adults aged 35-64; annual screening even at an unrealistic 6 patients per hour, 35 hours per week, and 48 weeks per year would employ 100 examiners full time. There are only 40 full-time equivalent dermatologists. There are some 2400 general practitioners: screening by them would mean each general practitioner devoting four percent of his or her time to such screening.

A second main option is self-screening, that is providing subjects in the population with information allowing them to assess their own skin, and perhaps those of family members and close friends, and then seeking the advice of a health professional if suspicious findings emerge. The issues here are very similar. While such a method appears attractive because it would avoid the cost implications of the professional examination, the procedure is hardly simple, and the response to it in a general population has not been tested. There would be a similar situation as applies to breast self-examination, in that the completeness and thoroughness of self-examination would need to be considered. It is possible that the test would be more acceptable to subjects, and to the health care system in terms of costs, than regular physician examination. The main problems of course are in terms of validity and reproducibility, which are unknown, and in the effects of such a programme on further visits to doctors, hospital referrals, and biopsies, in comparison to any benefit in terms of the early diagnosis of melanoma.

2.3   Identification of Precursor Lesions

Efforts in this area have of course concentrated on dysplastic naevi, although it is still not clear to what extent dysplastic naevi can be regarded as a precursor state of melanoma, as distinct from a risk indicator.   It is clear primarily from the NIH family studies in the United States that subjects with a family history of melanoma plus a personal history of dysplastic naevi have an extremely high subsequent risk of melanoma (Greene et al, 1985). In an assessment based on the published material up to 1987 (which may need to be updated), the importance of this group, in terms of the whole problem, appears to be small (Elwood, 1989). There have been 14 families studied, each having at least two members with melanoma, and the results relate to the frequency of melanoma in other family members.   The most important group is composed of family members who had dysplastic naevi.   This group has a relative risk of 148 and a prospectively measured absolute risk of 7.2 percent over 8 years.   This is based on 77 subjects, 398 person-years of follow-up (average 5.2 years per subject), and four observed melanomas versus 0.027 expected. The eight year cumulative risk has a large standard error: the 95 percent two-sided confidence limits are from 0.14 percent to 14 percent.   Further data have been published in less detail (Tucker and Bale, 1988), and a reassessment of this evidence is due.

The central issue here is the prevalence in the whole population of individuals with the combination of a family history of two or more relatives with melanoma and the presence of dysplastic naevi.   The NIH group estimated this as 0.014 percent of the population (Kraemer et al, 1983), and their data gave an incidence rate of melanoma of 1005/100,000 per year (approximately 1 percent) in such subjects (Greene et al, 1985).   Consider a population of 1 million in a high-risk area, giving in total some 200 new cases of melanoma per year.   There will be 0.014 percent;   that is, 140 high-risk subjects, who will have an expected number of 1.4 melanomas, using the NIH rate.   Thus, while the identification and surveillance of such subjects may be important for research and may be useful for those subjects, it will not make a major impact on the whole problem of melanoma.   Thus we have not stressed it in the New Zealand melanoma control strategy (Elwood et al, 1988).   These conclusions could, of course, change as better information concerning the risks, and particularly the prevalence, of this and other high-risk states becomes available. More recent reviews do not provide any better data on prevalence (Tucker and Bale, 1988; Elder, 1988).

Identification and surveillance of high-risk subjects should be considered on an individual basis.   In this regard, further results from the NIH and other studies are useful.   No increased risk has been seen in members of these families who did not themselves have dysplastic naevi;   therefore, the risk group is composed of members of families with at least two persons affected with dysplastic naevi.   Patients who have already had a melanoma are at an increased risk of subsequent new tumours, and, if they also have this strong family history and dysplastic naevi, their risk is very high: 33 percent at 8 years (Greene et al, 1985).   However, such subjects should already be under good follow-up for their first melanoma.

2.4 High-risk Subjects: Other Risk Markers

A considerable number of other risk markers for melanoma can be considered. These include a family history of melanoma in at least one relative, which gives a relative risk of 2-5 (Tucker, 1988), and the presence of dysplastic naevi without a family history of melanoma, which confers a relative risk of around 7 (Kraemer et al, 1986; Tucker, 1988). These, however, are lower than the risks given by several other simpler measures. Epidemiologic studies of melanoma have involved interviewing and examining patients and unaffected control subjects in their own homes, using a lay or nurse interviewer. In these circumstances, only a very limited examination is possible, and reliable and simple methods have been developed. These can be shown to be as good at defining high-risk subjects as some more complex methods, such as those involving whole body examination by dermatologists and assessments of dysplastic naevi.

We have reviewed available studies in regard to their application to the New Zealand situation (Elwood, 1989) and some results are shown in Table 2. Thus, in two UK studies, the risks of melanoma in subjects who (a) had three or more palpable naevi on the upper arm, assessed by a lay interviewer, or (b) had 50 or more naevi greater than 2mm in diameter on the whole body, assessed by a dermatologist, were in absolute terms very similar. In Australia, subjects who (a) had five or more palpable naevi on the arm, assessed by a nurse interviewer, and those who (b) had two or more naevi of 2mm or greater diameter on the arm, assessed by a physician, had similar risks.

Table 2 suggests that a simple method, based on a limited examination by a lay person, or even on a self-reporting basis, may be as valuable at identifying high-risk subjects as a time consuming full examination by a dermatologist. However, whether any of these methods is a good enough risk indicator to be used on a large scale is unclear. Applying the Australian criteria of five or more raised moles isolates 7 percent of the population who have 28 percent of the melanomas, but a ten year risk of only 1.8 percent. Thus in terms of a population of 1 million, identification of 70,000 subjects and surveillance for ten years might lead to the early diagnosis of melanoma in 1,260 subjects; 68,740 would have had the surveillance unnecessarily. Whether this balance is acceptable will depend on the resources available. A useful analogy is the treatment of mild hypertension. The ten year risk of a cardiovascular death in mildly hypertensive subjects in a large Australian trial was 2.6 percent (Management Committee, 1980), similar to the melanoma risk in a high risk group. The treatment of mild hypertension requires anti-hypertensive drugs and regular visits to a general practitioner; it may be comparable in terms of time and cost to the institution of regular skin surveillance by general practitioners. However if surveillance of such high risk people could be carried out effectively by an occasional visit to a general practitioner or other health professional, supplemented by teaching in self-examination, the costs might be considerably less than those currently accepted for the control of mild hypertension, with perhaps a greater benefit.

Table 2 Application of data on risk markers to a high-risk population, with an annual melanoma incidence rate of 45 per 100,000, as applies to adults age 35-69 in New Zealand (from Elwood, 1989)

Indicator and source	Prevalence in community (%) [a]	Relative risk [b]	Incidence in high-risk subjects: Annual per 100,000	Percent, over 10 years	Percent of melanomas in high-risk group
Whole-body examinations by specialists:					
1+ atypical naevi					
Sydney [c1]	7.1	6.6	213	2.1	34
> 50 naevi >2mm					
Scotland [c2]	4.6	9.2	289	3.0	32
1+ naevi with an irregular					
edge, Scotland [c2]	1.0	37.5	1236	11.6	27
Arm examination by general physician:					
2+ naevi >2mm left arm					
Queensland [c3]	25	15.8	152	1.6	84
Arm examination by lay examiner or nurse:					
5+ palpable naevi on arms,					
West Australia [c4]	7.0	5.1	178	1.8	28
Multiple naevi on limbs,					
(women only), Sydney [c5]	2.4	3.5	150	1.5	8
3+ palpable naevi on arms,					
Nottingham [c6]	4.8	14.4	365	3.6	41
Subjects response to questioning:					
> 15 moles on body,					
(interview) Nottingham [c6]	6.0	6.7	225	2.2	30
> 100 moles on body,					
(questionnaire) New York [c7]	2.7	2.7	117	1.2	7

Footnotes:

a, given by frequency of marker in the unaffected control group in the original study.

b, risk in those with, compared to those without, the risk marker (odds ratio). Calculated from the raw data where possible, as it is the crude ratio which is relevant.

c, References: 1. Nordlund et al, 1985; 2. Swerdlow et al, 1984; 3. Green et al, 1985; 4. Holman and Armstrong, 1984; Armstrong et al, 1986; 5. Beral et al, 1983; 6. Elwood et al, 1986; 7. Dubin et al, 1986.

A more extensive analysis using the Western Australia case-control study (English and Armstrong, 1988) shows that while the number of naevi was the major predictor of risk, additional discrimination power was given by four other variables; arrival in Australia before 10 years of age, history of non-melanoma skin cancer, time spent outdoors in summer between ages 10 and 24, and family history of melanoma. However, the reproducibility of the more complex questions outside the context of a well designed case-control study using trained interviewers is doubtful, and the difference in performance of the chosen model over a one-factor model is moderate. Thus the suggested five factor model isolated, from an independent sample of 111 case-control pairs, 16 percent of controls and 54 percent of melanoma patients; the single factor of "5 or more raised naevi on the arms" isolated 8 percent of controls and 50 percent of cases, although on all the available data the figures were 7 percent of controls and 28 percent of cases [Table 2]. For screening purposes, simplicity and reproducibility are paramount, and the extra information given by the more complex model suggested may not be a valuable addition in wider application.

3. RECOMMENDATIONS

Currently, screening programmes, as distinct from attempts to improve early diagnosis, cannot be recommended for melanoma on a general population basis, primarily because the specific tests to be used have not been defined and their validity and performance characteristics have not been assessed. On the basis of its overall frequency, seriousness, and the evidence that chronologically earlier diagnosis is likely to result in considerably improved survival, melanoma can however be considered a prime candidate for screening and early diagnosis programmes. This suggests that there is a high research priority to develop and validate particular tests for early diagnosis of melanoma, and for the identification of high risk subjects who might benefit from organised surveillance.

Acknowledgements
I thank Drs Robin Marks, Bill McCarthy, Rod McLeod, and Bob MacLennan for giving useful information.

REFERENCES

Armstrong BK, de Klerk NH and Holman CDJ: Etiology of common acquired melanocytic nevi: constitutional variables, sun exposure, and diet. JNCI, 1986; 77:329-335.

Beral V, Evans S, Shaw H and Milton G: Cutaneous factors related to the risk of malignant melanoma. Br J Dermatol, 1983; 109:165-172.

Burr ML and Elwood PC: Research and development of health promotion services-screening. In: Holland WW, Detels R, Knox G, (eds.). Oxford Textbook of Public Health, volume 3. Oxford, 1985, pp373-384.

Dubin N, Moseson M and Pasternack BS: Epidemiology of malignant melanoma: pigmentary traits, ultraviolet radiation, and the identification of high risk populations. In: Gallagher RP, (ed.). Epidemiology of Malignant Melanoma. Recent results in cancer research, Vol 102. Springer-Verlag, Heidelberg, 1986, pp38-55.

Elder DE: Dysplastic naevus syndrome - biological significance. Seminars in Oncology, 1988; 15:529-540.

Elwood JM: Epidemiology and control of melanoma in white populations and in Japan. J Invest Dermatol, 1989; 92:214S-221S.

Elwood JM, Cooke KR, Coombs BD, Cox B, Hand JE and Skegg DCG: A strategy for the control of malignant melanoma in New Zealand. NZMJ, 1988; 101:602-604.

Elwood JM and Gallagher RP: The first signs and symptoms of melanoma: a population based study. In: Elwood JM, (ed.). Naevi and Melanoma: Incidence, Interrelationships and Implications; Pigment Cell no 9. Basel, Karger, 1988, pp118-130

Elwood JM, Williamson C and Stapleton PJ: Malignant melanoma in relation to moles, pigmentation, and exposure to fluorescent and other lighting sources. Br J Cancer, 1986; 53:65-74.

English DR and Armstrong BK: Identifying people at high risk of cutaneous malignant melanoma: results from a case-control study in Western Australia. Br Med J, 1988; 296:1285-1288.

Fitzpatrick TB, Rhodes AR, Sober AJ and Mihm CM Jr: Primary malignant melanoma of the skin: the call for action to identify persons at risk; to discover precursor lesions; to detect early melanomas. In: Elwood JM, (ed.). Naevi and Melanoma: Incidence, Interrelationships and Implications; Pigment Cell no 9. Basel, Karger, 1988, pp110-117.

Friedman RJ, Rigel DS and Kopf AW: Early detection of malignant melanoma: the role of physician examination and self-examination of the skin. Ca, a Cancer Journal for Clinicians, 1985; 35:130-151.

Giles GG, Armstrong BK and Smith LN: Cancer in Australia. Australian Institute of Health, Canberra 1982.

Green A: Incidence and reporting of cutaneous melanoma in Queensland. Aust J Derm, 1982; 23:105-109.

Green A, MacLennan R and Siskind V: Common acquired naevi and the risk of malignant melanoma. Int J Cancer, 1985; 35:297-300.

Greene MH, Clark WH Jr, Tucker MA, Kraemer KH, Elder DE and Fraser MC: High risk of malignant melanoma in melanoma-prone families with dysplastic nevi. Ann Intern Med, 1985; 102:458-465.

Holman CD and Armstrong BK: Pigmentary traits, ethnic origin, benign nevi, and family history as risk factors for cutaneous malignant melanoma. JNCI, 1984; 72:257-266.

Kraemer KH, Greene MH, Tarone R, Elder DE, Clark WH Jr and Guerry DIV: Dysplastic naevi and cutaneous melanoma risk. Lancet, 1983; ii:1076-1077.

Kraemer KH, Tucker M, Tarone R, Elder DE and Clark WH Jr: Risk of cutaneous melanoma in dysplastic nevus syndrome Types A and B. N Engl J Med, 1986; 315:1615-1616.

MacKie RM and Doherty VR: Educational activities aimed at earlier detection and treatment of malignant melanoma in a moderate risk area. In: Elwood JM, (ed.). Naevi and Melanoma: Incidence, Interrelationships and Implications; Pigment Cell no 9. Basel, Karger, 1988, pp140-152

MacLennan R: A national cancer prevention policy for Australia. Australian Cancer Society, volume 2 1987.

Management Committee: The Australian therapeutic trial in mild hypertension. Lancet 1:1261-1267, 1980

McLeod GR: Control of melanoma in high-risk populations. In: Elwood JM, (ed.). Naevi and Melanoma: Incidence, Interrelationships and Implications; Pigment Cell no 9. Basel, Karger, 1988, pp131-139.

New Zealand Department of Health: New Zealand Health Goals and Targets. Wellington, 1989, p30.

Nordlund JJ, Kirkwood J, Forget BM, Scheibner A, Albert DM, Lerner E and Milton GW: Demographic study of clinically atypical (dysplastic) nevi in patients with melanoma and comparison subjects. Cancer Res, 1985; 45:1855-1861.

South Australian Cancer Registry: Epidemiology of Cancer in South Australia: incidence, mortality and survival 1977-1984, incidence and mortality 1984. South Australian Health Commission, Australia, Adelaide, 1986.

Swerdlow AJ, English J, MacKie RM, O'Doherty CJ, Hunter JAA, and Clark J: Benign naevi associated with high risk of melanoma. Lancet, 1984; ii:168.

Tucker MA: Individuals at high risk of melanoma. In: Elwood JM, (ed.). Melanoma and Naevi: Incidence, Interrelationships and Implications; Pigment Cell No 9. Basel, Karger, 1988, pp95-109.

Tucker MA and Bale SJ: Clinical aspects of familial cutaneous malignant melanoma. Seminars in Oncology, 1988; 15:542-548.

Whitehead SM, Wroughton MA, Elwood JM, Davison J and Stewart M: Effects of a health education campaign for the earlier diagnosis of melanoma. Br J Cancer, 1989; 60:421-425.

26 Screening for Melanoma in the UK

R. ELLMAN

Cancer Screening Evaluation Unit, Institute of Cancer Research Section of Epidemiology, Sutton, Surrey, U.K.

1 INTRODUCTION

Two factors have led to interest in screening for melanoma. The first is that the possibility of detecting the disease while it is easily curable seems high. The second is that, though the disease is rare, accounting for 1113 deaths (19.5 per million population) in the UK in 1984, both its incidence and mortality have increased steeply over the last 40 years. A rise in affluence, leading to more holidays taken abroad, changing fashions in clothing and sunbathing, and the use of sun lamps are the probable explanation.

Incidence rates have been increasing more steeply than mortality rates but this may, in part, be due to increased ascertainment. An improvement in survival rates is largely attributable to diagnosis at an earlier stage rather than to discovery of more effective treatments.

2 STRATEGIES FOR REDUCING MELANOMA MORTALITY

Primary prevention of melanoma should obviously be encouraged, but advice to avoid intense exposure to ultra-violet light, though uncontentious, is little heeded by young people.

The rarity of melanoma makes professional screening, meaning repeated whole body examination after baseline photography, inappropriate for mass application. It has, however, been suggested that six-monthly examination is appropriate for individuals at high risk of melanoma because they have dysplastic naevi and a family history of melanoma (Greene et al, 1984). In Britain the number of such people is not known and there has been no systematic effort to provide professional screening for them.

The alternative is to promote awareness of melanoma risk and encourage self-examination. Information that cancer can arise in moles and that changing moles should be reported to a doctor is now included in general health education courses and literature. In addition, publicity campaigns can be mounted and this is the main strategy which has been employed in Britain.

MacKie et al (1989) have recently suggested another approach: that people should be informed about their personal risk of melanoma by the use of a chart which divides people into four risk groups, taking into account gender, freckles, benign naevi, atypical naevi and previous episodes of sunburn. The validity of the relative risk coefficients requires testing on an independent sample, and the prevalence of the risk factors in a large and representative sample of the UK population would need to be discovered before endorsing this selective programme.   A selective approach is appropriate if a high proportion of melanomas occur in a small, easily defined sector of the population.

2.1 Health Education Campaigns and Pigmented Lesion Clinics

Information on early efforts to promote public and professional education about melanoma is fragmentary.   A pigmented lesion clinic (PLC) was started in Southampton (Southampton Melanoma Group, 1986) in 1981. Its purpose was to reduce delays in referral and an information pack was distributed to general practitioners (GPs). Over a period of three years and nine months 75 melanomas were discovered at the clinic. The mean thickness, as measured by the Breslow method, 2.42 mm, was not significantly lower than among patients referred elsewhere, or seen in Southampton in the previous five years; it was concluded that efforts to minimize delays between the patient presenting to a GP and excision of the tumour at hospital do not improve prognosis. A campaign to educate the public as well as GPs, involving broadcasts and distribution of posters, took place in the Bristol area in 1983 but its impact was not evaluated.

2.2   The Glasgow Campaign

In 1985 a more ambitious programme was mounted in Glasgow (Doherty and MacKie, 1988). The main purpose was to increase public knowledge about the disease, since a previous study in Glasgow had shown that the main reason for delay in presentation was ignorance (Doherty and MacKie, 1986). General practitioners were fully briefed in the first four months of the year, and all 650 received a specially prepared booklet 'An illustrated guide to early malignant melanoma' (MacKie, 1986). A weekly PLC had been in existence for many years and, until the campaign, gave immediate appointments to all, provided they had a GP referral.

Distribution of leaflets and posters was organized and a press release issued to local and national Scottish radio, television and newspaper services during May, with a request to maximize publicity in June. The publicity given to the campaign in all kinds of programmes and articles was such that it must have reached a very wide cross-section of the public, not only in Glasgow but in Scotland as a whole and even in England.

The campaign had an immediate effect on the workload of all dermatology departments in Glasgow, even though the majority of extra patients were referred to the PLC. It also had an effect in other Scottish cities. Questionnaires filled in by patients with pigmented lesions in Edinburgh showed that the publicity had been noted as much there as in Glasgow, though in Dundee it had been less influential. Plans to use Edinburgh as a control district were thereby thwarted.

Melanoma registries have been maintained by the Scottish Melanoma Group. In 1985 these showed a 28% increase in cases in the West of Scotland, the region including Glasgow, over the number detected in 1984. The increase was largely confined to lesions under 1.5 mm which showed a 46% increase, but in 1986 the number of thick melanomas over 3.5 mm, which had previously been fairly constant, also rose by 23% so that it is perhaps misleading to describe this as a "statistically significant fall in the proportion of thick lesions" (Doherty and Mackie, 1988). Hopefully longer follow-up will find a reduction in late stage incidence but this is not certain.

2.3 The CRC Campaign

A larger programme involving seven centres (Table 1) was next initiated by the Cancer Research Campaign (CRC). It was inspired by the experience of the Glasgow campaign and the basic elements - namely PLCs, preliminary GP education, summer publicity campaigns, and monitoring of attendance and melanoma detection - were the same.

Table 1 CRC Campaign

Centre	Target Populations
Exeter	300,000
Leicester	860,000
Edinburgh	700,000
Southampton	410,000
Nottingham	610,000
St. George's Hospital London	530,000
King's College Hospital, London	212,000

A CRC Malignant Melanoma Campaign Education Coordinator was appointed to supervise distribution of publicity material and conduct studies on health education.

Each centre organized a programme of GP education during the first half of 1987. Posters and leaflets were designed after consultation with consumer groups. They depicted a mole dressed as Sherlock Holmes and showed close-up photographs of moles to illustrate the suspicious signs of melanoma. Mackie's checklist of seven danger signs and symptoms was included, and advice was given on avoiding sunburn. The posters and leaflets were distributed to doctors' surgeries and to libraries, pharmacies, travel agents and beauticians. Despite the pictures of melanomas they were considered attractive and non-threatening.

A press release on the campaign was issued to national media by the CRC, and to local media by the centres themselves for a launch on July 8th, 1987. Some centres also conducted publicity campaigns in the two following years, but it was agreed not to mount another national campaign because of the strain the first campaign had put on services; by 1988 the PLCs were already filled to capacity and it was felt that there was sufficient attention given to melanoma by the media to make solicited programmes and articles unneccesssary.

PLCs were held weekly in each centre. They were additional to regular dermatology clinics, and some received support for extra staff from the CRC. Patients required a GP's letter of referral but appointments were either immediate or after considerably shorter delays than in ordinary dermatology clinics, only exceeding an average of four weeks in one centre. In Southampton the dermatologists diverted all referrals for pigmented lesion to the PLC irrespective of the dermatologist to whom they were addressed, whereas in other centres the PLC saw only those directly referred.

It was originally envisaged that demonstration of an increase in the number of melanomas detected and reduction in the proportion of thick melanomas would provide adequate evidence that the campaign was beneficial.

Eligibility for participation in the campaign depended on a centre's possession of a melanoma register covering the preceding five years. But beyond stating that records should include the Breslow thickness of the lesions no stipulations were made on the content of these registers.

Monitoring of control centres was discussed but rejected. The arguments against the proposal included concern that the effects of the health education campaign would be widespread throughout Britain and hence that comparisons would lead to under-estimation of its true value, and secondly a belief that it would be difficult and perhaps unethical to dissuade doctors interested enough to keep adequate records from mounting their own local campaigns during the period of follow-up.

The immediate effect of publicity was measured by counting referrals to the dermatology clinics involved during the six months before and the six months after the campaign launch. The effect on general practice workloads was monitored by asking a sample of GPs in each district to note the number of patients attending because of pigmented lesions and to record whether, in each case, the patient was referred to a dermatologist. As the period monitored followed the professional education period, the proportion referred is a measure of the appropriateness of self-referrals and of the GP's response to an increased attendance rate, rather than a measure of the effectiveness of professional education.

The PLCs were required to fill in a standard proforma on each patient attending the clinic. In addition to the normal identification details, the patients were asked to fill in questions on publicity they had seen, persons from whom advice had been sought, and the length of time since they first noticed change or new appearance of a mole. The doctor filled in details about the lesion including site, size and presence or absence of the seven danger signs and symptoms of MacKie's checklist (1986). The final diagnosis for those biopsied was also entered. The campaign, working with a small budget, at first relied on existing staff at the CRC's Clinical Trials Centre to enter the data on computer, but in 1990 the partially computerized data were transferred to the Cancer Screening Evaluation Unit and a part-time research assistant was employed to assist in searching for missing data. The PLC records will provide information about the characteristics of patients attending the clinics and their lesions, attendance rates, biopsy rates and melanoma prevalence among PLC attenders.

2.4 Population-Based Analysis

The defined populations for purposes of reporting incidence will be based on Health Authority District figures. Some centres have collected information on Health District residents who have been referred with pigmented lesions to other dermatologists, but in other centres referral rates will be based on the PLC figures alone and will consequently underestimate referral rates.

The completeness of melanoma registers is also variable at present. Some centres include cases sought from cancer registries, nearby laboratories and other dermatologists, but others are incomplete. Dermatologists' melanoma registers and cancer registries tend to be complementary in that cancer registries, which rely on hospital discharge records, tend to miss melanomas excised without hospital admission, while dermatologists tend to miss advanced cases which are referred to plastic or general surgeons. Linkage between all pathology laboratories and cancer registries has yet to be introduced in the UK but should improve melanoma registration in the future.

2.5 Mortality Data

The Cancer Screening Evaluation Unit proposes to monitor mortality from melanoma in the campaign districts and compare it with mortality in other health districts, which, though they may have been affected by media publicity given to the 'Mole Watch' campaign, have not been otherwise involved.

Six regional cancer registries covering the campaign districts will be requested to provide copies of death certificates mentioning melanoma, and information about place of residence and date of diagnosis. Cases will be sorted, by district of residence at the time of diagnosis, into those of campaign areas and those of areas acting as comparison districts. The cumulative mortality from melanoma of the two groups for cases diagnosed from July 1987, when the publicity campaign began, will be compared over a period of least seven years.

The populations of the seven campaign districts total over three million, and the remainder of the regions total at least four times as many. Estimates based on incidence and survival figures for the pre-trial period indicate that the cumulative number of deaths for cases aged 20-74 years will be adequate to give 80% power of detecting a 20% reduction in melanoma mortality if follow-up is continued for seven years. Such sample size calculations are, however, of limited value as the melanoma incidence rates and the survival rates are both rising. Since a true effect may be underestimated if the publicity on melanoma has affected the comparison populations, it would be valuable to demonstrate as significant even a more modest difference. Longer follow-up would be justified, provided districts maintain a PLC and continue to promote education on melanoma more vigorously than the comparison districts. Some centres plan to do so.

2.6   Pathological Definition and Consistency

The setting up of a Pathology Panel is still under discussion. Its objective would be to promote a more consistent use of terminology and, by reviewing cases arising from the campaign, or at least a sample of them, to discover the level of inter-observer consistency. A similar exercise in Western Australia, confined to melanoma cases, found 6% of original diagnoses to be false (English et al, 1986), reported excellent consistency among the six experienced pathologists on Breslow thickness measurement, but only moderate consistency on Clark level and histogenetic type (Heenan et al, 1984). Consistency in distinguishing melanomas from borderline lesions (dyplastic naevi) is important and cases in borderline categories should be included. The importance of distinguishing between invasive and non-invasive melanomas will be increased if recent findings of Moore et al (1990) are confirmed. They report that factors such as moles, skin type and colouring, which are associated with risk of invasive melanoma, are not associated with increased risk of non-invasive melanoma and suggest that many of the non- invasive melanomas which are detected with greater frequency as awareness increases may not be progressive. At present the international coding system (ICD, Ninth Revision) classifies invasive melanoma separately from other skin neoplasms but does not separately classify in-situ melanomas. This has led to inconsistencies between registries in the categories which they include in incidence figures.

2.7   Published Findings from the CRC Campaign Centres

Public knowledge of melanoma   A postal survey of knowledge and attitudes towards moles was conducted in early 1987, while professional education was going on but before the publicity campaign was launched. Manchester and Cardiff, which were not involved in the campaign, as well as three of the campaign districts, Nottingham, Southampton and Edinburgh, were included and the same questionnaire was sent out to a new sample a year later so that before and after comparisons could be made. The samples, each of 250 adults, were randomly selected from electoral registers. The pre-campaign findings (Newman et al, 1988) have been published showing that there was a 63% response rate and that 26% of respondents knew the word 'melanoma' (though a greater proportion knew that moles can become malignant) while 28% had already seen some publicity about moles or skin cancers.

Workload generated by the CRC Campaign   Three of the centres participating in the CRC Campaign have published findings (Nicholls, 1988; Whitehead et al, 1989; Graham-Brown et al, 1990) from which the following notes are drawn. Comparisons need to be treated with caution as the method of analysis is not uniform.

GP and PLC attendance   GP consultation rates rose fourfold in the first three weeks of the campaign in Leicester and, averaged over longer periods, had approximately doubled in Nottingham and Southampton. GPs in Southampton referred 39% of their patients with pigmented lesions to a dermatologist during the campaign, whereas in the pre-campaign period they referred 53%. The increase in GP workload (to, at most, three cases per GP per week) caused no problems but the increased attendance at PLCs necessitated extra sessions and caused the waiting time for appointments to lengthen in Nottingham.

The number of patients seen in the PLC rose from an average of 10 per week to 54 per week in Nottingham during the first three months, and from 12 to 55 per week in Leicester. Attendance at other dermatology clinics was little affected. Nottingham, commenting on the sex ratio of referrals, observed that the proportion of male patients, especially older men, increased after publicity although they were still outnumbered 1.6: 1 by women.

Biopsy   After the campaign started, 25% of PLC patients attending in Nottingham, and approximately 16% in Leicester, had a biopsy or other minor operation. The increased demand was met by an extra minor operations session, but in Nottingham there were no special operation sessions and about half of the patients waited three months. Presumably in some cases the objective of biopsy was cosmetic rather than diagnostic.

Melanoma   Leicester and Nottingham have also reported on melanomas though the post-campaign periods covered were less than a year. In Nottingham the total number with primary cutaneous melanoma among residents of the health district was 25 in the first six months. In Leicester 67 cases were diagnosed from specimens examined in Leicestershire hospitals over the first nine months. In both places the figures include in-situ superficial spreading melanomas. Leicester reported a significant rise in incidence compared with the previous four years, but the rise in Nottingham was small and consistent with the trend in previous years. Table 2 shows that Nottingham and Leicester, like Glasgow, have experienced a shift towards a lower proportion of poor prognosis melanomas, but this has been due to a rise in the number of thin and in-situ cases rather than to a reduction in advanced cases. Leicester, but not Nottingham, observed some further shift after the campaign and in both centres the proportion of thick melanomas appeared lower than in Glasgow in 1985 and 1986. The completeness of ascertainment and comparability of definitions and methods of analysis must be improved and larger numbers examined before valid conclusions can be drawn.

Criteria for referral   Nottingham reported that only 39% of patients attending the PLC fulfilled MacKie's criteria for referral. The sensitivity, 91.3% judged on 23 cases, and specificity, 62.1%, of the criteria were moderately good. The authors concluded that the criteria needed refining but that they should be emphasized in GP education.

Delay in presentation of melanoma   Among melanoma patients in Nottingham no improvement in delay was detected: 87% reported a delay of at least three months, 48% of

Table 2 The proportion of thick melanomas found before and after publicity campaigns

Year	Glasgow Total (1.5+mm)	Nottingham Total (1.5+mm)	Leicester Total (1.5+mm)
1979	124 (60%)		
1980	132 (61%)		
1981	123 (65%)		
1982	120 (62%)		
1983	154 (61%)	43 (70%)	
1984	158 (56%)	27 (48%)	24 (58%)
1985 ---•	195 (48%)	34 (44%)	35 (46%)
1986	230 (48%)	[63 (35%)]*	[76 (39%)]
1987 ---•		[25 (36%)]	[67 (30%)]

Footnotes:

---• indicates when publicity programmes were launched.

* The brackets indicate that figures for 1986 and 1987 in Nottingham and Leicester refer to periods before and after the campaign launch and not to calender years.

----

a year or more and in only three patients was recognition of the melanoma attributed to the campaign. Problems of recall inaccuracy, especially for an ill-defined change, plus the fact that publicity may lead to earlier awareness of subtle changes as well as to a quicker response when crude changes are discovered, make the interpretation of delays difficult. Other melanoma studies have failed to find an overall correlation between delay and prognosis (Temoshok et al, 1984).

2.8 Economic Aspects

The main effect of the programme was a large increase in attendance of patients with pigmented lesions of which 96% were benign. A cost benefit analysis is not possible without knowledge of long-term outcome, and it would be difficult in view of the trends occurring outside campaigns to decide on a suitable control population to calculate this. The average cost per case detected at a PLC clinic during a campaign can, however, be compared with the cost per case detected in the conventional way and this is currently under investigation in Glasgow.

The opportunity costs of running campaigns and introducing PLCs must also be considered. The demand on PLCs has exceeded the allocated resources in the immediate post-campaign period.   Other patients with skin diseases which, though not life-threatening, can substantially reduce the quality of life have presumably suffered delays in treatment, some waiting for months whilst patients with minor pigmented lesions are seen within a few days.

3   CONCLUSION

The Glasgow and CRC campaigns were undoubtedly effective in making the public more aware of the risk of melanoma and prompting referral. It is important, however, that effort should be put into demonstrating a true benefit in terms of reduced mortality or morbidity since there is, as yet, no evidence from any other studies that mortality or the incidence of advanced melanoma are significantly reduced by such campaigns.

Whether or not further deliberate education campaigns are mounted, GPs and dermatologists are likely to face increasing demand for attention to pigmented lesions. Research must therefore also be directed toward enabling GPs to reduce the number of unnecessary referrals, and towards reducing the costs of outpatient investigations by controlling biopsy rates and perhaps by employing nurse-specialists to sort out and reassure those who can safely be discharged without seeing the dermatologist.

REFERENCES

Doherty VR and MacKie RM. Reasons for poor prognosis in British patients with cutaneous malignant melanoma. BMJ, 1986; 292: 987-9.
Doherty VR and Mackie RM. Experience of a public education programme on early detection of cutaneous malignant melanoma.   BMJ, 1988; 297: 388-390.
English DR, Heenan PJ, Holman CD'AJ et al. Melanoma in Western Australia 1975-1976 to 1980-81: trends in demographic and pathological characteristics. Int J Cancer, 1986; 37: 209-215.
Graham-Brown RAC, Osborne JE, London SP et al.   The initial effects on workload and outcome of a public education campaign on early diagnosis and treatment of malignant melanoma in Leicestershire. Br J Dermatol, 1990; 122: 53-59.
Greene MH, Clark WH, Tucker MA et al. Managing the dysplastic naevus syndrome. Lancet, 1984; 84, i: 166-167.
Heenan PJ, Matz LR, Blackwell JB et al. Interobserver variation in the classification of cutaneous malignant melanoma in Western Australia. Histopathology, 1984; 8: 717-729.
Mackie RM. An Illustrated Guide to the Recognition of Early Malignant Melanoma. Edinburgh, Blackwood Pillans & Wilson, 1986.
MacKie RM, Freudenberger T & Aitchison TC. Personal risk-factor chart for cutaneous melanoma. Lancet, 1989; ii: 487-490.
Moore DH, Schneider JS and Sagebiel RW. Discordance of risk factors for invasive and non-invasive melanoma. Lancet, 1990; 335: 1523-1524.

Newman S, Nichols S and Freer C. How much do the public know about moles, skin cancer and malignant melanomas? The results of a postal survey. Comm Med, 1988; 10: 351-357.

Nichols S. Effect of a public campaign about malignant melanoma on general practitioner workload in Southampton. BMJ, 1988; 296: 1526.

Southampton Melanoma Group. Effects of rapid referral on thickness of melanomas. BMJ, 1986; 293: 790

Temoshok L, DiClemente RJ, Sweet DM et al. Factors relating to patient delay in seeking medical attention for cutaneous malignant melanoma. Cancer, 1984; 54: 3048-3053.

Whitehead SM, Wroughton MA, Elwood JM et al. Effects of a health education campaign for the earlier diagnosis of melanoma. Br J Cancer, 1989; 60: 421-425.

27 Screening for Melanoma/Skin Cancer in the United States

H. K. KOH, A. C. GELLER, D. R. MILLER and R. A. LEW

Boston University Schools of Medicine and Public Health, Boston, MA, U.S.A.

1 INTRODUCTION

Screening has great theoretical potential for the control of melanoma/skin cancer, but to date, few data exist on its true efficacy. In the United States, a national effort initiated by the American Academy of Dermatology (AAD) in 1985 has screened more than 260,000 persons and should produce more relevant data in the near future. We will review the rationale for screening for melanoma/skin cancer, present the data available to date, and raise questions and project trends for the future.

2 THEORETICAL CONSIDERATIONS

Screening for melanoma/skin cancer is theoretically attractive, as the disease is prevalent and causes considerable morbidity and mortality, its natural history is known, early treatment can reduce morbidity and mortality, and an acceptable, safe, noninvasive, and presumably reliable screening test exists (Miller, 1985).

The rising incidence of melanoma/skin cancer is a growing public health concern in the United States (Glass and Hoover, 1989). The projection of 27,600 cases for 1990 ranks melanoma as the ninth most common cancer (Silverberg et al., 1990). Melanoma incidence has doubled every decade since the 1930s, rising faster than any other cancer rate, except that for lung cancer in women (Kopf et al., 1982). Mortality from melanoma also has increased, with more than 6,000 deaths projected for 1990 (Silverberg et al., 1990); in addition, the mean age of persons who die of melanoma is decreasing, contributing to increasing years of potential life lost (Albert et al., 1990).

Nonmelanoma skin cancer (NMSC) (basal cell epithelioma and squamous cell carcinoma) is the most common form of cancer in the United States, with an estimated 600,000 new cases diagnosed each year (Silverberg et al., 1990). Although rarely fatal, NMSC can cause substantial morbidity, especially when local aggressive spread causes extensive tissue destruction on the face.

Numerous cooperative studies on prognostic factors have described the natural history of melanoma. Early, thin lesions are associated with excellent survival rates, whereas thicker, late lesions have a much higher chance of metastasis and death (Table 1). For NMSC, slow, steady, local growth and invasion are the rule, with certain subsites, such as the scalp, retroauricular areas, and nasolabial folds, associated with a poorer prognosis.

Table 1 Prognosis in melanoma

Stage	5-Year Survival Rate (%)
Stage I (confined to skin),	
Depth of lesion in mm:	
<0.76	99
0.76 - 1.49	95
1.50 - 2.49	84
2.50 - 3.99	70
>4.00	44
Stage II (lymph nodes)	30
Stage III (distant metastases)	<10

Early treatment can substantially reduce morbidity and mortality. For melanoma, the detectable preclinical phase, which corresponds to the noninvasive radial-growth phase, has been estimated to last months or even years. Dysplastic nevi, identifiable precursors to melanoma, can be present for about 2 years before full transformation into cancer (Rigel et al., 1989). NMSC grows even more slowly, and has easily-recognized precursors such as actinic keratoses.

Finally, visual inspection of the skin by a qualified observer should be an ideal cancer screening test, inasmuch as it is rapid, painless, and noninvasive and requires no special technology. Although some dermatologists question the practicality of total-body skin examination, citing patient embarrassment and lack of provider time as potential disadvantages, preliminary data suggest high patient acceptance of a total skin examination for cancer screening purposes (Koh et al., 1989). The confirmatory diagnostic procedure, skin biopsy, is relatively noninvasive and quick.

Screening for melanoma therefore defines a potentially broad set of activities (Roush et al., 1990). On the one hand, a person may conduct a casual self-examination, perhaps limited to areas of the body of greatest cosmetic interest; on the other hand, a person at high risk may undergo systematic monthly examinations of the entire skin surface by a skin cancer specialist (Roush et al., 1990). Melanoma screening can take place in many settings: in special screening sessions by a dermatologist, as part of an individual's routine preventive health care by a family physician, at the worksite, or in health fairs.

3 METHODOLOGIC CONSIDERATIONS

The optimal measure of the efficacy of screening for cancer is the reduction of mortality (Miller, 1985). However, for melanoma, a prospective trial that can demonstrate reduced mortality may require follow-up of several hundred thousand people over many years. An appropriate intermediate endpoint may be a change in the measured Breslow depth (thickness in millimeters) at diagnosis, since a significant and sustained shift from thick to thin lesions following the introduction of screening programs can suggest the effectiveness of early detection programs. Several groups outside the United States have demonstrated such changes following public and professional education programs (Roush et al., 1990).

To date, no randomized controlled trials have tested screening for melanoma/skin cancer. Other methods of evaluation that do not involve randomization exist but are more prone to bias (Koh et al., 1989). These methods include (1) verifying whether morbidity and mortality rates drop after the introduction of a screening program, (2) comparing rates of advanced disease or death in persons who are screened with those who are not, (3) employing a retrospective case-control study to determine whether the lack of screening increased the risk of the development of advanced disease or death, and (4) correlating the use of screening and the incidence of the disease among several populations (or among the same population at different times).

In studies of aggregate populations and time trends in relation to screening programmes, the ratio of mortality rates to incidence rates in the general population has generally declined over the decades (Roush et al., 1990) and the relative 5-year survival rates have improved substantially in recent years (Silverberg et al., 1990). These changes correspond to improved professional and public knowledge of melanoma/skin cancer as the incidence increases, greater attention to the possibility of cure with early detection, and the identification of precursor lesions, such as the dysplastic nevus. Because the treatment of metastatic melanoma has had negligible advances during this period, these observations imply a benefit of early detection; however, they may be complicated by lead-time bias, "pseudodisease" (i.e., in situ lesions), and other confounding effects (Roush et al., 1990).

A case-control comparison represents a promising approach to studying the efficacy of screening. However, one difficulty with such a comparison is that the risk factors for the occurrence of melanoma (and, consequently, risk factors for death from the cancer) may stimulate a higher rate of surveillance among the population that eventually gives rise to the cases (Roush et al., 1990); hence, statistical adjustment must be made for melanoma risk factors (e.g., family history, numbers of nevi, and nontanning skin) when comparing prior skin surveillance in the lethal melanoma cases with population controls. A population-based case-control study to examine the efficacy of screening for melanoma is now in progress in Connecticut (Berwick, 1989). The study focuses on types of self-examination of the skin but also includes the efficacy of a physician examination and surveillance as evidenced by prior biopsy of a mole.

3.1 The Visual Examination as a Cancer Screening Test
The visual examination is the only screening test for melanoma/skin cancer. Although dermatologists regard the visual examination as an accurate means of detecting

melanoma/skin cancer, few data exist on its validity, that is, its sensitivity and specificity, or on its predictive value.

The sensitivity and specificity of clinical evaluations for skin cancer in hospital settings have been reported in several studies (Koh et al., 1989; Kopf et al., 1975). The results vary according to the type of screener and the time and site of the study, but estimates of the sensitivity for melanoma detection average about 75%, with a specificity of about 98%. One dermatologist, Ervin Epstein, notes with admirable candor that his batting average for diagnosing melanoma is "only 0.400 (40%), great for an outfielder but gruesome for a clinician." (Epstein, 1984) The predictive value of a positive test has a wide range, from 38% to 80%. Results from skin cancer specialists in a hospital setting show high values for all three parameters: sensitivity, specificity, and positive predictive value of 77%, 99%, and 80%, respectively (Kopf et al., 1975). Preliminary studies have documented poorer recognition of malignancies by nonspecialists in simulated patient situations (e.g., recognition of tumors on slides) but not for actual clinical situations (Cassileth et al., 1986).

Koh et al (1990) offer the only predictive value and estimated sensitivity figures derived from screening by dermatologists, obtained from the national screening programs sponsored by the American Academy of Dermatology. By following positive screenees from the 2,560 persons screened for melanoma/skin cancer in 1986 and 1987 in Massachusetts, they found a predictive value for melanoma of 35 to 40% and an estimated sensitivity of 97% (assuming false-negative rates equivalent to the population incidence rate). The direct sensitivity and the specificity could not be measured, because screen-negative persons were not followed. The high estimated sensitivity seems to reflect the caution of screeners in this setting in labeling a questionable lesion as melanoma to hasten its removal. These figures must be confirmed by more data and follow-up data on screen-negative persons in future studies. Whether such accuracy for melanoma screening can be matched by nondermatologist physicians, nurse clinicians, or paraprofessionals is unclear (White and Faulkenberry, 1985). However, these values appear to be in keeping with the screening test parameters for breast and cervical cancer (Miller, 1985; U.S. Preventive Services Task Force, 1989).

4 REVIEW OF PUBLISHED MELANOMA/SKIN CANCER SCREENING DATA

At least 12 published studies examine melanoma/skin cancer screening in the United States. Table 2 summarizes these studies with regard to several important aspects of cancer screening. Although each study has unique merits and collectively they establish the feasibility and potential for screening, most of the major screening issues in melanoma/skin cancer remain incompletely addressed. As yet, no information exists regarding whether screening leads to decreased morbidity or mortality from melanoma/skin cancer.

Table 2   Published studies of melanoma/skin cancer screening (Modified from Koh et al., 1989)

Study (First author) /Year	Location of Screen	Type of Screener	Number of Screenees	Follow-up of Screenees*
Weary, 1971	Health department building (rural)	MD	548	No
Lynch, 1973	Mobile house trailer	MD, RN	3040	No
Kanof, 1974	State fair	MD	418	No
Zagula-Mally, 1974	Household visits (rural)	RN	978	Yes**
Loeffel, 1975	County fair	D	605	No
Biro, 1978	Church/Lion's Club	MD	232	?
Rigel, 1986	Manhattan (New York)	D	2239	Yes***
Snow, 1986	Wisconsin	D	477	Yes
Olsen, 1987	Dayton, Ohio	D	983	No
Field, 1987	Michigan	D	6340	No
Long, 1988	Rhode Island	D	200	No
Koh, 1990	Massachusetts	D	2560	Yes****

D = Dermatologists
MD = General Physicians
RN = Nurses

* Follow-up of screenees to determine pathologically-confirmed outcome.
** Nonmelanoma skin cancer only.
*** Melanoma only.
**** Melanoma, nonmelanoma skin cancer, and precursor lesions.

In 1971, Weary published the first American skin cancer screening study. He conducted skin and oral cancer detection clinics in rural Virginia and, with dermatologic colleagues, examined the light-exposed skin of 548 farmers and ranchers. Although malignant or premalignant lesions were found in 21.6%, no melanomas were found. In this important first study, Weary demonstrated that skin cancer screening is feasible and inexpensive. Other screening efforts ensued. Lynch et al.(1973) described a novel approach, the use of a mobile house trailer as the screening site, thus enhancing access to screening. Physicians and nurses screened 3,040 people for a variety of cancers, with particular attention paid to exposed skin sites. Although 51 presumed and histologically confirmed skin cancers were found and treated, biopsy results were not available on "many."

The study by Kanof (1974) represents another creative attempt at outreach, with screening done at a state fair. Of the 600,000 persons who visited the North Carolina State Fair during a 10-day period, general physicians and dermatologists examined the light-exposed skin of 418. Clinically suspicious lesions included 27 skin cancers (1 melanoma and 26 nonmelanoma skin cancers) (5.8%) and 99 precancerous lesions (23.6%). The major expense was $200 for the booth rental. No estimates are provided for compliance with referral, follow-up with biopsy, sensitivity, specificity, or ultimate impact on morbidity or mortality.

Zagula-Mally et al (1974) conducted screening in rural Tennessee, believing that people in this area experience a greater delay in seeking appropriate evaluation and therapy than those in urban areas. Nurses visited households, and screened the exposed skin of 978 white persons. They found 48 lesions suspicious for cancer, 43 of which were verified clinically by a dermatologist. Seventeen of these 43 (39.5%) persons visited their physicians specifically to inquire about their skin lesions after being advised to do so. Ten of the 17 lesions were surgically removed, and pathology reports were available on 9 (6 nonmelanoma skin cancer and 3 nonmalignant lesions). Thus, a gross predictive value of 66.7% (6/9) for NMSC can be calculated for this small series.

Loeffel and Watson (1975) also held skin cancer screening sessions at a county fair and in their examinations of 605 persons, they found 60 lesions that were clinically suspicious for nonmelanoma skin cancer and 96 that were possibly precancerous.

In examining the light-exposed skin of 232 people in New York, Biro and Price (1978) found that 26.7% had a malignant or premalignant skin cancer, including one melanoma. They gave no data on the sensitivity and specificity of the screen. In a brief subsequent report, Biro et al (1987) summarized data from 15 separate sessions held in Brooklyn over 10 years. In all, these researchers screened 877 persons and found 96 basal cell epitheliomas, 6 squamous cell carcinomas, and 1 nodular melanoma. It is not clear whether all these lesions were verified by biopsy. Biro and Price remarked that screening creates an "excellent training opportunity for residents in family practice, as well as for those in dermatology," but they did not comment on the proficiency of such personnel to carry out screening.

The National Melanoma/Skin Cancer Screening Program was initiated in 1985 by the AAD. In this campaign, the AAD asked members to hold annual free screenings for melanoma/skin cancer. The AAD has infused substantial funds to publicize the screenings, distribute educational materials and a standardized screening form, and encourage participation. This effort has been enthusiastically received by the American public and supported by former President Reagan, among others. The program has grown steadily since its inception. In 1985, an estimated 32,000 people were screened, and 1316 suspected skin cancers, including 97 suspected melanomas, were found. In 1989, the number screened increased to 78,486 persons, and approximately 593 suspected melanomas were found. A total of 260,745 persons were screened over the five year period (Table 3).

Table 3   1985-1989 results from National AAD melanoma/skin cancer screening*

	Number Screened	Precancerous Lesions	Malignant Melanoma	Basal Cell Ca	Squamous Cell Ca	Total Lesions Detected
1985	32,000	2,479	97	1,056	163	3,795
1986	41,486	10,366	262	3,049	398	14,075
1987	41,649	9,136	257	2,798	302	12,493
1988	67,124	14,494	435	4,457	474	19,860
1989	78,486	21,887	593	6,266	761	39,507
Total	260,745	58,362	1,644	17,626	2,098	89,730

* All diagnoses are clinical diagnoses made at the screen and <u>not</u> biopsy-proved.

To date, however, there has been little attempt to contact participants after the screen to confirm diagnoses and determine yield (follow-up). Rigel et al (1986) reported the results from the 1986 Manhattan (New York) program, concentrating exclusively on the yield of biopsy-proved melanomas. Of the 2239 persons screened by dermatologists, 14 cases of melanoma were verified by biopsy. It is important to note that this report also appears to be the first published account of an attempt to perform a total skin examination of most patients. The authors note that a complete skin examination was more likely to detect melanomas than a partial examination.

Snow and Cripps (1986) reported on 477 persons screened in the 1986 Wisconsin Program. One melanoma and 25 NMSC were confirmed by biopsy. Olsen et al. (1987) report on the efforts of the Dayton, Ohio, dermatologic community, which screened 983 participants and referred 356 (36%) for possible skin malignancy. The screen attracted a preponderance of female participants (64%), and complete examination was possible in only 39%. The authors present a detailed discussion of methods for publicizing a screening program.

Field et al (1987) present statewide data from Michigan over a 2-year period. This study of 6340 screenees represents the largest number reported to date, although no follow-up information is available. Field notes that most (102/177) dermatologists in the state participated in the screening. Long (1988) reported the experience of screening in a health maintenance organization (HMO) setting.

Koh et al. (1990) have recently published an evaluation of 2560 persons screened for melanoma/skin cancer in Massachusetts in 1986 and 1987 as part of the AAD program. By following the positive screenees in this group, 9 melanomas, 91 NMSC, and 39 dysplastic nevi were found. Of the melanomas, four were in situ and one had metastasized to the groin (Stage II disease). While the yield of cancers appears high, the effects of possible pseudodisease and harvesting of prevalent cases may play a role, and further follow-up in these and other settings is critical.

Koh et al. (1990c) have begun an attempt to document confirmed melanomas from the national AAD screening efforts. In a first preliminary report, most of 30 melanomas detected were found to be less than 0.75 mm thick, which compares favorably to the distribution in the Connecticut Tumor Registry and national SEER data; however, survival could not be determined in this non-randomized study.

5   OTHER OPPORTUNITIES FOR SKIN CANCER SCREENING

While the AAD's annual free skin cancer screening by dermatologists will and should continue, it represents only one type of screening, that is, episodic screening performed by dermatologists on self-selected persons. Other types of programs will be needed to reduce morbidity and mortality from this disease. A number of possibilities must be explored.

5.1 Screening as Part of a Routine Physical Examination or Multiphasic Screening

The integration of a skin examination into a routine physical examination by primary-care providers may be the best strategy for reducing skin cancer morbidity and mortality. Screening in this way serves as an add-on to ongoing multiphasic screening by primary-care providers. Opportunities for such screening exist, inasmuch as approximately 85% of the population of the United States sees a physician every 2 years and routine physical examinations are among the 10 most common reasons for seeing a physician (Fletcher, 1984). In addition, primary-care physicians already manage many skin problems. Dermatologic complaints constitute about 7% of all ambulatory patient visits, yet dermatologists see only a third of these disorders (Stern & Gardocki, 1983). Preliminary data from a Massachusetts survey (Koh et al., 1990b) show that about 25% of melanomas are currently first detected by physicians and only a small fraction by dermatologists; most of the remaining melanomas were first detected by the patients themselves. The health-care use patterns of persons with melanoma and those at high risk for melanoma are not well characterized.

Experts differ on the value of a routine skin examination for the early detection of melanoma/skin cancer. The American Cancer Society recommends a physical examination of the skin every 3 years for persons 20 to 40 years of age and annually for those over 40.

Ackerman (1985) recommends that all types of physicians, as well as nurses, paramedical personnel, and medical students, be taught to recognize melanoma. Because many melanomas affect the back, some believe that chiropractors, physical therapists, and others also should be trained. In contrast, the Canadian Task Force on the Periodic Health Examination regards a routine skin examination as optional (Canadian Task Force on the Periodic Health Examination, 1979). Others fear that examinations by nondermatologists lack a high enough level of sensitivity and specificity in detecting skin cancers. The U.S. Preventive Services Task Force (1989) has recently recommended routine screening for skin cancer for persons at high risk.

Finally, even if physicians could agree on screening guidelines, it is not clear whether they would follow such guidelines on a regular basis. Evidence shows that internists do not always follow agreed upon screening tests for other cancers. Also, the little data available suggests that primary-care physicians lack the time and the training to recognize melanoma and other common dermatologic disorders.

5.2 Screening at the Workplace
Health promotion activities at the workplace have the potential of conveniently reaching many persons. Such efforts in the United States began in 1986 under the auspices of the Skin Cancer Foundation and the Mutual Life Insurance Company of New York, whereby 10,000 employees in 20 corporations, nonprofit organizations, and government agencies in New York City were scheduled to be screened. A report of the results from these efforts is pending.

5.3   Screening at Health Fairs
In 1985, Berwick (1985) reviewed the experience of screening at health fairs, noting that almost 2 million Americans visit them regularly. Of 940 health fairs surveyed in 1983, at least 4 (0.4%) offered screening for skin cancer. Preliminary statistics at one of those sites showed that abnormal findings were seen in 5.5% of 1382 people screened (Berwick, 1985).

5.4   Self-Screening
Although publicity increasingly encourages skin self-examination, as with breast and testicular self-examination, no evidence indicates that this type of activity actually results in early detection. The ongoing case-control study by Berwick in Connecticut should add data in this regard (Berwick, 1989). Some physicians recommend that self-examination of the skin start at age 25 and continue as part of a lifetime program of preventive medicine. One article shows explicit directions for examining the skin, including the use of mirrors to examine parts of the body that are otherwise difficult to see (Friedman et al., 1985).

5.5   Targeted Screening
Targeting screening efforts to high-risk persons improves the predictive value of a screening test. The use of data from population-based cancer registries across the United

States may help locate areas where screening will be more efficient. If such data can identify towns with a high incidence of advanced disease, then early detection programs in these areas may save lives.

Screening family members of melanoma patients makes sense, as those persons are at increased risk (Lew et al., 1985). In particular, patients with familial melanoma and multiple dysplastic nevi have a risk of melanoma several hundred times over the general population. In the family kindreds followed by Greene and colleagues in Philadelphia, deaths from melanoma ceased after the onset of surveillance of the family members since all subsequent melanomas were found at an early stage (Roush et al., 1990; Greene et al., 1985; Masri et al., 1990). Schneider et al. (1987) present evidence that active surveillance improves melanoma prognosis at Lawrence Livermore National Laboratory.

Finally, those who choose to attend voluntary AAD melanoma/skin cancer screenings are likely to include many high-risk persons. This was shown in a preliminary analysis of 1116 screenees in Massachusetts which found 86% had at least one risk factor for melanoma/skin cancer and 78% had at least two risk factors (Koh et al, 1990a). These results suggest that persons attending the screening in Massachusetts were, for the most part, at increased risk for the disease and appropriately selected themselves to be screened.

6   CONCLUSION

While screening for melanoma/skin cancer is theoretically appealing, few data exist to evaluate its effectiveness. Given the rising incidence and mortality rates of melanoma, and with no cure for metastatic disease in sight, the need to improve the efficacy of screening is great. The AAD screening programme, with the number of screenees involved, offers an opportunity to obtain critical data. In the absence of a randomized controlled trial, other design measures with continued tracking of incidence and mortality rates are critical to assessing whether screening for melanoma/skin cancer saves lives.

Acknowledgement
Supported in part by National Cancer Institute Grant #5K07CA01380-02. Dr. Koh is a recipient of the Preventive Oncology Academic Award from the National Cancer Institute.

REFERENCES
Ackerman AB. No one should die of malignant melanoma (Editorial). J Am Acad Dermatol 1985; 12:115-116.
Albert V, Koh H, Geller A, et al. Years of potential life lost: Another indicator of the impact of cutaneous malignant melanoma on society. J Am Acad Dermatol 1990 (in press).
Berwick D. Screening in health fairs. JAMA 1985; 254:1492-1498.
Berwick M. Personal communication, 1989.
Biro L, Price E. Skin Cancer screening in urban community. NY State J Med 1978; 78:753-755.

Biro L, Price E, Brand AJ. Skin cancer detection clinics. J Am Acad Dermatol 1987; 16:406-407.

Canadian Task Force on the Periodic Health Examination. The periodic health examination. Can Med Assoc J 1979; 121:1193-1203.

Cassileth BR, Clark WH, Luck ET, et al. How well do physicians recognize melanoma and other problem lesions? J Am Acad Dermatol 1986; 14:555-560.

Epstein E. Thoughts on melanoma. Dermatol Clin 1984; 2:171-183.

Field SI. Melanoma/skin cancer screening in Michigan. J Am Acad Dermatol 1987; 16:637-41.

Fletcher S. The periodic health examination and internal medicine: 1984. Ann Intern Med 1984; 101:866.

Friedman RJ, Rigel DS, Kopf AW. Early detection of malignant melanoma: The role of physician examination and self-examination of the skin. CA 1985; 35:130-151.

Glass AG, Hoover RN. The emerging epidemic of melanoma and squamous cell skin cancer. JAMA 1989; 262:2097-2100.

Greene MH, Clark WH, Tucker MA, et al. High risk of malignant melanoma in melanoma-prone families with dysplastic nevi. Ann Int Med 1985; 102:458-465.

Kanof E. Experience with a skin cancer detection clinic at a state fair. NC Med J 1974; 35:159-161.

Koh HK, Caruso A, Gage I, et al. Evaluation of melanoma/skin cancer screening in Massachusetts: Preliminary results. Cancer 1990; 65:375-379.

Koh HK, Geller AC, Miller DR, et al. Who is being screened for melanoma/skin cancer? Characteristics of persons screened in Massachusetts. J Am Acad Dermatol 1990a (in press).

Koh HK, Geller AC, Miller R, et al. Who detects melanoma? Patterns from a population-based survey. 1990b (submitted).

Koh HK, Lew RA, Prout MN. Screening for melanoma/skin cancer: Theoretic and practical considerations. J Am Acad Dermatol 1989; 20:159-175.

Koh HK, Norton LA, Geller AC, et al. Confirmed melanomas in the 1989 melanoma/skin cancer screening program sponsored by the American Academy of Dermatology 1990c (submitted).

Kopf A, Mintzis M, Bart R. Diagnostic accuracy in malignant melanoma. Arch Dermatol 1975; 111:1291-1292.

Kopf A, Rigel D, Friedman R. The rising incidence and mortality rates of malignant melanoma. J Dermatol Surg Oncol 1982; 8:760-761.

Lew RA, Koh HK, Sober AJ. Epidemiology of cutaneous melanoma. Dermatol Clin 1985; 3:257-269.

Loeffel E, Watson W. Screening for skin cancer at a county fair. West J Med 1975; 122:123-126.

Long TP. Skin cancer screening in an HMO. HMO Practice 1988; 2:84-88.

Lynch H, Lynch J, Kraft C. A new approach to cancer screening and education. Geriatrics 1973; 28:152-157.

Masri GD, Clark Jr WH, Guerry IV D, et al. Screening and surveillance of patients at high risk for malignant melanoma result in detection of earlier disease. J Am Acad Dermatol 1990; 22:1042-1048.

Miller AB, ed. Screening for Cancer. Orlando, FL: Academic Press, 1985.

Olsen TG, Feeser TA, Conte ET, et al. Skin cancer screening - A local experience. J Am Acad Dermatol 1987; 16:637-641.

Rigel DS, Friedman RJ, Kopf AW, et al. Importance of complete cutaneous examination for the detection of malignant melanoma. J Am Acad Dermatol 1986; 14:857-860.

Rigel DS, Rivers J, Kopf A, et al. Dysplastic nevi: Markers for increased risk for melanoma. Cancer 1989; 63:386-389.

Roush GC, Berwick M, Koh HK, et al. Screening for melanoma. In: Cutaneous melanoma, 2nd ed, C Balch. JB Lippincott: Philadelphia, Pennsylvania, 1990 (in press).

Schneider JS, Sagebiel RW, Moore DH, et al. Melanoma surveillance and earlier diagnosis. Lancet 1987; i: 1435.

Silverberg E, Boring C, Squires T. Cancer statistics, 1990. CA 1990; 40:9-26.

Snow SN, Cripps D. Skin cancer prevention and detections; results of a free screening program in Madison, Wisconsin. Wisconsin Med J 1986; 85.

Stern RS, Gardocki GJ. Office-based care of dermatologic disease. J Am Acad Dermatol 1983; 14:286-93.

U.S. Preventive Services Task Force. Guide to Clinical Preventive Services: An Assessment of the Effectiveness of 169 Interventions. Williams & Wilkins: Baltimore, Maryland, 1989.

Weary P. A two-year experience with a series of rural skin and oral cancer detection clinics. JAMA 1971; 217:1862-3.

White LN, Faulkenberry JE. Screening by nurse clinicians in cancer prevention and detection. Curr Probl Cancer 1985; 9:1-42.

Zagula-Mally ZW, Rosenberg EW, Kashgarian M. Frequency of skin cancer and solar keratoses in a rural southern county as determined by population sampling. Cancer 1974; 34:345-9.

28 The Dysplastic Naevus Syndrome: Implications for Screening

V. R. DOHERTY

Department of Dermatology, Western Infirmary, Glasgow

1 INTRODUCTION

In 1978 Clark and colleagues described the features of a newly recognised type of naevus occurring in two melanoma prone families named B and K. They noted that some members of the kindreds had large numbers of unusual looking moles which they termed the B-K mole syndrome (Clark, 1978). Other workers described similar moles and familial melanoma and coined the name FAMMS syndrome (Familial Atypical Multiple Moles Melanoma Syndrome) (Lynch, 1980). More recently the more widely used term dysplastic naevus syndrome was introduced (DNS).

Similar moles have been described in individuals with family histories of dysplastic moles, in individuals with personal but not family histories of melanoma and in individuals with neither. This has led to the sub-classification of DNS. Multiple dysplastic naevi have also been reported in association with ocular melanoma (Albert, 1985). Much attention has since been directed at the histological and clinical characteristics of these naevi.

2 CLINICAL FEATURES

Dysplastic naevi (DN) differ in several ways from the common, benign acquired naevus (AN). (Table 1).

Table 1: Clinical features of Acquired and Dysplastic naevi

	Acquired naevi	Dysplastic naevi
Size	<7mm	>7mm
Shape	Symmetrical	Asymmetric
Pigmentation	Uniform	Variable
Inflammation	Absent	Present
Number	30-50	Several hundred
Distribution	Spare doubly covered sites	All sites
Incidence	100%	2-6%

2.1 Size
ANs tend to attain a maximum size of 7mm in diameter. DNs are usually larger than 7mm.

2.2 Shape
ANs tend to have a symmetrical shape, usually round or oval. DNs are of irregular outline and are asymmetric.

2.3 Margin
ANs usually have a distinct edge clearly demarcating the lesion from the surrounding skin. DNs characteristically blend into the adjacent normal skin and have a blurred edge.

2.4 Pigmentation
The colour of ANs is very variable - from flesh-coloured to brown to almost black. Individual ANs do not show instructional variation in pigmentation.
DNs show both intra and inter- lesional variation in pigmentation.

2.5   Distribution
ANs can occur on any part of the body but usually spare the doubly covered sites like buttocks and breasts and the scalp. DNs occur on all sites .

2.6   Onset
ANs appear in childhood with a peak at puberty. They usually stop appearing after age 30. Characteristically they diminish in numbers after age 50 becoming fibrotic and/or pedunculated. DNs appear throughout both childhood and adult life and do not appear to decrease in numbers with age.

2.7   Numbers
Most people have between 20 and 50 ANs in their young adult life. Patients with DNs may have anything from a few to hundreds of these lesions.

3   SUB-CLASSIFICATION OF DNS
The syndrome has been subdivided into four main types according to the presence or absence of personal and/or family histories of melanoma and dysplastic naevi. The classification is listed in Table 2.

4   HISTOLOGICAL FEATURES
Elder and colleagues described the main features of dysplastic naevi as follows; lentiginous melanocytic hyperplasia, cytological atypia, lamellar fibroplasia and lymphoid infiltrate (Elder, 1982). An alternative histological classification has been suggested more recently (Seywright, 1986). Many workers feel that typical histology must be seen in at least 2 macroscopically dysplastic naevi before a diagnosis of DNS can be made (Clark, 1978).

Table 2: Sub-classification of DNS

Types	History of:	
	Dysplastic naevi	Melanoma
A	+ (-)	- (-)
B	+ (+)	- (-)
C	+ (-)	+ (-)
D	+ (+)	+ (+)

Signs in brackets () refer to family history.

Early work suggested that clinical dysplasia always correlated with histological dysplasia (Kelly, 1985). More recent studies (Klein, 1990) have failed to confirm this correlation. Immunohistochemical techniques and cytomorphometry have also been employed to give a more objective measure of melanocytic atypia (Bergman, 1988).

5 EPIDEMIOLOGY
Approximately a third of patients with melanoma will have at least one dysplastic naevus (Elder, 1980). Likewise 2-5% of the population of the USA have such lesions (Crutcher, 1984). Only 1% of healthy controls in a melanoma case-control study had more than three clinically atypical naevi (MacKie, 1989). One study of workers in a chain of British shops reported a prevalence of multiple DNs of 1.3% in 2000 healthy individuals (Curley, 1989).

6 GENETICS
Several studies have suggested that DNS associated with familial melanoma may be inherited in an autosomal dominant manner (Greene, 1985; Bergman, 1986). Others suggest that DNS and familial melanoma may represent the pleiotropic effects of a single, highly penetrant gene behaving in an autosomal dominant manner (Bale, 1986) or chromosome instability (Caporoso, 1987). Various workers have attempted to localise the DNS gene and this matter remains undecided at present (Tucker, 1989; van Hareingen, 1989).

7 MELANOMA RISK
Along with congenital naevi DNs are recognised as precursors of malignant melanoma (MM) by many workers and as a marker of increased MM risk by most others (Greene, 1985). The precursor theory is supported by two main observations. Firstly histologically diagnosed MMs can occur in contiguity with a histological DN (Rhodes, 1983). Secondly, on clinical grounds, centres which use serial photography to follow their DNS patients have excised changing, clinically diagnosed DNs and found these to be histological MMs (Rigel, 1989). It has then been argued that the MM arose in the pre-existing DN.

There is considerable overlap between the clinical and histological features of DNs with that of the early MM. The diagnosis of DNs and to a much lesser extent MMs on both histological and clinical grounds is somewhat subjective. For obvious reasons it is impossible to completely prove or disprove either of the above observations.

The risk of MM in the setting of familial DNS appears very high. It has been estimated at 100% for individuals in the DNS- D1/ D2 type over a lifetime.. The risk in the other types is significantly smaller . Genetic studies suggest that DNS patients are at risk not only of MM but also of other cancers including those of the breast, lung and pancreas (Lynch, 1983). A more recent study of DNS families found no evidence to suggest that they are at increased risk of other types of cancer (Greene, 1987).

8 MANAGEMENT OF THE DNS PATIENT
Individuals at very high risk with large numbers of DNs are best followed up by serial photography at regular intervals.Any changing lesion should be excised and submitted for histological evaluation. In addition close family members should be examined to see if they too have DNs. In our experience it is worth examining the whole family rather than relying on the patient to select those he says have "moles".

Prophylactic excision of DNs may be helpful if the patient has very few lesions or for lesions on difficult to monitor sites like the scalp. It must be remembered, however, that not all the MMs seen in these patients arise on pre-existing naevi. Likewise it is recognised that dysplastic naevi continue to appear well into adult life and thus, even if they are all removed prophylactically, new ones are likely to appear (Barnes, 1987).

The most important part of the management of DNS patients is education. They must become familiar with the clinical appearance of MM and must learn to monitor their own skin regularly. Appropriate advice on sensible sun-exposure should be given.

If in the future the genetic basis of DNS is more clearly delineated it might be possible to select out the high risk family members by these techniques.

9 SCREENING
The relative rarity of DNS in the community and the unknown risk of malignancy in types A-C makes it an unlikely target for mass population screening at present. If an attempt at identifying the high risk type were to be made it would seem logical to make it a part of a more widely based skin cancer screening or early detection programme. Most centres currently involved in early MM diagnosis are reporting the referral of individuals with unusual mole patterns to designated pigmented lesion clinics.

At present considerable educational effort has been made to familiarise the medical profession and the public with the DNS in the USA and Australia. Like MM education it has been carried out using illustrated leaflets, posters, radio and television. As yet I am not aware of any separate DNS screening programmes being underway. In Britain it would be likely that any DNS screening would take place through general practitioner referral of selected individuals to a specialist pigmented lesion clinic. This would require an additional section in current melanoma education ventures aimed at general practitioners.Public education on recognition of DNs would also need to be included in population based education on melanoma.

Screening for DNS would have many similarities to MM screening. The screen itself, i.e. a full skin examination, is non-invasive and requires no specialised equipment. Patients could be taught self examination techniques.

The most important factor in screening would be the early detection of the very high risk DNS patient. Currently these individuals usually are identified only when they or a close family member develop a melanoma.It is likely that the numbers of these high risk patients will be small and would certainly not justify a separate screening programme from MM itself. However they are identified it would seem logical to offer such individuals advice on sensible sun exposure though it is not known whether this would necessarily reduce their melanoma risk.

As with all possible screening efforts, before embarking on a DNS screening programme due attention would have to be given to the cost to benefit ratio. Much more work needs to be done before such an evaluation can be made for British DNS patients.

REFERENCES

Albert DM, Chang MA, Lamping K et al. The dysplastic naevus syndrome; a pedigree with primary melanomas of the choroid and skin. Ophthalmology, 1985; 92: 1728-34.

Bale SJ, Chakravarti A and Greene MH. Cutaneous malignant melanoma and familial dysplastic naevi: evidence for autosomal dominance and pleiotropy. Am J Hum Genet, 1986; 38: 188-96.

Bale SJ, Dracopoli NC Tucker MA et al . Mapping the gene for hereditary cutaneous malignant melanoma- dysplastic naevus to chromosome 1p. N Engl J Med, 1989; 320: 1367-72.

Barnes LM and Nordlund JJ. The natural history of dysplastic nevi. Arch Dermatol, 1987; 123: 1059-61.

Bergman W, Ruitert DJ Scheffer E et al. Melanocytic atypia in dysplastic naevi. Cancer, 1988; 61: 1660-66.

Clark WH, Reimer RR, Greene M, et al. Origin of familial melanoma from heritable melanocytic lesions; "The B-K mole syndrome". Arch Dermatol, 1978;5: 85-7.

Crutcher WA and Sagabiel RW. Prevalence of dysplastic naevi in a community practice. Lancet, 1984; 1: 729.

Curley RK, Cox J, Taylor FG and Marsden RA. The prevalence of dysplastic naevi; an epidemiological survey.(Abstract). Presented at 2nd World Conference on Malignant Melanoma in Venice 1989.

Elder D ,Goldman LI,Goldman SC et al. Dysplastic naevus syndrome: a phenotypic association of sporadic malignant melanoma. Cancer, 1980; 46: 1787-94.

Elder DEN,Greene MH,Guerry D et al. The dysplastic nevus syndrome: Our definition. Am J Dermatopathol, 1982; 4: 455-60.

Greene MH, Clark WH,Tucker MA et al. High risk of malignant melanoma in melanoma prone families with dysplastic naevi. Ann Int Med, 1985; 102: 458-465.

Greene MH, Clark WH,Tucker MA et al. Precursors to malignant melanoma in "Malignant Melanoma-Consensus Conference " JAMA, 1984; 251: 1864-1866.

Greene MH, Clark WH,Tucker MA et al. The Familial Dysplastic Naevus Syndrome. New Eng J Med, 1985; 312: 91-7.

Greene MH, Tucker MA , Clark WM et al . Hereditary melanoma and the dysplastic naevus syndrome; the risk of cancers other than melanoma. J AM Acad Dermatol, 1987; 16: 792-7.

Kelly JW. Crutcher WA and Sagebiel RW. Clinical diagnosis of dysplastic naevi. J Am Acad Dermatol, 1986; 14: 1044-1052.

Klein LJ and Barr RJ. Histologic atypia in clinically benign naevi. J Am Acad Dermatol, 1990; 22: 275-82.

Kopf A, Goldman RJ, Rivers JK et al . Skin Types in dysplastic naevus syndrome. J Dermatol Surg Oncol, 1988; 14:827-31.

Kraemer KH , Greene MH, Tarone R et al. Dysplastic naevi and melanoma risk. Lancet, 1983; ii: 1076-77.

Lynch HT, Fusaro RM, Danes BS et al. A review of hereditary malignant melanoma including biomarkers in familial atypical multiple mole melanoma sundrome. Cancer Genet Cytogenet, 1983; 8: 325-58.

Lynch HT,Fusaro RM, Pester J et al. Familial atypical multiple mole-melanoma (FAMM) syndrome:Genetic heterogeneity and malignant melanoma. BR J Cancer, 1980; 42: 58-70.

MacKie RM,Freudenberger TF and Aitchison TC. Personal risk-factor chart for cutaneous melanoma. Lancet, 1989; ii : 487-90.

Rhodes AR, Melski JW, Sober AJ et al. Increased intra epidermal melanocyte frequency and size in dysplastic melanocytic naevi, superficial apreading melanoma, nevocellular nevi and solar lentigines. J Invest Dermatol, 1983; 80: 452-9.

Rigel DS,Rivers JK,Kopf AW et al. Dysplastic Naevi: Markers for increased risk for melanoma. Cancer, 1989; 63: 386-389.

Seywright M, Doherty VR and Mackie RM. Proposed alternative terminology and subclassification of o called dysplastic naevi. J Clin Path, 1986; 39: 189-94.

Slue W, Kopf A and Rivers J. Total body photographs of dysplastic naevi. Arch Dermatol, 1988; 124: 1239-43.

van Haeringen A, Bergman W, Nelen MR et al Exclusion of the DNS locus from the short arm of chromosome 1 by linkage studies in Dutch families. Genomics, 1989; 5: 61-4.

29 Summary of Discussion on Screening for Melanoma of the Skin

Malignant melanoma is a candidate site for screening as the disease is increasing in incidence in many populations and there are major differences in long term survival in terms of lesion thickness. The only screening test which has been proposed is visual examination of the skin. This is relatively simple and non-invasive though relatively non-specific, and if used on a wide scale such testing could involve a substantial time commitment on the part of many health professionals.

Campaigns aimed at encouraging limitation of sun exposure, use of sun-screens, self-examination and prompt response to early suspicious signs have occurred in many parts of the world. Some programmes also encourage professional screening by offering free skin checks. For none of these programmes is there as yet any evidence for reduction in mortality in the population. Nor have the programmes been organized on a population basis, rather they have been based on general advertising, presumably with largely health conscious individuals responding. Nevertheless, programmes that increase public awareness should not be discouraged, but fully evaluated.

It was questioned whether it was possible to perform a randomised trial of screening for melanoma in areas with major public awareness programmes. If the intervention was directed at specific individuals to encourage compliance with screening, the effect of the campaign would have to be carefully considered in determining the sample size for the trial. A trial would not be precluded, however. In the absence of a trial, the effect of screening for melanoma could only be evaluated using indirect measures.

The sensitivity and specificity of the skin examination are unknown. Sensitivity is difficult to assess in programmes encouraging mass self-examination. However, programmes can and should monitor specificity, costs and compliance with follow-up. It is uncertain who can best perform examinations and which is the appropriate target population. The fundamental issue is whether the programmes can reduce mortality from the disease. Only then will it be possible to determine whether the thickness of the lesion can be used as an intermediate endpoint. At present there is insufficient information available to primary care practitioners to enable them to make informed decisions on who should be referred for further evaluation.

It is clear that the role of the dysplastic naevus syndrome (DNS) in the natural history and screening for melanoma is controversial. It is not known whether this is a true precursor lesion or a high risk indicator. The syndrome occurs in 2-8% of the melanoma-free population, and in about one-third of melanoma patients. However, the clinical and histologic features are not generally agreed upon.

State of the Art on Screening for Prostate Cancer

Screening for prostate cancer cannot be recommended at present as public health policy. There are strong contraindications for any screening on a large scale, given the problem of over-treatment.

Recommendations for Research
Obtain data on the sensitivity and specificity of the tests proposed on those cancers that will progress to clinical disease, the morbidity and mortality from treatment for early stage prostate cancer and the resulting quality of life of those treated.

If the above data are satisfactory, perform large scale randomized controlled efficacy and effectiveness trials as a prerequisite before screening for prostate cancer is introduced as public health policy. These trials should collect data on the quality of life of those with screen detected disease in comparison to the controls, as well as on mortality as the definitive endpoint.

30 Issues in Screening for Prostate Cancer

A.B. MILLER

Department of Preventive Medicine and Biostatistics, University of Toronto, Toronto, Ontario, Canada

1 INTRODUCTION

Prostate cancer is the leading cancer in incidence in men in the United States and second (after lung) in Canada, and in Canada and the United States, second in importance (to lung) in cancer mortality (National Cancer Institute of Canada, 1990; Silverberg et al, 1990). However, it is a condition that has a steep rise of incidence with increasing age relatively late in life, therefore it has less importance as a cause of Potential Years of Life Lost, in Canada being number 3 after lung and colorectal cancer (National Cancer Institute of Canada, 1990). Nevertheless, like many cancers it can be an important cause of morbidity, and there is increasing interest in the possibility of screening for prostate cancer using the digital rectal examination (DRE) and/or prostatic ultrasound, as well as other potential screening tests such as that for a prostate specific antigen (PSA). There are, however, insufficient data available as to whether these are valid and effective screening tests, and therefore a major trial is proposed in North America (Prorok et al, this volume).

It is clear, however, that there are many obstacles in the way of an effective screening programme for a disease that is a relatively unimportant cause of premature mortality. Not only has an acceptable and valid screening test to be available but there must also be an acceptable and effective treatment for the preclinical lesions found as a result of screening. This problem is particularly acute for prostate cancer because of the increasing frequency of latent prostatic carcinoma with increasing age and the not inappreciable morbidity and mortality of the radical procedures usually used to treat prostate cancer.

2 THE VALIDITY OF THE SCREENING TESTS FOR PROSTATE CANCER

In this section I shall consider the data available on the sensitivity and specificity of some of the screening tests that have been proposed. Part of the difficulty is that there are few studies that have been performed in screening circumstances and it is by no means certain that inferences that might be drawn from clinical series will be replicated in a screening programme. In the accompanying paper some data are provided from US series (Prorok et al, this volume). One series has recently been studied in Toronto comprising 317 men referred for prostatic ultrasound on whom a DRE and a PSA were also performed. Unfortunately we do not know the denominator from which these referrals were drawn.

Nevertheless it is possible to derive some indication of the sensitivity of the tests and the positive predictive value of the tests under clinical circumstances. Table 1 summarises the findings.

Table 1   Summary of results of Toronto clinical series

Test	Sensitivity	PPV
Digital rectal examination (DRE)	88%	46%
Prostate specific antigen (PSA)	88%	62%
Ultrasound (US)	86%	36%
DRE+PSA*	89%	41%

* With US used as a diagnostic test

Even though this was a series derived from ultrasound referrals, it would seem that ultrasound alone had the lowest sensitivity and positive predictive value (PPV). DRE and PSA used alone had equivalent sensitivity, but PSA had better PPV than DRE. The addition of PSA to DRE with ultrasound used to detemine a biopsy if either alone was negative marginally increased sensitivity but at a cost of a reduced PPV. In this series, therefore, the PSA seems to be the best screening test and ultrasound the worst.

This must be considered, however, together with from the conclusion of Thompson and Fair (1989) who, after a review of the findings from their own studies and those of others stated "Although serum tumor markers [such as PSA] have tremendous appeal for mass screening, application of statistical methods suggest that: (a) most patients with localised carcinoma of the prostate would remain undetected, (b) most cases of carcinoma of the prostate detected would have progressed beyond local disease, and (c) the vast majority of patients with positive tests would be subjected unnecessarily to expensive and potentially morbid diagnostic procedures. At this time, serum tumor markers can not be advocated for mas screening for carcinoma of the prostate."

A study of the DRE has recently been completed in Linköping, Sweden in which 1,163 men age 50-69 were independently examined by two observers, a family physician and a urologist (Pedersen et al, 1990). Of 45 men suspected as having cancer of the prostate, cancer was confirmed in 13. This works out as a prevalence of cancer of 11.2 per 1,000, with a PPV of the test of 29% and a specificity of the order of 97.2%. Assuming approximately equal numbers of men in each of the age groups 50-54, 55-59, 60-64 and 65-69 the expected annual incidence in Sweden of cancer of the prostate is around 1.26 per 1,000 (Gunnarsen and Ericsson, 1987). Thus the detection rate on first examination was about 9 times the expected annual incidence which is a much larger excess than would be expected by analogy with other sites, suggesting either that symptomatic men preferentially volunteered, or that a large number of latent cancers were detected. Extrapolating that to the age group planned for the North American trial (60-74) suggests that the detected prevalence might be of the order of 24.6 per 1,000 (based on data from Ontario, (Dale et al, 1987)). If one then assumes that the PPV in screening circumstances would be of a similar order to that in Sweden for the DRE, but scale it down for the combination of DRE and PSA as in the Toronto clinical series, you end up with a fourfold table for each 1,000 men examined of the order of Table 2.

Table 2   Validity of DRE+PSA as screening tests for prostate cancer (with ultrasound as a diagnostic test)

		Prostate cancer		
		Present	Absent	Total
Tests	Positive	25	72	97
	Negative	4	899	903
	Total	29	971	1000

Sensitivity: 86.2%, Specificity: 96.2%, PPV: 25.8%

3 THE MORBIDITY FROM TREATING LATENT PROSTATE CANCER

It is well recognised that cancer of the prostate is frequently found at autopsy, especially in elderly men. Although it is not certain that either the DRE or the PSA will be particularly sensitive to such lesions, the previous section suggests they may be, and that if prostatic ultrasound is used as a diagnostic test, a substantial proportion of the cancers found, especially at the upper end of the age range likely to be included in screening, will be found to have such lesions. This is a particular example of overdiagnosis bias, the tendency for screening to detect abnormalities labelled as cancer that would never have presented in the absence of screening, one of the four biases that can cause an artifactual increase in survival from cancers found on screening.

One possible effect of therapy for latent cancer of the prostate in elderly men is that the costs of the treatment in terms of post-operative mortality could easily overwhelm any possible benefit from the screening from delayed mortality for a few. Chodak and Schoenberg (1989) pointed out that if 30% of 25 million men over the age of 50 had a prostate cancer detected and excised, the 1% operative mortality rate would yield 75,000 deaths, or 45,000 more than would be expected to die from prostate cancer.

4 THE COSTS ASSOCIATED WITH SCREENING

The major cost associated with any screening programme is the cost of the screening tests. However an additional factor is the cost of the investigation and management of the false positives found on screening. This is a major concern of Health Maintenance

Organizations, who may, for example, be unable to collaborate in clinical trials of screening unless the granting agency agrees to pick up the costs of the examinations and treatment generated over and above the norm by the trial. Table 2 suggests that there could be as many as 7 false positives for every 100 men screened, all of whom would require ultrasound, and perhaps as many as a half prostatic biopsy. That is a not inconsiderable load for any HMO, not to mention the extra morbidity and anxiety for the participants.

Chodak and Schoenberg (1984) estimated that the cost of screening by the DRE was approximately $6,300 per case detected, which they felt was favourable compared to the costs of breast and cervix screening. However, it is inappropriate to base cost estimates on "per case detected". It seems likely that for prostate cancer screening, the cost per person-year of life saved would be very much greater than for breast or cervix screening.

5 THE ETHICAL ISSUE
The crucial distinction between screening and normal medical diagnosis and care is that the encounter is not originated by the individual who is the subject of screening, rather the provider of screening initiates the process (Miller, 1988). The screener believes that as a result of screening, the health of the community will be better. It is not possible to be certain that the health of everyone offered screening will be better, but at the very least the screener has an obligation to reduce to the minimum the possibility that individuals will receive harm. Clearly these conditions can not yet be met for screening for prostate cancer, and therefore screening for this condition should only be offered in the context of a properly designed experiment with validly constituted informed consent forms.

6 CONCLUSION
Prostate cancer is an important disease in elderly men but because of the problems discussed in this paper it will only be appropriate to evaluate the effectiveness of screening programmes for prostate cancer by well designed randomised trials. Such trials will have to be completed, however, before a recommendation on including screening in programmes of cancer control could be developed. We must be at least a decade away from such a recommendation.

REFERENCES
Chodak GW, Schoenberg HW. Early detection of prostate cancer by routine screening. J Am Med Assoc 1984; 252:3261-3264.
Chodak GW, Schoenberg HW. Progress and problems in screening for carcinoma of the prostate. World J Surg 1989; 13:60-64.
Dale D, Nemes M, Weir H et al. Cancer incidence in Ontario, 1978-82. In: Muir C, Waterhouse J, Mack T et al (eds). Cancer incidence in five continents, Volume V. Lyon, (IARC Scientific Publications no 88), 1987, p 262.

Gunnarson T, Ericsson J. Cancer incidence in Sweden, 1978-82. In: Muir C, Waterhouse J, Mack T et al (eds). Cancer incidence in five continents, Volume V. Lyon, (IARC Scientific Publications no 88), 1987, p 618.

Miller, AB. The ethics, the risks and the benefits of screening. Biomed & Pharmacother. 1988; 42:439-442.

National Cancer Institute of Canada: Canadian Cancer Statistics 1990. Toronto, Canada, 1990.

Pedersen KV, Carlsson P, Varenhorst E et al. Screening for carcinoma of the prostate by digital rectal examination in a randomly selected population. Br Med J 1990; 300:1041-1044.

Silverberg E, Boring CC, Squires TS. Cancer Statistics, 1990. Ca 1990; 40:9-26.

Thompson IM, Fair WR. Screening for carcinoma of the prostate: efficacy of available screening tests. World J Surg 1989; 13:65-70.

31 Available Screening Tests for Prostate Cancer

J. H. M. BLOM

Department of Urology, Erasmus University and Academic Hospital,
Dr. Molewaterplein 40, 3015 GD Rotterdam, The Netherlands

1 INTRODUCTION

Prostate cancer contributes in a significant way in most countries of the western world to premature deaths in males (Zaridze et al, 1984). In The Netherlands and other western countries prostate cancer is the third most frequent malignancy in men, after lung and colorectal cancer and is the second cause of death from cancer in men (Central Bureau of Statistics, 1979). In The Netherlands in 1984, 1,782 men died from prostate cancer, accounting for 9.2 % of the total deaths from cancer in men (Central Bureau of Statistics, 1986). In the United States prostate cancer is the second most common malignancy in males and the third most common cancer cause of death in men older than the age of 55 years (Catalona et al, 1986). Five year survival figures for localized tumours vary between 65 and 85%, whereas only 15-20% of patients who present with metastatic disease will be alive after 5 years (Catalona et al, 1986).

Early diagnosis offers the only chance for cure. Unfortunately, approximately 50% of patients present with clinically advanced disease at initial diagnosis (Murphy et al, 1982). If we are to reduce the mortality from prostate cancer, we will have to detect it while it is still localized to the prostate and therefore potentially curable. Therefore we must be able to detect the disease before it is symptomatic. This can only be done by identifying screening methods that can be effectively employed in those asymptomatic patients considered most at risk.

The options for screening for prostate cancer include examining the prostate gland by digital rectal examination, imaging the gland by transrectal ultrasonography, and/or examining the serum for tumour markers. Each of these tests will be discussed in the present paper.

2 DIGITAL RECTAL EXAMINATION

Rectal examination is capable of detecting suspicious lesions within the prostate. Several investigators have stated that the percentage of patients with localized prostate cancer could be increased by performing a routine digital rectal examination on asymptomatic men (Gilbertsen, 1971; Thompson et al, 1984; Chodak et al, 1984). Chodak et al (1989) investigated the effect of routine digital rectal examination on the stage of cancer at diagnosis. In a 6 year time period 4160 rectal examinations were performed on 2131 men. In 144 men a prostate biopsy was performed because an induration of the prostate gland was felt, and 36 malignant tumours were detected. One patient, who refused prostate biopsy died of prostate cancer within one year. Thus, the positive predictive value of the digital examination was 25.7%. Of the 37 cases 1 had stage A disease, while the tumours of 25 patients were stage B. Thus, in this study 70% of the patients had a tumour which was clinically localized to the prostate. Of the 25 patients who had stage B disease 18 underwent an operation. Pathological examination of the operation specimens revealed that only 9 tumours (50%) were localized to the prostate. The other 9 tumours showed extension beyond the confines of the gland. Similar observations were made by Thompson et al (1984), who reported that of 17 prostate cancers found on routine digital examination, 2 had already metastasized at the time of diagnosis. Of the 9 patients who were staged surgically, 6 already had tumour growth beyond the confines of the prostate. Thus, of 17 prostate carcinomas at least 8 (47%) were already beyond the limits of curability. Apparently digital rectal examination is able to detect cancers earlier, but the proportion of patients that present with an advanced stage remains approximately 50%.

Another question is whether the digital rectal examination should be repeated every year. Chodak et al (1989) offered an annual rectal examination to 2,131 men on entry into the study and discovered 32 of the 37 prostate cancers during the first examination, i.e. 1.5% of the men examined. In the second and further examinations 0 to 0.4% of those examined were found to have prostate cancer. The conclusion of Chodak et al was that digital rectal examination may be of little use for screening for prostate cancer. There are several reasons why digital rectal examination may not be an appropriate screening test for prostate cancer. In the first place apparently only 35% of the men found to have carcinoma of the prostate had a tumour that was pathologically confined to the gland. Secondly, only 20-25% of the clinically detected tumours are stage A (Murphy et al, 1982). These tumours were not detected by rectal examination, but incidentally found after prostatectomy for presumed benign disease. Thus, digital rectal examination is capable of detecting only a relatively small number of patients with a tumour in a curable stage.

3 TRANSRECTAL ULTRASONOGRAPHY

The rapid improvement of transrectal ultrasonography has resulted in considerable enthusiasm for the use of this diagnostic test to improve early detection of prostate cancer. Since the initial screening report by Watanabe et al (1980) a number of reports have demonstrated that transrectal ultrasonography is capable of detecting localized prostate cancer in asymptomatic men who have a normal digital rectal examination. Several investigators have examined the value of transrectal ultrasonography in screening for prostate cancer (Chodak et al, 1986; Lee et al, 1989; Cooner et al, 1990). Chodak at el, (1986) reported on 216 men who were investigated by transrectal ultrasonography and digital rectal examination. Prostate cancer was suspected by transrectal ultrasonography in 19 of 22 cases; in 3 cases the cancer was regarded benign. So, the sensitivity of transrectal ultrasonography was 86.4%. Lee et al (1989) reported their experience with 784 patients evaluated by transrectal ultrasonography and digital rectal examination in a screening programme. A total of 22 cancers were detected, 20 by transrectal ultrasonography and 10 by digital rectal examination; thus the detection rate of prostate cancer by the former was twice that of the latter (2.6% vs. 1.3%). Cooner et al (1990) performed transrectal ultrasonography in 1807 referred men. Transrectal ultrasonography showed a suspicion for cancer in 835 patients and a biopsy was performed in all of them; 263 cancers were detected, a detection rate of 14.6% (Table 1)

Table 1   Prostate Sonography - DRE correlation (Cooner et al, 1990)

	No.	+ TRUS	+ biopsies	PPV of TRUS	positive biopsies
DRE +	565	470	203	43.2%	35.9%
DRE -	1242	365	60	16.4%	4.8 %
TOTAL	1807	835	263	31.5%	14.6%

(DRE : digital rectal examination; TRUS : transrectal ultrasonography;
PPV : positive predictive value)

In the remaining 972 patients no sonographically suspicious area could be identified. Digital rectal examination revealed suspicious areas in 123 prostates. Biopsies yielded 6 cancers that were not detected sonographically. The positive predictive value of digital rectal examination alone was 4.9%. The positive predictive value of transrectal ultrasonography alone was 31.5%. These data show clearly that evaluation of men using transrectal ultrasonography detects prostate cancer more often than does digital palpation.

Of 1242 patients with negative findings on digital rectal examination 365 patients had positive findings on transrectal ultrasonography; biopsies showed prostate cancer in 60 of them. This indicates that the value of transrectal ultrasonography is increased when suspicious findings are present on digital rectal examination.

4 SERUM PSA LEVELS
More than 50 years ago Alexander and Ethel Gutman (Gutman et al, 1938) observed an elevated acid phosphatase activity in the serum of patients with metastatic prostate cancer. For many years acid phosphatase was the main serum parameter for monitoring metastatic disease. For screening purposes serum acid phosphatase is not very useful. In 10-30% of the patients with metastatic prostate cancer serum acid phosphatase is not elevated, while

slight elevations of serum acid phosphatase are found in benign prostatic hypertrophy, prostate infarction and after prostatic massage (Wajsman et al, 1979).

In 1979 Wang et al (1979) isolated the prostate specific antigen (PSA). PSA is not cancer-specific, it is specific for prostatic epithelium. Both PSA and prostatic acid phosphatase (PAP) are present in normal prostate tissue. In the serum of healthy young men low concentrations of PSA are measured. The normal range of PSA in the serum for men without prostatic disease (benign prostatic hyperplasia or prostate cancer) is 0.0 to 4.0 ng/ml (Oesterling et al, 1988). Elevated concentrations are found in the serum of men with benign prostatic hyperplasia and with prostate cancer. Bentvelsen et al (1990) compared the PSA values of 162 men with untreated prostate cancer with the PSA levels of 187 men with benign prostatic hyperplasia and 127 men older than 50 years of age without prostatic disease. The results of their study are summarized in Table 2:

Table 2 Serum PSA levels in normal men, patients with benign prostatic hyperplasia and patients with prostate cancer. (Bentvelsen et al, 1990)

Group	No.	PSA > 5.0 ng/ml		PSA >10.0 ng/ml
Normal	127	3	(2.4%)	-
Benign prostatic hyperplasia	187	77	(41.2%)	37 (19.8%)
Prostate cancer	162	131	(80.9%)	118 (72.8%)

These observations imply that on the basis of PSA levels alone a high number of men without prostate cancer will be identified as being suspicious. The same observation was made by Cooner et al (1990), who found that of 236 men with a PSA level higher than 10.0 ng/ml only 137 (58.1%) were found to have prostate cancer.

The combination of transrectal ultrasonography and PSA determination improves the detection of cancer. In Cooner's series (Cooner et al, 1990) prostate cancer was detected in 4.8% of the patients with negative digital findings. When PSA levels were normal (below 4.0 ng/ml) the detection rate was only 2.1%. This proportion rose to 28.1% when PSA levels were above 10.0 ng/ml. Nevertheless, out of 146 patients with suspicious findings on transrectal ultrasonography and on digital rectal examination with a serum PSA level higher than 10.0 ng/ml, 112 had proven prostate cancer. Thus 34 patients (23.3%) did not have proven cancer in spite of all three positive findings.

5 CONCLUSION

With the combination of digital rectal examination, transrectal ultrasonography and PSA levels it is possible to increase the detection rate of prostate cancer in a significant way. However, several questions remain to be answered, such as "Will the small nodules be the least harmful ones and the larger nodules the tumours that will threaten the patient?" In other words: "Does early detection of prostate cancer in an earlier stage of the disease indeed improve survival?"; "Can screening for prostate cancer be cost-effective?"; "Is screening using digital rectal examination, transrectal ultrasonography and PSA feasible?" Certainly, a large amount of work has to be done before the value of screening for prostate cancer is determined.

REFERENCES

Bentvelsen FM, Bogdanowicz JFAT, Oosterom R, Schröder FH. Een vergelijking tussen prostaat-zure-fosfatase en prostaatspecifiek antigeen bij de diagnostiek van het prostaatcarcinoom. Ned Tijdschr Geneeskd 1990; 134: 1596-1600.

Catalona WJ, Scott WW. Carcinoma of the prostate. In: Walsh PC, Gittes RF, Perlmutter AD, Stamey TA (eds). Campbell's Urology, Ed 5. Philadelphia: WB Saunders Co, 1986, pp 1463-1534.

Central Bureau of Statistics. Cancer: Morbidity and Mortality 1975/1976. Staatsuitgeverij, 's-Gravenhage, 1979.

Central Bureau of Statistics. Compendium of health statistics of the Netherlands 1986. Staatsuitgeverij, 's-Gravenhage, 1986.

Chodak GW, Keller P, Schoenberg HW. Assessment of screening for prostate cancer using the digital rectal examination. J Urol 1989; 141:1136-1138.

Chodak GW, Schoenberg HW. Early detection of prostate cancer by routine screening. JAMA 1984; 252: 3261-3264.

Chodak GW, Wald V, Parmer E, Watanabe H, Ohe H, Saitoh M. Comparison of digital examination and transrectal ultrasonography for the diagnosis of prostatic cancer. J Urol 1986; 135:951-953.

Cooner WH, Mosley BR, Rutherford Jr CL, Beard JH, Pond HS, Terry WJ, Igel TC, Kidd DD. Prostate cancer detection in a clinical urological practice by ultrasonography, digital rectal examination and prostate specific antigen. J Urol 1990; 143:1146-1154.

Gilbertsen VA. Cancer of the prostate gland. Results of early diagnosis and therapy undertaken for cure of the disease. JAMA 1971; 215:81-84.

Gutman AB, Gutman EB. An "acid" phosphatase occurring in the serum of patients with metastasizing carcinoma of the prostate gland. J Clin Invest 1938; 17: 473-478.

Lee F, Torp-Pedersen ST, Siders DB, Littrup PJ, McLeary RD. Transrectal ultrasound in the diagnosis and staging of prostatic carcinoma. Radiology 1989; 170: 609-615.

Murphy GP, Natarajan N, Pontes JE, Schmitz RL, Smart CR, Schmidt JD, Mettlin C. The national survey of prostate cancer in the United States by the American College of Surgeons. J Urol 1982; 127:928-934.

Oesterling JE, Chan DW, Epstein JI, Kimball Jr AW, Bruzek DJ, Rock RC, Brendler CB, Walsh PC. Prostate specific antigen in the preoperative and postoperative evaluation of localized prostatic cancer treated with radical prostatectomy. J Urol 1988; 139:766-772.

Thompson IM, Ernst JJ, Gangai MP, Spence CR. Adenocarcinoma of the prostate: results of routine urological screening. J Urol 1984; 132:690-692.

Wajsman Z, Chu TM. Detection and diagnosis of prostate cancer. In: Murphy GP (ed). Prostatic Cancer. Littleton, Massachussetts: PSG Publishing Company, Inc., 1979, pp 111-128.

Wang MC, Valenzuela LA, Murphy GP, Chu TM. Purification of a human prostate specific antigen. Invest Urol 1979; 17:159-163.

Watanabe H, Date S, Ohe H, Saitoh M, Tanaki S. A survey of 3,000 examinations by transrectal ultrasonography. Prostate 1980; 1:271-278.

Zaridze DG, Boyle P, Smans M. International trends in prostatic cancer. Int J Cancer 1984; 33:223-230.

32 Evaluation of Screening for Prostate, Lung, and Colorectal Cancers: The PLC Trial

P. C. PROROK, D. P. BYAR, C. R. SMART, S. G. BAKER
and R. J. CONNOR

Division of Cancer Prevention and Control, National Cancer Institute, Bethesda, MD, USA

1 INTRODUCTION

Prostate, lung, and colorectum are the three major cancer sites in males in the U.S. Together they accounted for 54 percent of new cancer cases and 57 percent of cancer deaths in 1988. There were an estimated 99,000 new cases of prostate cancer, 100,000 new cases of lung cancer, and 71,000 new cases of colorectal cancer with 28,000 prostate cancer deaths, 93,000 lung cancer deaths, and 29,600 colorectal cancer deaths. Death rates for prostate and colorectal cancers have remained relatively constant for many years, while the death rate from lung cancer has continued to rise (American Cancer Society, 1988). Thus any successful screening program for these three cancers could possibly have a major impact on overall cancer mortality in the U.S. Unfortunately, the guidelines for such a screening program are not well defined. No screening test for any of the three sites has been clearly established as efficacious. Furthermore, there is controversy in the U.S. within the clinical and public health communities regarding the value of screening for these cancers. The combination of circumstances is such that carefully conducted studies are necessary to determine the value of screening for these sites. A randomized trial is being considered for this purpose. This paper describes the basic design features of this trial. A detailed discussion of the background and rationale for the trial appears in Appendix I.

2 PROJECT DESCRIPTION

The proposed project is a two-armed randomized clinical trial of 16 years duration involving 100,000 males aged 60-74 at entry. These men will be randomized to two arms each containing 50,000 participants. Individuals in the control group will receive their usual medical care. Individuals in the group randomized to screening will receive screening examinations for prostate, lung, and colorectal cancers and examinations of the mouth, neck, and skin according to the following frequency and duration:

>   Digital rectal examination - initial, then annual x 3
>   PSA (serum prostate specific antigen) - initial, then annual x 3
>   Chest x-ray - initial, then annual x 3
>   Flexible sigmoidoscopy - initial, then at 3 years
>   Exams of the mouth, neck and skin - initial, then annual x 3.

There are three major objectives of this trial. They are to determine in males aged 60-74 at entry to the study whether:

(1) screening with digital rectal examination plus PSA can reduce mortality from prostate cancer;

(2) screening with flexible sigmoidoscopy plus digital rectal examination can reduce mortality from colorectal cancer; and,

(3) screening with chest x-ray can reduce mortality from lung cancer.

Secondary objectives fall into two categories:

(1) to assess screening variables other than mortality for each of the interventions including sensitivity, specificity, and positive predictive value, as well as incidence, stage, and survival experience of cancer cases.

(2) to store blood samples for use in future studies of prostate, lung, and colorectal cancers.

The organisation and duration of the study are expected to adhere to the following timetable:

Years 1-2:	Protocol development and pilot studies
Years 3-5:	Recruitment and initial screening of subjects
Years 6-8:	Follow-up and completion of screening
Years 9-15:	Further follow-up
Year 16:	Final follow-up and data analysis

The general plan is to establish up to 10 screening centres, each of which must be capable of randomizing 10,000 or more subjects to the study. Proposals will be solicited from military and veterans' hospitals, health maintenance organisations, cancer centres, and university or other groups who are capable of putting together the necessary staff and facilities to recruit subjects, conduct the screening, and follow-up all randomized participants for at least ten years after entry.

In addition, a single contract will be awarded for a Study Coordinating and Data Management Centre which will be responsible for receiving and processing data from the screening centres in all phases of the study, and will also provide logistical support for meetings and other activities required by the project. Another single contract will be awarded to an organisation capable of performing all PSA determinations, and of storing blood samples from selected screened individuals.

The study is designed to have high statistical power for detecting decreases in mortality separately for prostate cancer, lung cancer, and colorectal cancer. Subjects with lesions suspicious for lung cancer on x-ray will receive further work-up according to a protocol to be developed during the pilot phase (see below). Subjects with colorectal polyps or suspected cancer detected by digital rectal exam or by flexible sigmoidoscopy will undergo biopsy and removal of the polyps and biopsy of other lesions followed by further work-up, possibly including barium enema studies and/or colonoscopy, according to the protocol worked out in the pilot phase.

Although transrectal ultrasound will not be used as an initial screening modality for prostate cancer in this study, it is proposed that it be used in the diagnostic work-up of subjects suspicious for prostate cancer. A possible scheme is the following, where all biopsies are to be ultrasonically guided:

```
Rectal +, PSA +  ────►  Biopsy

Rectal +, PSA - ⎫          Ultrasound +  ────►  Biopsy
                ⎬ <
Rectal -, PSA + ⎭          Ultrasound -  ────►  No biopsy

Rectal -, PSA -  ────►  No biopsy
```

The examinations of the mouth for oral cancer, neck for enlarged lymph nodes due to head and neck cancer, and the skin for skin cancer and malignant melanoma are included because it is believed that the opportunity to have these examinations performed will increase initial compliance as well as provide a further incentive for return visits. It is recognized that with the proposed sample size there will not be adequate statistical power to evaluate the possible benefits from screening for these sites. Nevertheless, information will be obtained about the yield of these cancers and performance of the tests. This information could be useful in the design of future studies.

2.1 Endpoints
For screening modalities directed at each of the three major cancer sites (prostate, lung, and colorectum), cancer-specific mortality for that site will be the primary endpoint. In addition, cancer incidence, stage shift and case survival will be monitored to help understand and explain the results, and to aid in protocol modification decisions, possibly including early termination.

2.2 Pilot Phase
A. *Protocol Development* During the first six months of the pilot phase the study investigators shall jointly develop a detailed protocol including but not limited to the following major subjects:
   (1) Eligibility requirements for participants,
   (2) How screened individuals are to be notified of screening results and encouraged to seek further work-up of suspicious or positive results,
   (3) A procedure for recall of participants screened negative to maximize attendance at scheduled repeat screens,

(4) Work-up of participants with suspicious or positive screens -- what further tests are required and in what sequence,

(5) A mechanism for providing appropriate therapy for cancers (or other lesions) detected by the screening program. Staging and therapy should be standardized to the extent possible,

(6) Procedures for establishing and monitoring quality control of the screening examinations,

(7) Procedures for follow-up of all randomized individuals, monitoring of compliance with screening, determining cancer incidence, and ascertaining cause of death.

B. Pilot Studies Before the full scale screening trial can be undertaken, certain pilot studies will be necessary. The major activities to be carried out during the pilot phase are summarized below:

(1) Test acceptability of the randomization procedure by randomizing at least 300 individuals per screening centre.

(2) Work out the detailed logistics by actually performing the screening examinations. It is assumed that each screening encounter for any one participant will take place during a single visit lasting no more than three hours.

(3) Assess background level of usage of each screening modality by appropriate surveys in each centre's population catchment region and among the 300 randomized individuals at each screening centre.

(4) Test in actual practice all the data forms and procedures developed during the first year of the pilot phase.

(5) Establish facilities and procedures to collect, ship, and store blood samples from screened participants and conduct such procedures for the 150 individuals randomized to the screened group.

Each screening centre will identify recruitment sources and strategies appropriate to the local situation. Randomization of individuals will begin at six months as soon as the protocol is completed and the screening procedures are set up. One approach to randomization is to prepare a list of potential participants who will then be randomized to screened or control groups before seeking their consent to participate in the study. Randomization of 300 men at each screening centre and initial screening for those individuals assigned to screening will be accomplished in the second six months of the study. If the proportion of men who agree to be screened is too low, or the prevalence of screening in the control group is too high, to maintain adequate statistical power, then other approaches to recruitment and randomization will have to be tried in a second year of pilot testing. However, should the randomization turn out to be acceptable, then full scale recruitment can begin in the second year. The approximately 3000 individuals randomized during the pilot phase will be treated as a vanguard group and will be included with the population recruited later in the full scale trial.

2.3   Recruitment and Screening

If recruitment during the second six months of the pilot phase is concluded satisfactorily in the opinion of the Policy Advisory and Data Monitoring Panel (see below), then full scale recruitment will begin in the second year. However, as noted above, if recruitment is not satisfactory, a second year of pilot studies will be required. Each screening centre will be required to randomize a minimum of 10,000 subjects to the trial during the third through fifth year of the study (or the second through fourth year if the full scale trial is begun after the first year of pilot studies). After recruitment is complete, further screening will be required for three years and annual determination of cancer incidence and of deaths among study subjects will be needed for the remaining years of the trial. However, before embarking on this phase of the study, a second decision point will occur at the end of the recruitment phase when the Policy Advisory and Data Monitoring Panel will be requested to evaluate the progress to-date, including recruitment experience and compliance rates, and to recommend whether or not the trial should proceed as planned.

2.4   Policy Advisory and Data Monitoring Panel

In order to assist in study overview, a Policy Advisory and Data Monitoring Panel will be formed consisting of outside experts with experience in mass screening, clinical trials, appropriate medical specialties, medical ethics, biostatistics, and other appropriate disciplines. It will be the responsibility of this panel to review the results of pilot studies, the protocol developed during the pilot phase, plans for subject recruitment, and any other questions pertinent to the conduct of the trial. They will also consider any outside events, such as the results of other screening trials which might impinge on the appropriateness of the groups randomized in this study. They will review any suggested protocol changes and may also suggest such changes as appropriate. As the trial progresses, their function will include data monitoring to determine whether significant benefit or harm has been demonstrated for any of the screening modalities.

2.5   Sample Size Calculations

Sample sizes were calculated using the method suggested by Taylor (1972) modified to allow for arbitrary magnitude of screening impact, arbitrary sample size ratio between screened and control groups, and arbitrary levels of compliance in the screened and control groups. Let N_c be the number of individuals randomized to the control group, and N_s the number randomized to the screened group, with $N_s = fN_c$. For $0 \leq r \leq 1$, assume the study is designed to detect a $(1-r) \times 100\%$ reduction in the cumulative disease-specific death rate over the duration of the trial. Also let P_c be the proportion of individuals in the control group who comply with the control group intervention and P_s be the proportion of individuals in the screened group who comply with the screened group intervention. The total number of disease-specific deaths needed for a one-sided α-level significance test with power $1-\beta$ is then

$$D = \frac{\left\{ (Q_1 + f\, Q_2)\, Z_{1-\alpha} - \sqrt{Q_1 Q_2}\, (1+f)\, Z_\beta \right\}^2}{f\, (Q_1 - Q_2)^2},$$

where $Q_1 = r + (1-r)P_c$ and $Q_2 = 1 - (1-r)P_s$. The number of participants required in the control group is $N_c = D/\{(Q_1 + fQ_2)\,R_cY\}$, where Y is the duration of the trial from entry to end of follow-up in years, and R_c is the average annual disease-specific death rate in the control group expressed in deaths per person per year.

Calculation of N_c requires an estimate of R_c. The estimation procedure is illustrated for prostate cancer for white males. Similar calculations can be done for the other sites using the data in Table 1. Because those recruited for the screening trial are expected to be healthier than the general population, the usual cancer mortality rate obtained from national or registry data will over-estimate the mortality rate of the participants, at least for the early part of the trial. For a 10 year prostate cancer screening trial with men entered between the ages of 60 and 74, it is assumed that for the first two years the control group mortality rate is 25 percent of the usual rate, for the next three years it is 50 percent of the usual rate, and for the last five years it equals the usual rate. The usual mortality rate was estimated by the unweighted average prostate cancer mortality rate for men 65 to 79. This age range was used to adjust for aging over the 10 years of the trial. The usual mortality rates from national data (National Cancer Institute, 1987) are shown in Table 1. The estimated rate for this example is $R_c = 103.763 \times 10^{-5}$.

Table 1 Cancer mortality rates per person per year ($\times 10^{-5}$), estimated using 1981-1985 data.

Age	Prostate White males	Prostate Black males	Colorectum White males[1]	Lung White males[2]
50-54	3.6	10.9	20.8	91.1
55-59	11.5	32.1	40.3	165.4
60-64	30.0	80.4	66.1	251.3
65-69	68.7	173.0	105.4	364.1
70-74	134.3	325.6	158.7	463.7
75-79	241.7	490.6	219.5	527.4
80-84	391.8	774.3	296.8	522.1
85+	588.8	899.6	384.2	417.6

[1] Rates for black males are very similar.
[2] Average rate for black males in age group 65-79 is approximately 13 percent higher.

Required sample sizes for the PLC trial are displayed in Table 2. These were calculated assuming a 10 year trial using a one-sided 0.05 level test, a power of 0.8 or 0.9, $P_c = P_s = 1$

and possible mortality reductions of 5, 10, 15, 20, 25 or 30 percent in a screened group compared to an equal sized control group (f=1). These sample sizes are based on mortality rates for white males. For black males, the sample sizes for colorectal cancer are virtually identical, for lung cancer about 13 percent smaller, and for prostate cancer less than half. Thus, participation of black males will increase the trial's power for prostate and lung cancer.

It is felt that the smallest mortality reduction of public health significance which it is reasonable to attempt to detect in this trial is approximately 20 percent for prostate and colorectal cancers, and approximately 10 percent for lung cancer. Using Table 2, this leads to a sample size of 50,000 men in each arm of the study so as to achieve a high power (about .9 or greater) of finding such mortality reductions if they exist (see Table 3).

Table 2   Number of males age 60-74 at entry needed in each arm of a screening trial

Mortality reduction (%)

Site	Power	5	10	15	20	25	30
Prostate	.9	643,832	156,686	67,692	**36,954**	22,911	15,382
	.8	464,844	113,150	48,902	26,712	16,575	11,140
Lung	.9	211,269	**51,415**	22,213	12,126	7,518	5,048
	.8	152,535	37,129	16,047	8,765	5,439	3,656
Colorectum	.9	592,041	144,082	62,247	**33,981**	21,068	14,145
	.8	427,451	104,048	44,969	24,563	15,241	10,244

Table 3   Power against various mortality reduction alternatives assuming 50,000 males per study arm

Mortality reduction (%)

Site	5	10	15	20	25	30
Prostate	.20	.50	.81	**.96**	.996	.999
Lung	.41	**.89**	.997	.999	.999	.999
Colorectum	.21	.53	.84	**.97**	.998	.999

It is recognized that compliance will not be perfect in either randomized group. Contamination or drop-in will occur in the control group ($P_c < 1$) and non-compliance or drop-out is to be anticipated in the screened group ($P_s < 1$). Non-compliance includes those who refuse to participate when first contacted. The target mortality reductions of 20 percent for prostate and colorectal cancers and 10 percent for lung cancer mentioned above are therefore to be interpreted as effects which the study seeks to detect *in the presence of* whatever non-compliance and contamination exist in the populations. This implies that if there were perfect compliance, the mortality reductions would be greater since they would not be diminished by non-compliance.

One can assess the relationship between true effect size and level of non-compliance by examining Tables 4 and 5 which show what the mortality reductions with perfect compliance would have to be in order to realize a 20 percent (Table 4) or 10 percent (Table 5) mortality reduction for various levels of non-compliance in the screened and control groups. For example, from Table 4, if 80 percent of men in the screened group are examined by flexible sigmoidoscopy (P_S = .8) while 20 percent of control group individuals are so screened (P_C = .8), then the mortality reduction from such screening would have to be at least 31 percent with perfect compliance for there to be a 20 percent effect in the presence of non-compliance.

Table 4 Percent mortality reduction when compliance is 100 percent in both groups, as a function of P_C and P_S, based on a mortality reduction of 20 percent in the presence of non-compliance

$P_C \backslash P_S$	0.5	0.6	0.7	0.8	0.9	1.0
0.5	200	100	67	50	40	33
0.6	90	71	53	42	34	29
0.7	77	56	43	36	30	26
0.8	59	45	37	31	27	24
0.9	48	39	32	28	24	22
1.0	40	33	29	25	22	20

Table 5 Percent mortality reduction when compliance is 100 percent in both groups, as a function of P_C and P_S, based on a mortality reduction of 10 percent in the presence of non-compliance

$P_C \backslash P_S$	0.5	0.6	0.7	0.8	0.9	1.0
0.5	200	67	40	29	22	18
0.6	71	42	29	23	19	16
0.7	43	30	23	19	16	14
0.8	31	24	19	16	14	12
0.9	24	20	16	14	12	11
1.0	20	17	14	12	11	10

3 ESTIMATED COSTS

The following cost estimates were used for the screening procedures: sigmoidoscopy–$40.50; single view chest x-ray–$20.00; PSA determination–$10.00; digital rectal exam–$2.50; screening of mouth, neck, and skin–$2.50. These costs are assumed to include salaries for medical personnel and to reflect equipment and overhead costs. Screening centre costs for years 1 and 2 of the pilot phase were set at $1.0 and $1.5 million. In addition, $1.5 million per year (including indirect costs) was allocated to cover other screening centre expenses in years 3-16 such as data coordination, quality control, training, follow-up, and death ascertainment. The budget for the Study Coordinating and Data Management Centre was set at $0.5 million per year for years 1-16. The estimated costs per year of the trial follow.

		(cost in millions) unadjusted	adjusted for 5% inflation per year	
FY	1	$ 1.50	$ 1.50	Pilot work and protocol development
FY	2	$ 2.00	$ 2.10	Pilot work and protocol development
FY	3	$ 3.25	$ 3.58	Recruitment, screening, and follow-up
FY	4	$ 3.84	$ 4.45	Recruitment, screening, and follow-up
FY	5	$ 4.42	$ 5.37	Recruitment, screening, and follow-up
FY	6	$ 4.42	$ 5.64	Screening and follow-up
FY	7	$ 3.84	$ 5.15	Screening and follow-up
FY	8	$ 3.25	$ 4.57	Screening and follow-up
FY	9	$ 2.00	$ 2.95	Follow-up
FY	10	$ 2.00	$ 3.10	Follow-up
FY	11	$ 2.00	$ 3.26	Follow-up
FY	12	$ 2.00	$ 3.42	Follow-up
FY	13	$ 2.00	$ 3.59	Follow-up
FY	14	$ 2.00	$ 3.77	Follow-up
FY	15	$ 2.00	$ 3.96	Follow-up
FY	16	$ 2.00	$ 4.16	Final analysis and close-out of study

Sub-total		**$ 42.52**	**$ 60.57**	
Blood storage:		$ 2.00	$2.00	Freezers and supplies
		$ 0.35	$ 0.49	Parts and maintenance ($25K per year x 14 years)
Sub-total		**$ 2.35**	**$ 2.49**	
TOTAL		**$ 44.87**	**$ 63.03**	

Appendix I. BACKGROUND AND RATIONALE

I.1 Prostate Cancer Screening

The digital rectal examination is the test most often mentioned for prostate cancer screening, but recently two other test procedures have become available: transrectal ultrasound and prostate-specific antigen (Scardino, 1989). Although the digital rectal examination has been used for many years, careful evaluation of this modality has yet to take place. Several observational studies have been reported which examined process measures such as sensitivity as well as case survival data, but without appropriate controls and with no adjustment for lead time and length biases (Gilbertsen, 1971; Jenson, Shahon, and Wangensteen, 1960).

Chodak and Schoenberg, 1984 reported on 811 unselected patients from 50 to 80 years of age who underwent rectal examination and follow-up. Thirty-eight of 43 patients with a palpable abnormality in the prostate agreed to undergo biopsy. The positive predictive value of a palpable nodule, i.e., prostate cancer on biopsy, was 29 percent (11/38). Further evaluation revealed that 45 percent of the cases were stage B, 6 percent stage C, and 18 percent stage D. More recent results from the same investigators revealed a 25 percent positive predictive value with 68 percent of the detected tumors clinically localized (Chodak, Keller, and Schoenberg, 1989). Some additional investigators (Donohue, Fauver, Whitesel, et al, 1979; Gilbertsen,1971; Thompson, Ernst, Congai, et al, 1984; Thompson, Rounder, Teague, et al, 1987) also reported a high proportion of localized disease when prostate cancer is detected by routine rectal examination. In contrast, Wajsman and Chu (1979) reported that even with annual rectal examination, only 20 percent of cases are localized at diagnosis. More recently, a report appeared concerning screening of 1163 randomly selected men aged 50-69. Forty-five men were suspected of having prostate cancer, with 13 cancers actually found (Pedersen, Carlsson, Varenhorst, et al, 1990).

A recent review of the literature (Resnick, 1987) summarized the data on rectal examination for detection of prostate cancer as follows: sensitivity 55 to 69 percent, specificity 89 to 97 percent, positive predictive value 11 to 26 percent, negative predictive value 85 to 96 percent. Clearly, the rectal examination depends on the skill and experience of the examiner. However, it is inexpensive, non-invasive, non-morbid, and can be taught to non-professional health workers. What remains to be determined is whether routine annual screening by rectal examination reduces prostate cancer mortality.

Imaging procedures have also been suggested as possible screening modalities for prostate cancer. Prostatic imaging is possible by ultrasound, computerized tomography, and magnetic resonance imaging. From the early experience to date, each modality has relative merits and disadvantages for distinguishing different features of prostate cancer. Ultrasound has received the most attention to date, having been examined by several investigators in observational settings (Chodak and Schoenberg, 1989; Chodak, Wald,

Parmer, et al, 1986; Clements, Griffiths, Peeling, et al, 1988; Cooner, Mosley, Rutherford, et al, 1988; Lee, Littrup, Torp-Pedersen, et al, 1988; Lee, Torp-Pedersen, Littrup, et al, 1989; McClennan, 1988; Torp-Pedersen, Littrup, Lee, et al, 1988). The experience has been summarized by Waterhouse and Resnick (1989) who report that ultrasound has a low sensitivity and specificity with regard to the values necessary for screening. Sensitivity ranged from 71 to 92 percent for prostatic carcinoma and 60 to 85 percent for subclinical disease. Specificity values ranged from 41 to 79 percent, and positive predictive values in the 30 percent range have been reported. The sensitivity and positive predictive value for ultrasound appear to be better than for rectal examination. However, the relatively low specificity, the invasiveness and cost of the procedure preclude routine screening for prostate cancer by ultrasound or other current imaging techniques. Further refinement and controlled evaluation of this technique is needed to assess its role in screening.

A potentially more promising screening test is measurement of prostate-specific antigen (PSA). This procedure too has been examined in several observational settings, both for initial diagnosis of disease and as a tool to monitor for recurrence after initial therapy (Cooner, Mosley, Rutherford, et al, 1988; Lange, Ercole, Lightner, et al, 1989; Lee, Torp-Pedersen, Littrup, et al, 1989; Oesterling, Chan, Epstein, et al, 1988; Seamonds, Yang, Anderson, et al, 1986; Stamey, Kabalin, McNeal, et al, 1989; Stamey, Kabalin, Hay, et al, 1987). Parameter estimates for this test include sensitivity in the range of 70 percent and positive predictive values of 26-52 percent (Scardino, 1989). The potential value of the test appears to lie in its simplicity, lack of invasiveness, and lower cost relative to ultrasound; therefore, it may be a valuable adjunct to digital rectal examination. However, the possibility of identifying an excessive number of false positives in the form of benign prostatic lesions requires that the test be carefully evaluated.

To attempt to resolve questions surrounding the relative merits of the three tests, data were obtained on 1,788 men seen in Dr. William Cooner's clinic in Mobile, Alabama. All subjects had a rectal examination, PSA determination (Hybritech, normal ≤ 4.0), and a 7 mHz ultrasound examination. Dr. Cooner's group biopsied most of the subjects with positive results on ultrasound (U+) plus a few other subjects.

Lee, Torp-Pedersen, and Littrup (1989) have recently reported similar data on a series of U+ subjects who also had digital rectal exams (DRE) and PSA determinations (Yang, normal ≤ 2.6). The two studies are in very good agreement about the positive predictive value of the biopsy recommendation based on rectal exam plus PSA in U+ subjects. The pertinent results are given in the following table:

	Dr. Cooner's study			Dr. Lee's study		
	Biopsies	Cancer	Rate	Biopsies	Cancer	Rate
Rectal+, PSA+	235	151	.64	89	63	.71
Rectal+, PSA-	166	23	.14	23	6	.26
Rectal-, PSA+	134	41	.31	92	31	.34
Rectal-, PSA-	177	12	.07	44	2	.05

From these results it is apparent that the rate of cancer among U+ subjects in whom the rectal and PSA exams are normal is extremely low, not justifying the performance of ultrasound exams on everyone as a primary screening test.

Rigorous evaluation of any prostate cancer screening modality is mandatory because the natural history of the disease is so variable and appropriate treatment is not clearly defined (Johansson, Andersson, Krusemo, et al, 1989; Miller, 1989; Scardino, 1989). The incidence of prostate cancer found at autopsy steadily increases for each decade after age 50, and many of these lesions are clinically silent. Some progress has been made in predicting the biologic behavior of these tumors, but despite improved understanding of the biologic potential of prostate cancer as it relates to histologic grade and tumor volume, the necessity to treat or diagnose a given case of prostate cancer cannot be proved at this time. Given the possibility of unnecessary morbidity associated with diagnosis and treatment of many such lesions, careful evaluation of prostate cancer screening is needed.

I.2 Lung Cancer Screening

Chest x-ray and sputum cytology are the two modalities that have been suggested as screening tests for lung cancer. Attempts to evaluate these modalities were begun over 20 years ago. The studies include: (i) the Philadelphia Pulmonary Neoplasm Research Project (Boucot and Weiss, 1973), a non-randomized, uncontrolled study begun in 1951; (ii) the Veterans Administration study (Lilienfeld, Archer, Burnett, et al, 1966), a non-randomized, uncontrolled study performed from 1958 to 1961; (iii) the South London Lung Cancer Study (Nash, Morgan, and Tomkins, 1968), a non-randomized, uncontrolled study done in 1955 to 1963; (iv) the North London Cancer Study (Brett, 1968; Brett, 1969), a randomized study with industrial firms randomized between screening and no screening done in the early 1960s; and (v) the Kaiser Foundation Health Plan multiphasic screening trial (Dales, Friedman, and Collen, 1979; Friedman, Collen, and Fireman, 1986), a controlled trial with annual chest x-ray, spirometry, and medical questionnaire as part of the multiphasic screening begun in 1964. None of these studies demonstrated a significant impact of screening. The type of result obtained is illustrated by the South London study which showed an increase in the survival of screen-detected cases compared with other cases found in the same geographical region, but without adjustment for self-selection bias, lead time bias, overdiagnosis bias, or length bias (Cole and Morrison, 1980; Prorok and Connor, 1986). It should also be noted, however, that these studies typically were small and for most, follow-up was short so that any small to moderate size effect or any long-term effect was not likely to be demonstrated.

More recent studies include a randomized trial in Czechoslovakia (Kubik and Polak, 1986; Kubik, Parkin, Khlat, et al, 1990) and a case-control study in the German Democratic Republic (Ebeling and Nischan, 1987). As with some earlier studies, the randomized groups in the Czechoslovakian study were screened with x-ray and cytology at two different frequencies, semi-annual versus every three years, so that there was no unscreened control group. There was no difference in deaths between the two groups. The case-control study retrospectively evaluated chest x-rays originally used for control of tuberculosis. No effect of screening was seen, with the relative risk of lung cancer death being close to one, and no trend observed with number of tests or interval of testing.

Three other randomized controlled trials have recently ended. One trial, the Mayo Lung Project (Fontana, 1984; Fontana, 1985; Fontana, 1986) was initiated in 1971 for males 45 years or older who were heavy smokers. Mayo Clinic patients found to be free of lung cancer on initial screening were randomized either to a group that was offered cytologic and radiologic screening every four months or to a group that was not offered such screening. The other two studies, conducted at the Johns Hopkins University Hospital (Levin, Tockman, Frost, et al, 1982; Stitik and Tockman, 1978; Stitik, Tockman, and Khouri, 1985; Tockman, Frost, Stitik, et al, 1985) and at Memorial-Sloan Kettering Cancer Centre (Melamed, Flehinger, Zaman, et al, 1981; Melamed, Flehinger, Zaman, et al, 1984), solicited volunteers through local organisations, driver's license lists, media announcements, and other sources. In these two studies, both the study group and control group were offered annual chest x-ray, while the study group was also offered sputum cytology every four months. At the Mayo Clinic, cytology and radiology screening were compared with only advice to be screened annually with both modalities, while the other two centres assessed the additional value of cytology over and above the annual x-rays. In the Mayo Clinic study, cases found in the arm screened by sputum cytology and x-ray tended to be diagnosed in earlier stages than those in the control arm. However, there was no significant reduction in lung cancer mortality between the screened group and the control group in any of these trials.

At this point there is no solid evidence that screening for lung cancer can reduce lung cancer mortality. Sputum cytology has not been shown to be effective as an adjunct to annual chest x-ray. There is evidence from all three studies that screening with chest x-ray plus sputum cytology does improve stage at diagnosis and case survival rate relative to cases diagnosed through usual care, but even when this occurred there was no reduction in lung cancer mortality.

The Mayo study is the only one of the three which is pertinent to the proposal to study annual x-ray in the present trial because the use of screening x-rays differed in the two arms. Several reservations can be noted about the Mayo study finding however. First, the study was designed to detect a 50 percent reduction in lung cancer mortality, and as such the sample size of 10,000 men was insufficient to demonstrate a small but important reduction of 10-15 percent. Secondly, at the time the study was terminated there were still some 40 excess cases of lung cancer in the screened group. Whether these cases represent overdiagnosis or a source of screening benefit which would only be seen with longer follow-up is not known. Thirdly, it has been stated that some 50 percent of men in the control group received an annual chest x-ray (Fontana, 1986). To the extent that these were screening x-rays, the level of contamination may have been sufficient to obscure any small to moderate size benefit. A further factor possibly obscuring benefit in the Mayo study, and the Czechoslovakian study as well, is that a prevalence screen was conducted on the entire trial population before randomization, and any prevalence lung cancers found were excluded from the randomized study. Thus any effect on lung cancer mortality from a prevalence screen cannot be ascertained in these studies.

The concern about insufficient size of previous studies of chest x-ray screening is illustrated in the following table:

Power to detect various screening effects in previous studies of chest x-ray screening for lung cancer

Study	Mortality reduction (%)				
	10	20	30	40	50
Philadelphia	.14	.32	.59	.85	.98
VA	.16	.38	.69	.92	.99
South London	.14	.31	.57	.83	.97
North London	.16	.39	.70	.93	.995
Kaiser	.12	.27	.50	.76	.94
Czechoslovakia	.16	.39	.71	.93	.996
Mayo	.21	.54	.88	.99	.999

The uncertainty in interpretation of results from completed studies, and the apparent widespread clinical perception that the annual chest x-ray is of some value lead one to conclude that a clear difference of opinion exists regarding the value of annual chest x-rays. Whether a small but important benefit exists can only be demonstrated reliably by a properly designed randomized trial.

I.3 Colorectal Cancer Screening

Digital rectal examination, sigmoidoscopy, and occult blood testing have been suggested for colorectal cancer screening because they are relatively simple, rapid, and inexpensive. While these tests are in use by many private physicians and as part of screening programs in various parts of the world, none has received a definitive evaluation and the evidence of benefit for each is at best uncertain.

Digital rectal examination and rigid sigmoidoscopy were both part of the multiphasic screening program carried out by the Kaiser Foundation and some consider the results of this study to be evidence of the effectiveness of these tests (Guidelines, 1980). Approximately 5,000 individuals were allocated to a study group urged to receive an annual multiphasic checkup, and a comparable number served as controls. After 11 years, the screened group experienced a colorectal cancer death rate of 1.0 per 1,000 compared to a rate of 3.3 per 1,000 in the control group (Dales, Friedman, and Collen, 1979; Friedman, Collen, and Fireman, 1986). The observed decrease in colorectal cancer mortality in this study could be a real effect resulting from screening by digital rectal examination and sigmoidoscopy. However, this conclusion has been questioned for several reasons (Morrison, 1985). For example, some cancers were detected in an investigation of anemia resulting from the multiphasic examination as well as by the two tests. Furthermore, some 30 different causes of death were investigated, and among these the cumulative mortalities observed for lymphohematopoietic cancer and suicide were similar in size but opposite in direction to the values for colorectal cancer. Thus, it is possible that chance or some unrecognized bias was responsible for part or all of the observed mortality difference. Further, in a recent re-analysis the investigators found that rates of sigmoidoscopy were low in both groups (control - 25%, screened - 30%), that there was only a slight excess of exposure to sigmoidoscopy in the study group compared to the control group, and that there was not an appreciable difference in removal of colorectal polyps between groups. They concluded that the results are inconclusive with respect to sigmoidoscopy and should not be used as evidence either for or against sigmoidoscopy screening (Selby, Friedman, and Collen, 1988).

Two additional observational studies of sigmoidoscopy have been reported. One involved 21,000 subjects in Minnesota who underwent an annual physical examination that included sigmoidoscopy (Gilbertsen, 1974; Gilbertsen and Nelms, 1978). The second study followed 26,000 men and women in New York (Hertz, 1960). In the Minnesota study, any polyps discovered during screening were removed and the number of sigmoid cancers ultimately found was only 15 percent of the number expected based on statewide incidence rates. These data suggest that early cancers were detected, and that a major benefit of sigmoidoscopy is the removal of polyps before they have a chance to develop into cancer. All of the 13 cancers found were localized and none of the patients had died as of 1979. In 50 cancer patients identified by screening and followed over 15 years in the New York study, the five-year survival rate was reported to be near 90 percent.

The interpretation that screening was of benefit in these studies can be questioned on several grounds. Both studies are likely to be affected by self-selection bias of participants and by exclusion of certain individuals from the follow-up process. In the New York study, seven people with a history of symptoms and eight with previously diagnosed lesions were excluded, thereby automatically lowering the observed incidence and mortality rates. In the Minnesota study, cases found at the initial examination were excluded from the observed incidence, and only individuals without gastrointestinal symptoms were allowed to participate. Thus, data from a general population are not valid for comparison (Morrison, 1985). In addition, the reported survival data from both studies are affected by lead time and length biases, but no adjustment for these biases was attempted.

Several uncontrolled studies suggesting that the occult blood test leads to early detection have been reported (Fruchmorgen and Demling, 1980; Winawer, 1987, Winawer, Fath, Schottenfeld, et al, 1985). In addition, three controlled studies using occult blood tests for colorectal cancer screening have been conducted. A randomized trial in the United Kingdom involving 20,525 individuals reported a 36.8 percent compliance rate with the test. Of 13 cancers found in the screened group, nine were Dukes stage A and two Dukes B, while among the 10 cancers in the control group, four were Dukes B and the remainder more advanced. In view of the problems with staging as an outcome variable, it was concluded that a larger study is necessary to determine whether mortality rates can be reduced by such screening (Hardcastle, Farrands, Balfour, et al, 1983; Hardcastle, Armitage, Chamberlain, et al, 1986). The Strang Clinic of New York is conducting a non-randomized study involving some 12,000 screenees and 7,000 controls. The study is designed to test the effect of combining the stool guaiac test with annual sigmoidoscopy. Preliminary results show a shift toward earlier stage of diagnosis among the screened group, but no mortality data have been reported (Flehinger, Herbert, Winawer, et al, 1988). A randomized trial of the stool guaiac test began in 1974 at the University of Minnesota, where 48,000 persons were randomized into three groups, a control group, an annually screened group, and a biennially screened group. Preliminary results indicate a shift toward earlier stage cancers in the screened group compared to the controls (Gilbertsen, McHugh, Schuman, et al, 1980). Two additional randomized trials of occult blood screening were recently initiated (Kewenter, Bjork, Haglind, et al, 1988; Klaaborg, Madsen, Sondergaard, et al, 1986; Kronborg, Fenger, Olsen, et al, 1989).

Recent reviews of the status of colorectal cancer screening, particularly using an occult blood test, have concluded that no clear cut evidence of benefit exists and that data from ongoing studies are needed to clarify the situation (Frank, 1985; Simon, 1985). A Consensus Conference convened by the National Cancer Institute in 1978 reached the same conclusion (Consensus, 1979). Alternatively, both the NCI Working Guidelines for Early Cancer Detection, 1987 and the guidelines for a cancer-related checkup by physicians published by the American Cancer Society (Fink, 1983; Guidelines, 1980) recommend an annual digital rectal examination for persons over 39, an annual stool guaiac test starting at age 50, and sigmoidoscopy every three to five years beginning at age 50. In view of the uncontrolled nature of most reported studies and the difficulty in interpreting available data, evidence for effectiveness of screening for colorectal cancer is not conclusive.

Testing for occult blood in the stool to reduce colorectal cancer mortality is under study in five trials, and even if shown effective, the lack of specificity of the test could render its mass applicability questionable on cost-benefit grounds. The focus of this trial is therefore flexible sigmoidoscopy. The flexible procedure has been shown to be more acceptable to screenees than the rigid scope (Crespi, Weissman, Gilbertsen, et al, 1984; Winawer, Miller, Lightdale, et al, 1987) and the test appears to be very sensitive and highly specific for cancer. The need to address the impact of flexible sigmoidoscopy screening on colorectal cancer mortality has been discussed by several investigators (Chamberlain, Day, Hakama, et al, 1986; Neugut and Pita, 1988; Winawer, Miller, Lightdale, et al, 1987). Encouraging reports of the potential impact of this test come from modeling work of Eddy which suggests a mortality reduction of 25-40 percent (Eddy, Nugent, Eddy, et al, 1987). However, these results are subject to the assumptions in the methodology, so that conclusive results will only be obtained from a randomized trial.

REFERENCES

American Cancer Society. Cancer facts and figures - 1988. New York: American Cancer Society, 1988.

Boucot KR, Weiss W. Is curable lung cancer detected by semiannual screening? JAMA 1973; 224:1361-1365.

Brett GZ. The value of lung cancer detection by six-monthly chest radiographs. Thorax 1968; 23:414-420.

Brett GZ. Earlier diagnosis and survival in lung cancer. Br Med J 1969; 4:260-262.

Chamberlain J, Day NE, Hakama M, et al. UICC workshop of the project on evaluation of screening programmes for gastrointestinal cancer. Int J Cancer 1986; 37:329-334.

Chodak GW, Keller P, Schoenberg HW. Assessment of screening for prostate cancer using the digital rectal examination. J Urol 1989; 141:1136-1138.

Chodak GW, Schoenberg HW. Early detection of prostate cancer by routine screening. JAMA 1984; 252:3261-3264.

Chodak GW, Schoenberg HW. Progress and problems in screening for carcinoma of the prostate. World J Surg 1989; 13:60-64.

Chodak GW, Wald V, Parmer E, et al. Comparison of digital examination and transrectal ultrasonography for the diagnosis of prostatic cancer. J Urol 1986; 135:951-954.

Clements R, Griffiths GJ, Peeling WB, et al. How accurate is the index finger? A comparison of digital and ultrasound examination of the prostatic nodule. Clinical Radiology 1988; 39:87-89.

Cole P, Morrison AS. Basic issues in population screening for cancer. JNCI 1980; 64:1263-1272.

Consensus Conclusions and Recommendations. In: Brodie DR, ed. Screening and early detection of colorectal cancer. U.S. Department of Health, Education and Welfare, NIH Publication No. 80-2075, 1979, pp.1-3.

Cooner WH, Mosley BR, Rutherford CL, et al. Clinical application of transrectal ultrasonography and prostate specific antigen in the search for prostate cancer. J Urol 1988; 139:758-761.

Crespi M, Weissman GS, Gilbertsen VA, et al. The role of proctosigmoidoscopy in screening for colorectal neoplasia. CA–A Cancer Journal for Clinicians 1984; 34:158-166.

Dales LG, Friedman GD, Collen MF. Evaluating periodic multiphasic health check-ups: a controlled trial. J Chronic Dis 1979; 32:385-404.

Donohue RE, Fauver HE, Whitesel JA, et al. Staging prostatic cancer: a different distribution. J Urol 1979; 122:327-329.

Ebeling K, Nischan P. Screening for lung cancer - results from a case-control study. Int J Cancer 1987; 40:141-144.

Eddy DM, Nugent FW, Eddy JF, et al. Screening for colorectal cancer in a high-risk population. Results of a mathematical model. Gastroenterology 1987; 92:682-692.

Fink DJ. Facts about colorectal cancer detection. CA–A Cancer Journal for Clinicians 1983; 33:366-367.

Flehinger BJ, Herbert E, Winawer SJ, et al. Screening for colorectal cancer with fecal occult blood test and sigmoidoscopy: preliminary report of the colon project of Memorial Sloan-Kettering Cancer Centre and PMI-Strang Clinic. In: Chamberlain J, Miller AB, eds. Screening for gastrointestinal cancer. Toronto: Hans Huber, 1988, pp.9-16.

Fontana RS. Early detection of lung cancer: the Mayo Lung Project. In: Prorok PC, Miller AB, eds. Screening for cancer. I - general principles on evaluation of screening for cancer and screening for lung, bladder and oral cancer; vol 78. Geneva: International Union Against Cancer. UICC Technical Report Series, 1984, pp.107-122.

Fontana RS. Screening for lung cancer. In: Miller AB, ed. Screening for cancer. New York: Academic Press, 1985, pp.377-395.

Fontana RS. Screening for lung cancer: recent experience in the United States. In: Hansen HH, ed. Lung cancer: basic and clinical aspects. Boston: Martinus Nijhoff, 1986, pp.91-111.

Frank JW. Occult-blood screening for colorectal carcinoma: the benefits. Am J Prev Med 1985; 1:3-9.

Friedman GD, Collen MF, Fireman BH. Multiphasic health checkup evaluation: a 16-year follow-up. J Chronic Dis 1986; 39:453-463.

Fruchmorgen P, Demling L. Early detection of colorectal cancer with a modified guaiac test - a screening examination of 6,000 humans. In: Winawer S, Schottenfeld D, Sherlock P, eds. Progress in cancer research and therapy. Colorectal cancer prevention and screening; vol 13. New York: Raven Press, 1980, pp.311-315.

Gilbertsen VA. Cancer of the prostate gland: results of early diagnosis and therapy undertaken for cure of the disease. JAMA 1971; 215:81-84.

Gilbertsen VA. Proctosigmoidoscopy and polypectomy in reducing the incidence of rectal cancer. Cancer 1974; 4:936-939.

Gilbertsen VA, McHugh RB, Schuman LM, et al. Colon cancer control study: an interim report. In: Winawer S, Schottenfeld D, Sherlock P, eds. Progress in cancer research and treatment. Colorectal cancer prevention and screening; vol 13. New York: Raven Press, 1980, pp.261-266.

Gilbertsen VA, Nelms JM. The prevention of invasive cancer of the rectum. Cancer 1978; 41:1137-1139.

Guidelines for the cancer-related check-up: recommendations and rationale. CAA Cancer Journal for Clinicians 1980; 30:191-240.

Hardcastle JD, Farrands PA, Balfour TW, et al. Controlled trial of fecal occult blood testing in the detection of colorectal cancer. Lancet 1983; ii:1-4.

Hardcastle JD, Armitage NC, Chamberlain J, et al. Fecal occult blood screening for colorectal cancer in the general population. Results of a controlled trial. Cancer 1986; 58:397-403.

Hertz RE. Value of periodic examinations in detecting cancer of the colon and rectum. Postgrad Med 1960; 27:290-294.

Jenson CB, Shahon DB, Wangensteen OH. Evaluation of annual examinations in the detection of cancer. JAMA 1960; 174:1783-1788.

Johansson JE, Andersson SO, Krusemo UB, et al. Natural history of localised prostatic cancer. A population-based study in 223 untreated patients. Lancet 1989; i:799-803.

Kewenter J, Bjork S, Haglind E, et al. Screening and rescreening for colorectal cancer. A controlled trial of fecal occult blood testing in 27,700 subjects. Cancer 1988; 62:645-651.

Klaaborg K, Madsen MS, Sondergaard O, et al. Participation in mass screening for colorectal cancer with fecal occult blood test. Scand J Gastroenterol 1986; 21:1180-1184.

Kronborg O, Fenger C, Olsen J, et al. Repeated screening for colorectal cancer with fecal occult blood test. A prospective randomized study at Funen, Denmark. Scand J Gastroenterol 1989; 24:599-606.

Kubik A, Polak J. Lung cancer detection - results of a randomized prospective study in Czechoslovakia. Cancer 1986; 57:2427-2437.

Kubik A, Parkin M, Khlat M, et al. Lack of benefit from semi-annual screening for cancer of the lung: follow-up report of a randomized controlled trial on a population of high-risk males in Czechoslovakia. Int J Cancer 1990; 45:26-33.

Lange PH, Ercole CJ, Lightner DJ, et al. The value of serum prostate specific antigen determinations before and after radical prostatectomy. J Urol 1989; 141:873-879.

Lee F, Littrup PJ, Torp-Pedersen ST, et al. Prostate cancer: comparison of transrectal US and digital rectal examination for screening. Radiology 1988; 168:389-394.

Lee F, Torp-Pedersen S, Littrup PJ, et al. Hypoechoic lesions of the prostate: clinical relevance of tumor size, digital rectal examination, and prostate-specific antigen. Radiology 1989; 170:29-32.

Levin ML, Tockman MS, Frost JK, et al. Lung cancer mortality in males screened by chest x-ray and cytologic sputum examination: a preliminary report. Recent Results Cancer Res 1982; 82:138-146.

Lilienfeld A, Archer PG, Burnett CH, et al. An evaluation of radiologic and cytologic screening for the early detection of lung cancer: a cooperative pilot study of the American Cancer Society and the Veterans Administration. Cancer Res 1966; 26:2083-2121.

McClennan BL. Transrectal US of the prostate: is the technology leading the science? Radiology 1988; 168:571-575.

Melamed MR, Flehinger BJ, Zaman MB, et al. Detection of true pathologic stage I lung cancer in a screening program and the effect on survival. Cancer 1981; 47:1182-1187.

Melamed MR, Flehinger BJ, Zaman MB, et al. Screening for lung cancer. Results of the Memorial Sloan-Kettering study in New York. Chest 1984; 86:44-53.

Miller GJ. Histopathology of prostate cancer: prediction of malignant behavior and correlation with ultrasonography. Urology 1989; 33:18-26.

Morrison AS. Screening in chronic disease. New York: Oxford University Press, 1985.

National Cancer Institute. 1987 annual cancer statistics review, including cancer trends: 1950-1985. NCI, DCPC. NIH Publication No. 88-2789, 1987.

Nash FA, Morgan JM, Tomkins JG. South London lung cancer study. Br Med J 1968; 2:715-721.

Neugut AI, Pita S. Role of sigmoidoscopy in screening for colorectal cancer: a critical review. Gastroenterology 1988; 95:492-499.

Oesterling JE, Chan DW, Epstein JI, et al. Prostate specific antigen in the preoperative and postoperative evaluation of localized prostatic cancer treated with radical prostatectomy. J Urol 1988; 139:766-772.

Pedersen KV, Carlsson P, Varenhorst E, et al. Screening for carcinoma of the prostate by digital rectal examination in a randomly selected population. Br Med J 1990; 300:1041-1044.

Prorok PC, Connor RJ. Screening for the early detection of cancer. Cancer Invest 1986; 4:225-238.

Resnick MI. Editorial comments. In: Rattiff TL, Catalona WJ, eds. Genitourinary cancer. Boston: Martinus Nijhoff, 1987, pp.94-99.

Scardino PT. Early detection of prostate cancer. Advances in Urologic Ultrasound 1989; 16:635-655.

Seamonds B, Yang N, Anderson K, et al. Evaluation of prostate-specific antigen and prostatic acid phosphatase as prostate cancer markers. Urology 1986; 28:472-479.

Selby JV, Friedman GD, Collen MF. Sigmoidoscopy and mortality from colorectal cancer: the Kaiser Permanente multiphasic evaluation study. J Clin Epidemiol 1988; 41:427-434.

Simon JB. Occult blood screening for colorectal carcinoma: a critical review. Gastroenterology 1985; 88:820-837.

Stamey TA, Kabalin JN, McNeal JE, et al. Prostate specific antigen in the diagnosis and treatment of adenocarcinoma of the prostate. II. Radical prostatectomy treated patients. J Urol 1989; 141:1076-1083.

Stamey TA, Yang N, Hay AR, et al. Prostate-specific antigen as a serum marker for adenocarcinoma of the prostate. N Engl J Med 1987; 317: 909-916.

Stitik FP, Tockman MS. Radiographic screening in the early detection of lung cancer. Radiologic Clinics of North America 1978; 16:347-366.

Stitik FP, Tockman MS, Khouri NF. Chest radiology. In: Miller AB, ed. Screening for cancer. New York: Academic Press, 1985, pp.163-191.

Taylor WF, Fontana RS. Biometric design of the Mayo lung project for early detection and localization of bronchogenic carcinoma. Cancer 1972; 30:1344-1347.

Thompson IA, Ernst JJ, Congai MP, et al. Adenocarcinoma of the prostate: results of routine urological screening. J Urol 1984; 132:690-692.

Thompson IM, Rounder JB, Teague JL, et al. Impact of routine screening for adenocarcinoma of the prostate on stage distribution. J Urol 1987; 137:424-426.

Tockman MS, Frost JK, Stitik FP, et al. Screening and detection of lung cancer. In: Aisner J, ed. Lung cancer. New York: Churchill Livingstone, 1985, pp.25-39.

Torp-Pedersen ST, Littrup PJ, Lee F, et al. Early prostate cancer: diagnostic costs of screening transrectal US and digital rectal examination. Radiology 1988; 169:351-354.

Wajsman Z, Chu TM. Detection and diagnosis of prostatic cancer. In: Murphy GP, ed. Prostatic cancer. Littleton, MA: PSG Publishing, 1979.

Waterhouse RL, Resnick MI: The use of transrectal prostatic ultrasonography in the evaluation of patients with prostatic carcinoma. J Urol 1989; 141:233-239.

Winawer SJ. Screening for colorectal cancer. In: DeVita VT, Hellman S, Rosenberg SA, eds. Cancer principles and practice of oncology, second edition. Philadelphia: JP Lippincott 1987; 1:1-16.

Winawer SJ, Fath RB, Schottenfeld D, et al. Screening for colorectal cancer. In: Miller AB, ed. Screening for cancer. New York: Academic Press, 1985, pp.347-366.

Winawer SJ, Miller C, Lightdale C, et al. Patient response to sigmoidoscopy. A randomized, controlled trial of rigid and flexible sigmoidoscopy. Cancer 1987; 60:1905-1908.

Working guidelines for early cancer detection rationale and supporting evidence to decrease mortality. Early Detection Branch, DCPC, NCI. December, 1987.

33 Summary of Discussion on Screening for Cancer of the Prostate

Screening for prostate cancer is confronted by a number of questions including:

the sensitivity and specificity of the screening tests;

the appropriate treatment to be used for "early" disease;

the morbidity and mortality associated with the detection and treatment of non-progressive cancer;

the costs of screening;

the few potential years of life saved, given the age distribution of prostate cancer patients; and

the ethics of screening for the disease.

Post mortem studies have shown that many times more men have latent prostate cancer than will ever surface in life, so that uncovering and operating on these cancers would lead to great over-diagnosis and over-treatment. No data are available on the accuracy of any screening test in detecting with reasonable sensitivity and specificity those cancers that will progress to clinical disease.

The incidence of prostate cancer is greatest at oldest ages, where any possible extension of life following screening is likely to be short, while the quality of life for many may be low. Therefore in any research study it is important to assess the quality of life years that may be gained as well as other harms and benefits. One approach to limit poor quality of life gained might be to exclude people with severe cardiovascular or other disease who might suffer greater harm from radical surgery for prostate cancer than others.

State of the Art on Screening for Neuroblastoma

There is some suggestion from Japanese studies that screening for neuroblastoma can reduce mortality. There is a need to determine if the results from Japan can be replicated in other countries.

At present, screening for neuroblastoma in countries other than Japan cannot be recommended as public health policy.

Recommendations for Research
Complete the evaluation studies in the UK and North America.
Determine the optimum age to screen.

34 Neuroblastoma: Studies in Japan

T. SAWADA, T. MATSUMURA, Y. MATSUDA, and H. KAWAKATSU

Department of Pediatrics, Kyoto Prefectural University of Medicine
Kawaramachi, Kamikyoku, Kyoto, 602, Japan

1 INTRODUCTION

Neuroblastoma (NB) is the second most common malignant tumour of children and accounts for 10% of all cases of childhood cancer in Japan (Table 1) (Children's Cancer Association of Japan, 1987).

Table 1 Childhood Cancer in Japan (1969-1984)

Leukemia	8,459 (42.6%)
Neuroblastoma	2,052 (10.3%)
Brain tumour	1,827 (9.2%)
Malignant lymphoma	1,617 (8.1%)
Retinoblastoma	1,528 (7.7%)
Wilms' tumour	932 (4.7%)
Hepatoblastoma	591 (3.0%)
Rhabdomyosarcoma	548 (2.8%)
Testicular or ovarian tumour	481 (2.4%)
Bone tumour	281 (1.4%)
Others	1,537 (7.7%)
Total	19,853 (100%)

The incidence of NB in Japan is about 8.2 per million children (under 15 years of age) (Sawada et al., 1984), the same as in the US (Young and Miller, 1975), the UK (Jones, 1981) and Torino, Italy (Pastore et al., 1982).

The tumour originates from the adrenal glands or sympathetic ganglia and is diagnosed by a palpable abdominal mass, typical clinical symptoms such as leg pains, persistent high fever, exophthalmus, intractable diarrhoea or opsomyoclonus, etc., in addition to elevation of urinary vanillylmandelic acid (VMA) and homovanillic acid (HVA) levels (Sawada et al., 1971; Gitlow et al, 1970) and serum neurone specific enolase level (Ishiguro et al., 1983; Zelter et al., 1983). Patients with the tumour are treated intensively by surgery, chemotherapy and radiotherapy, but their prognoses are unfavourable because most patients are not discovered until progressive stages when the tumour is already palpable or causes overt symptoms. The most important prognostic factors for NB are age and stage of disease at diagnosis. The 2-year survival rate of patients was nearly 30% in Japan in 1979 (Sawaguchi et al., 1985) before the introduction of mass screening for NB, the same rate as in the Children's Cancer Study Group A report in 1971 (Breslow and McCann, 1971). Most NB patients under 1 year of age and/or with stage I, II or IVs have a good prognosis, but it is difficult to clinically detect NB masses in infants or at early stages because there are no characteristic symptoms. Early diagnosis is essential to improve the survival rate for NB patients, but most cases are not discovered until progressive stages.

As NB is a catecholamine producing tumour, similar to pheochromocytoma in adults, most cases demonstrate excessive excretion of VMA and HVA (Sawada et al, 1971; Gitlow et al., 1970).

In this paper, we present our recent results of NB Mass Screening (MS) during infancy in Japan and discuss some problems related to our MS program.

2 THE BACKGROUND OF NB MASS SCREENING IN JAPAN

In 1972, NB-MS for 3-year old children in Kyoto which aimed at the early detection of NB by a VMA spot test commenced, although this test was known to miss 25% of all NBs, the non-VMA secreting ones. Only one case was detected among 42,636 3-year old children, but he died from NB progression although his disease was confirmed to stage II (Sawada et al., 1978).

In 1974, NB-MS was initiated for 6-month-old infants in Kyoto. Four cases with asymptomatic NB were detected from 78,331 infants screened during the 6 year period from July, 1973, to September, 1979 (Sawada et al., 1982), which all had good prognoses. Thereafter, NB-MS in infancy was also initiated in 8 other districts in Japan, and NB was detected in 16 of the 281,939 infants screened (Sawada et al., 1984). Fifteen of these 16 infants with NB were cured. In 1986, the outcomes of 25 NB cases detected by MS were also reported to be favourable (Sawada et al., 1986).

In 1985, nation-wide MS was initiated throughout Japan with the financial support of the Japanese Government. In 1988, the Ministry of Health and Welfare recommended MS by the quantitative measurement of VMA, HVA and creatinine using HPLC (high performance liquid chromatography) to replace the qualitative VMA test to enable detection of non-VMA secreting NBs.

A summary of the events leading to the national programme is given in Table 2.

Table 2   The Background of Mass Screening for NB in Japan

1972: In Kyoto, a VMA spot test was distributed by local health centres for 3 year old children.
1974: In Kyoto, NB screening for 6 month old infants was initiated.
1977: Nagoya joins NB screening programme by a VMA dip test.
1980: Osaka joins NB screening programme by a VMA spot test.
1981: The NB-Mass Screening Study Group (NB-MSSG) was organized to evaluate the effectiveness of NB mass screening.
1985: Nation-wide NB mass screening was initiated.
1988: Quantitative screening (VMA, HVA and creatinine) using HPLC was recommended.

3 THE MASS SCREENING SYSTEM

A representative diagram of the screening system during infancy is shown in Figure 1 (Sawada et al., 1982). All 3-month-old infants receive physical examinations at local health centres under the Child Health Survey Program, at which time parents are given a screening set which contains a small urine container or a filter paper, a return-paid envelope and a prospectus that describes the MS program. Each mother is asked to mail a urine sample when her infant is 6-months old. If a sample shows a positive result, the infant is sent to a hospital for further physical examination, chest and abdominal X-rays and abdominal echogram. If a mass is detected, the infant is admitted to hospital and treatment is given soon. If a mass is not detected by further examination, the infant should be re-examined and follow-up should be continued until the infant reaches one year of age.

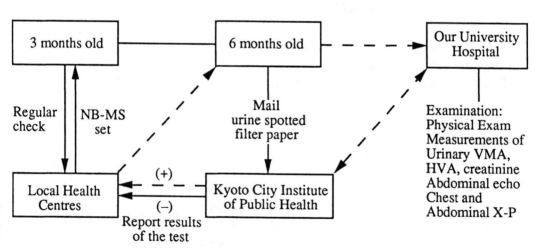

Figure 1 Neuroblastoma mass screening system

3.1 Results

A summary of the present status of the screening programme in Japan is shown in Table 3.

Table 3   Number of infants and incidence of NB detected by mass screening

Year	Number of births	Number of infants tested	Percentage tested	Number of NB infants	Incidence of NB
1984	1,469,923	124,870	8.5%	3	1/41,623
1985	1,425,043	834,536	58.6%	56	1/14,902
1986	1,374,666	997,643	72.6%	66	1/15,116
1987	1,332,491	1,024,841	76.9%	88	1/11,646
1988	?	1,036,740*	?	123	1/ 8,429
	4,018,630			342	1/11,750

*Qualitative 508,924, Quantitative 527,816

In 1985, 58.6% of all 6-month-old infants in Japan received MS and in 1987 the figure was 76.9%, or over one million infants. During the past 5 years, 342 cases were diagnosed as NB from about 4 million infants who received screening. The incidence of NB detected by nation-wide MS is 1/11,750 infants. Notably, since 1988, by monitoring quantitative VMA and HVA levels with HPLC, the number of NB cases detected has increased and 1 NB case has been detected for every 8,500 infants screened. By the end of 1989, the Japanese NB-MS Study Group had 337 registration case-cards for patients that were detected by the MS programme since its inception in Kyoto in 1974. Their analytical results (Sawada and the Committee on Neuroblastoma Mass Screening of the Japanese Childhood Cancer Research, 1987) follow.

3.2 Analysis of the 337 cases detected by NB-MS
The majority, 289 cases (85.8%), were diagnosed by 9 months of age (Table 4). Some mothers had forgotten to send the urine samples of their infants at 6 months of age.

Table 4   Age distribution at diagnosis

Age (months)	Number of Cases (percentage)	
5	1	(0.3%)
6	25	(7.4%)
7	108	(32.0%)
8	88	(26.1%)
9	67	(19.9%)
≥10	43	(12.8%)
Unknown	5	(1.5%)
Total	337	(100%)

Symptoms and physical findings   Only 5 cases (1.5%) were known to have had complaints before diagnosis. Case 1 had fever and anaemia, case 2 sweating, case 3 sweating and poor weight gain, case 4 had exophthalmos, typical for stage IV, and case 5 had respiratory disturbance by a mediastinal NB. For 9 cases (2.7%) it was not known whether or not symptoms were present.   Remarkably, 96% of the cases were asymptomatic.

Investigation showed that 293 (86.9%) of the cases had abdominal NB and 42 (12.5%) mediastinal NB.   At the initial physical examination, only 52% (152 cases) of the 293 abdominal NB cases were found to have an abdominal mass. In 42.3% (124 cases), abdominal masses were not found by the paediatric oncologist and in the remaining 17(5.7%) the presence or absence of a mass was not reported. None of the 42 mediastinal NB cases had indicative findings at the time of physical examination. There were two (0.6%) cases with cervical NB. Both had a palpable mass.

Urinary VMA and HVA and other markers Fourteen percent (48 cases) of these patients had measurements of under 24 ug VMA/mg creatinine. Several of these cases were detected by increased urinary HVA by HPLC. The remaining 86% showed excess VMA excretion into the urine, 23% (77 cases) had under 34 ug HVA/mg creatinine. Following the introduction of HPLC, patients with lower VMA or HVA levels have been detected. Other biochemical markers such as serum neuron specific enolase (NSE) and ferritin which are reported to be specific markers of NB are less sensitive than VMA and HVA for detecting NB at early stages. Serum NSE was measured in 234 of the 337 cases. The levels in 102 cases (42%) were under 14 ng/ml, 116 cases (55%) between 15 and 49 ng/ml, 13 cases (3%) between 50 and 99 ng/ml, and in only 3 cases, over 100 ng/ml.

Primary sites and histology There were no characteristic original sites and no characteristic histologies for these infant neuroblastomas. Abdominal NBs accounted for 87% and mediastinal NBs 12% of all tumours in this study. These figures were the same as in the US report (Pochedly, 1976) and Japanese reports (Committee of Malignant Tumour of Society of the Japanese Paediatric Surgeon, 1979), which consisted of a complete analysis of the total number of NB cases clinically detected before the introduction of NB-MS in Japan (Table 5).   Additionally, in the NB-MS results, there were 101 ganglioneuroblastomas (30%):   12 well differentiated, 26 composite, 57 poorly differentiated and 6 unclassified. Of the 227 neuroblastoma cases 193 (57%) were of the rosette-fibrillary type.

Weights of primary masses ranged from 3.0 g to 490 g; 58% of the patients (196 cases) had tumours under 50 g; however, 138 primary masses (41% of the cases) had unilateral or bilateral extension.

Table 5   Primary sites of NB in some series

Primary Sites	Our Study (1989)	Registry of Jap Paed Surg (1971-1976)	From textbook, Pochedly (1976)
Mediastinal	42(12%)	60(12%)	(15%)
Abdominal	293(87%)	403(82%)	(70%)
Adrenal	182(54%)	238(48%)	(66%)
Retroperitoneal	101(30%)	113(23%)	
Pelvic	10(3%)	20(4%)	(4%)
Others		32(7%)	
Others	2(1%)	12(2%)	(3%)
Unknown	0	20(4%)	(12%)
Total	337(100%)	495(100%)	1,303(100%)

The stage distribution The staging system used was that of Evans, D'Angio and Randolph (1971). Thirty-two percent (105 cases) were detected at stage I; 34% (116 cases) at stage II; and 9% (31 cases) at stage IVs. Conversely, only 8% (26 cases) were detected at stage IV. The stage distributions of the total number of NBs in the Registry of the Japanese Paediatric Surgeons (Committee of Malignant Tumour of Society of the Japanese Paediatric Surgeon, 1979; and Committee of Malignant Tumour of Society of the Japanese Paediatric Surgeon, 1989) and the CCSGA (Breslow and McCann, 1971) are shown in Table 6.

Table 6   Stage distribution

Stage	This study (1989)	Registry of Jap Paed Surg			CCSGA (1971)
		(1988)	(1987)	(1971-1976)	
I	105(32%)	33(17%)	28(20%)	42(9%)	21(9%)
II	116(34%)	42(21%)	23(16%)	52(11%)	35(14%)
IVs	31(9%)	8(4%)	16(11%)	38(8%)	27(11%)
III	57(17%)	40(20%)	32(22%)	83(17%)	27(11%)
IV	26(8%)	77(39%)	44(31%)	267(55%)	136(55%)
Unknown	2(1%)				
Total	337(100%)	200(100%)	143(100%)	482(100%)	246(100%)
I+II+IVs	252 (75%)	83 (42%)	67 (47%)	132 (27%)	83 (34%)

From 1971 to 1976, cases with favourable stages comprised 27% and stage IV cases were 55%, the same as the CCSGA results; but, in 1987, 3 years after initiation of NB-MS, NB cases with favourable stages had increased to 47% and stage IV cases had decreased from 55% to 31% for all NB in the Japanese registry.

Metastatic Sites Metastases were observed in 177 cases (53%). Lymph node metastases were observed in 154 cases (48%), ipsilateral in 102, bilateral in 40 and distant in 12. There were some cases which had widely spread metastases, 35 (10%) (5 suspicious and 30 positive) in the bone marrow, 24 (7%) in the liver (3 in one lobe and 21 in both), 6 in bones and 5 in other sites.

Outcome At the end of August, 1989, 328 cases (97%) were still alive and 7 cases (2%) had died, 3 cases with stage IV from progressive neuroblastoma and the remaining 4 (2 stage IVs, 1 stage III and 1 stage II) from surgical complications or unknown causes, but not neuroblastoma progression. One case refused treatment and another one could not be followed up. Out of the 83 stage III or IV cases, 78 (95%) are alive now and are expected to be cured.

4 DISCUSSION

4.1 Problems with the programme
Some major problems encountered during the NB-MS programme are as follows.

The screening method As a qualitative VMA test misses non-VMA secreting NB, it is better to screen for NB by quantitative VMA and HVA measurement using HPLC (Sato et al., 1986; Yoshikawa et al., 1987).

The System Careful selection of institutes and hospitals is important for good prognosis.

Timing The optimal timing and frequency for the screening must be determined.

Acceptance It is necessary to get good public acceptance of screening for childhood cancer. We should make a greater effort to give accurate public information and education about cancer.

Follow-up Future clinical evaluation should be continued and improvement in the survival rate for patients should be monitored.

Evaluation of cost-benefit.

4.2 The screening method
As the VMA spot test previously used misses non-VMA secreting NBs, it is desirable to screen for NB by quantitative VMA/HVA measurement using HPLC. Comparative studies

of the VMA spot test and the HPLC method in Kyoto are shown in Table 7. The number of cases detected by HPLC was 4 times higher than by the VMA qualitative test. Both Kyoto and Sapporo, where MS is being conducted by the HPLC method, have the same frequencies. The number of retests and false positive results have clearly decreased after the introduction of the HPLC method.

By the end of October 1989, 49 of the 57 regional administrations in Japan had already begun using the HPLC method. Six of the remaining 8 districts, which now use the qualitative VMA method, will start using HPLC in the near future. Some guidelines are recommended for the collection of urine samples and the assay of creatinine, VMA, and HVA (Sawada et al., 1988). For this program, concerning the decision for cut-off levels of VMA and HVA expressed per mg of creatinine, we consider levels over mean +2.5 SD to be abnormally high and indicative of NB. A urinary creatinine level below 8 mg/dl indicates a diluted urine sample, or a false positive result; and over 120 mg/dl, an overly concentrated urine sample, or a false negative result. These infants must be retested. A contaminated urine sample will be indicated by a low creatinine level and also requires a retest. Dietary restriction of food, recommended for the VMA spot test, is unnecessary

Table 7   Numbers of test, retest, false positive and NB cases in Kyoto and Sapporo

	Number tested	Number Retested	Positive Results	NB cases
A VMA spot test in Kyoto	118,116	6106 (5.2%)	99 (0.08%)	6 (1/19,686)
Nov 1985 – March 1988 (Kyoto) HPLC	30,941	769* (2.4%)	13** (0.04%)	7 (1/4,420)
April 1981 – Dec 1988 (Sapporo) HPLC	115,922	1056 (0.9%)	82** (0.07%)	21 (1/5,520)

* Lack of urine sample: 369 (1.2%)
   Diluted urine: 222 (0.7%)
   Positive ?:   178 (0.6%)
** False Positive: 0.02% in Kyoto and 0.05% in Sapporo.

because foods consumed during infancy have no effect on the separation of VMA and HVA on the chromatogram; however, it is better to record the name of any drugs an infant has been administered at the time the urine sample is taken.

A new technique for measurement of VMA and HVA using monoclonal antibodies of VMA and HVA has recently been developed. It is essential to determine whether it is useful for MS and applicable for field work, depending on time and accuracy factors, economical benefit, and so on (Yoshioka et al., 1987; Yokomori et al., 1989).

4.3 Optimal time and frequency for screening
The age distribution of clinically diagnosed NB patients before the introduction of NB-MS in Japan is shown in Figure 2.

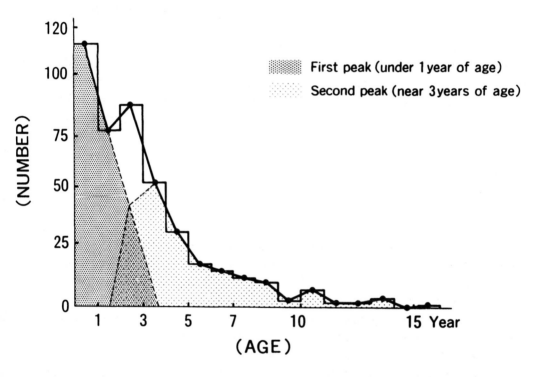

Figure 2 The age distribution curve for Neuroblastoma for 466 children in Japan before the initiation of Neuroblastoma Mass Screening.

There are 2 major peaks, a prominent peak approaching 1 year of age (early onset), and a second peak near 3 or 4 years of age (late onset). The pattern of age distribution of these peaks is the same as in the US (Miller, Fraumeni and Hill, 1968), the Netherlands (Voute, 1984), and Denmark (Carlsen, 1986). No report has been made on differences between the NB cases that occur in these two peaks, but a clear relationship between prognosis and age at diagnosis can be seen. The prognosis of NB cases that occur in the former peak is known to be favourable, but in the latter peak, unfavourable, based on clinical data and past experience. The age distribution shows that 53.7% of all NB cases belonged to the first peak and 46.3% to the later peak, or the 3 to 4 year age group. From this figure, it is obvious that not all NB cases can be detected by our screening programme at 6 months. At the present time, only NB cases in the first peak are being detected; however, as 97% of the cases detected by MS have been cured, it seems reasonable for this programme to begin screening at 6 months of age. Other findings which support screening at 6 months after birth are that metastases have been observed in 53% of these 337 cases, indicating that there is a strong tendency for primary tumours to demonstrate accelerated growth at an early age. Also since volumes of VMA and HVA excreted into the urine appear to become constant after 6 months of age (unpublished observation), the results should also be more reliable.

There is the important question that our programme may detect many NB which will spontaneously regress (Everson and Cole, 1966; Beckwith and Perrin, 1963; Gross, Farber and Martin, 1959; Evans et al., 1980). Although the incidence is still unknown, spontaneous regression has sometimes been observed in patients under 3-4 months of age with stage IV tumours, especially those with skin metastases and mediastinal NB in the older age group. NBs which will potentially regress spontaneously may be among those detected at 6 months screening. In the Kyoto area, the annual number of cases of NB increased from 2.80 to 3.27 after introduction of MS. Contrary to expectation, analytical results of the 337 cases detected by MS in Japan did not show an increased incidence of stage IVs and mediastinal NBs.

In the near future we hope to clarify this problem through further analysis of NB cases.

4.4 Long-term clinical evaluation and the effect on survival rates
Serial investigation of all NB deaths in Japan from death certificates showed a decrease in the number of NB deaths and the mortality from NB in Japan after introduction of NB-MS (Hanawa et al, 1990). The total number of NB deaths has decreased since 1985, the year nationwide NB mass screening commenced. Most notably, deaths in cases between 1 to 4 years of age have decreased, although in age groups 0, 5 to 9 and over 10 years of age, the number of deaths did not change. The mass screening in infancy programme has saved many NB patients aged 1 to 4 by early detection. The same number of deaths for patients over 5 years of age suggests that there has been little progress in chemotherapeutic treatment. The Kyoto study has had the same results (Sawada T, unpublished). The survival rates of all NB patients in this area improved from 17.1% (6/35) during the 12-year period from 1962 to 1974 before Ms initiation to 71.1% (35/49) during the 14-year period from 1974 to 1988 after MS initiation. The annual real number of NB deaths has decreased from 2.42 to 1.00, although the annual number of NB cases has increased from 2.80 before MS to 3.27 after MS. These data show that this screening programme is useful by increasing the number of NB patients cured.

Acknowledgements
We wish to thank the Japanese Childhood Cancer Association for permission to present data from the Neuroblastoma Mass Screening Study.

This study was supported by grants-in-aid for cancer research (1-29) and research of mass screening system from the Ministry of Health and Welfare of Japan.

REFERENCES

Beckwith JB, Perrin EV. In situ neuroblastoma: a contribution to the natural history of neural crest tumours. Am J Pathol 1963; 43:1089-1100.

Breslow N, McCann B. Statistical estimation of prognosis for children with neuroblastoma. Cancer Res 1971; 31:2098-2103.

Carlsen NLT. Epidemiological investigation on neuroblastomas in Denmark 1943-1980. Br J Cancer 1986; 54:977-988.

Children's Cancer Association of Japan. All Japan Children's Cancer Registration. Nozomo (Japanese) 1987; 68(6):6.

Committee of Malignant Tumour, Society of the Japanese Paediatric Surgeon. Registration of neuroblastoma, Wilms' tumour and hepatoblastoma during 6 years from 1971 to 1976. J Jpn Soc Paediatr Surg 1979; 15:507-515.

Committee of Malignant Tumour, Society of the Japanese Paediatric Surgeon. Annual report of the registration of childhood malignant tumours in 1987. J Jpn Soc Paediatr Surg 1989; 25:123-138.

Evans AE, Chatten J, D'Angio GJ, et al. A review of 17 IV-s neuroblastoma patients at the Children's Hospital of Philadelphia. Cancer 1980; 45:833-839.

Evans AE, d'Angio GJ, Randolph J. A proposed staging for children with neuroblastoma. Cancer 1971; 27:371-378.

Evans AE, Gerson J, Schnaufer. Spontaneous regression of neuroblastoma. Natl Cancer Inst Monogr 1976; 44:49-54.

Everson TC, Cole WH. Spontaneous Regression of Cancer. Philadelphia: Saunders, 1966, pp 11-87.

Gitlow SE, Bertani LM, Rausen A, et al. Diagnosis of neuroblastoma by qualitative and quantitative determination of catecholamine metabolites in urine. Cancer 1970; 25:1377-1383.

Gross RE, Farber S, Martin LW. Neuroblastoma sympatheticum. A study and report of 217 cases. Paediatrics 1959; 23:1179-1191.

Hanawa Y, Sawada T, Tsunoda A. Decrease in Childhood Neuroblastoma Death in Japan. Submitted, 1990.

Ishiguro Y, Kato K, Ito T, et al. Nervous system specific enolase in serum as a marker for neuroblastoma. Paediatrics 1983; 72:696-700.

Jones MP. The Manchester Children's Tumor Registry and its lessons. In: Kobayashi N (ed), Recent Advances in Managements of Children with Cancer. Tokyo: The Children's Cancer Association of Japan, 1981, pp 19-26,.

Miller RW, Fraumeni JF, Hill AJ. Neuroblastoma: Epidemiologic approach to its origin. Am J Dis Child 1968; 115:253-261.

Pastore G, Magnai C, Zenetl R, et al. Epidemiology of childhood cancer within province of Torino (Italy), 1967-1978. In: Rayband C, Clement R, Lebreuil G, et al. (eds), Paediatric Oncology. 1982, Amsterdam: Excerpta Medica, pp 372-374.

Pochedly C (ed). Neuroblastoma. Acton, Massachusetts: Publishing Sciences Group, 1976.

Sato Y, Hanai J, Takasugi N, et al. Determination of urinary vanillylmandelic acid and homovanillic acid by high performance liquid chromatography for mass screening of neuroblastoma. Tohoku J Exp Med 1986; 150:169-174.

Sawada T. Unpublished.

Sawada T and the Committee on Neuroblastoma Mass Screening of the Japanese Childhood Cancer Research. "Annual registration of the neuroblastoma cases detected by mass screening program - 1987." Annual Meeting of Childhood Cancer, November 28, 1987, Tokyo, 1987.

Sawada T, Hirayama M, Nakata T, et al. Mass screening for neuroblastoma in infants in Japan. Lancet 1984; ii:271-273.

Sawada T, Imashuku S, Takada H, et al. Early biochemical diagnosis of neuroblastoma in childhood. Gan No Rinshou (Japanese) 1971; 17: 727-739.

Sawada T, Kodama K, Mizuta M, et al. Laboratory techniques and neuroblastoma screening. Lancet 1988; ii:1134-1135.

Sawada T, Sugimoto T, Kidowaki T, et al. Incidence of neuroblastoma in Japan. Med Paediatr Oncol 1984; 12:101-103.

Sawada T, Takada H, Imashuku S, et al. Mass screening for early and immediate detection of neuroblastoma in childhood. Acta Paediatr Jpn 1978; 20: 55-61.

Sawada T, Takeda T, Tsunoda T, et al. Outcome of 25 neuroblastomas revealed by mass screening in Japan. Lancet 1986; i:377-378.

Sawada T, Todo S, Fujita K, et al. Mass screening for neuroblastoma in infancy. Am J Dis Child 1982; 136:710-712.

Sawaguchi S, Suganuma Y, Watanabe I, et al. Studies on the biological and clinical characteristics of neuroblastoma: evaluation of the survival rates in relation to stage and age of onset. J Jpn Soc Paediatr Surg (Japanese) 1985; 15:1119-1128.

Voute PA. Neuroblastoma. In: Sutow WW, Fernbach DJ, Vietti TJ (eds). Clinical Paediatric Oncology. St. Louis, Missouri: The Mosby Company, 1984, pp 559-587.

Yokomori K, Hori T, Tsuchida Y, et al. A new urinary mass screening system for neuroblastoma in infancy by using monoclonal antibodies against VMA and HVA. J Paediatr Surg 1989; 24:391-394.

Yoshikawa S, Okuda S, Ohe T, et al. Liquid chromatographic determination of vanillylmandelic acid and homovanillic acid by a column-switching technique involving direct injection of urine. J Chromatogr 1987; 421: 111-116.

Yoshioka M, Aso C, Tamura Z, et al. Preparation of monoclonal antibodies to vanillylmandelic acid and homovanillic acid. Biogenic Amines 1987; 4: 229-235.

Young YJL Jr, Miller RW. Incidence of malignant tumors in U.S. children. J Paediatr 1975; 86:254-258.

Zelter PM, Parma AM, Dalton A, et al. Raised neuron specific enolase in serum of children with metastatic neuroblastoma. Lancet 1983; ii:361-363.

35 Screening for Neuroblastoma

Background, preliminary experience in the North of England and proposals for an evaluative study

L. PARKER, A. W. CRAFT and G. DALE

Departments of Child Health and Clinical Biochemistry, University of Newcastle Upon Tyne

1 BACKGROUND OF PROPOSED RESEARCH

Neuroblastoma is a malignant tumour derived from the primitive neural crest and is one of the most common solid tumours in childhood. The incidence of neuroblastoma in the Northern Region is 1 in 10,580 live births; 8.6% of all childhood malignancies (Craft et al, 1987). Unfortunately there has been little improvement in prognosis for neuroblastoma over the past decade despite dramatic changes in the outlook for other forms of childhood cancer (Draper et al, 1982).

There have been 32 deaths from neuroblastoma in children under 6 years in the Northern Region since 1975. This accounts for 15% of all deaths from childhood cancer and 25% of non-leukaemia cancer deaths in this age group. There were 36 deaths from neuroblastoma in Great Britain in 1987, the latest year for which data are available (G. Draper, Personal communication).

Prognosis is dependent on age and stage at diagnosis (Evans et al, 1987). The European Neuroblastoma Study Group (ENSG) has collected data from most of the major treatment centres in Europe and their survival figures can be taken as representative of current best practice and outcome. Based on 304 cases diagnosed in 1982 and 1983, the five year disease free survival by age and stage is shown in Tables 1 and 2 respectively.

Table 1 Neuroblastoma. Five year disease free survival by age n-304 (ENSG data)

	Age		
	< 1 yr	1-5 yr	> 5 yr
5 year survival (%)	80	38	21

Table 2   Neuroblastoma. Five year disease free survival by stage;
n=304 (ENSG data)

	Stage				
	I	II	III	IV	IVs
5 year survival (%)	97	89	52	21	80

Overall the survival of children presenting after the age of 1 year is poor and mortality for those with advanced disease, ie. stage IV presenting after the first birthday, is over 80%. Recent studies have shown that the disease free survival (DFS) of Stage III and IV disease may be prolonged with very intensive chemotherapy and bone marrow transplantation, but even the most optimistic views are only a 20% DFS with a relatively short follow-up (Shafford, Rogers and Pritchard, 1984).

Using information on the average daily cost of bed occupancy in the Children's Cancer Ward at the Royal Victoria Infirmary, provided by the Newcastle Health Authority, together with an estimate of the number of in-patient days required on average for treatment of children with late stage neuroblastoma, it is currently estimated that the cost of treatment per child is around £45,000. This is derived from the average cost of £450 for one patient day in a paediatric oncology ward. This is similar to the cost estimated for a paediatric oncology bed in St. James' Hospital, Leeds (Bailey, personal communication). Survival in this group is as low as 9%, indicating an estimated cost of around £450,000 per life saved. Any potential costs of screening can therefore be viewed against this financial background.

Recently it has been suggested that stages I to IV represent the natural progression of the disease (Carlsen, 1988). This lends strong support to the concept that screening may indeed detect cases at an early stage before they progress to a more advanced incurable stage.

Some neuroblastomas may be present at birth but regress spontaneously, a condition described as in situ neuroblastoma (Beckwith and Perrin, 1963). This is evidenced clinically by the occasional finding of a calcified adrenal ganglioneuroma at routine autopsy in the elderly.

Neuroblastoma is unusual amongst childhood tumours in that there is an increased excretion of catecholamine metabolites including homovanillic acid (HVA) and vanillylmandelic acid (VMA) in over 90% of cases (Tuchman et al, 1987). These metabolites can be detected in the urine and act as biological markers for the presence of disease. It was formerly considered that a 24 hour urine collection was necessary for accurate quantification of VMA and HVA excretion. However, it has been shown that a random specimen of urine is adequate provided VMA and HVA measurements are related to creatinine content (Tuchman et al, 1987). The possibility of whole population screening for the early detection of neuroblastoma has been considered for many years but only recently have developments in technology made it a realistic proposition.

The Japanese, in particular Sawada (this volume), have pioneered the technique of screening for neuroblastoma using spot urine samples from babies at around six months of age. On the basis of the preliminary results from Kyoto, Tokyo and Sapporo City screening was implemented in the whole of Japan in April 1985. The first studies were reported by Sawada et al (1984) who collected urine on filter paper by blotting it on a wet nappy. They then used a qualitative method of analysis (La Brosse spot test) for VMA content only. This was a very crude screening test and of the first 282,000 babies studied, over 10,000 gave false positive results (the La Brosse spot test is known to give false positive results with dietary phenolic acids from, for example, vanilla and bananas). Sixteen cases of neuroblastoma were eventually confirmed giving a detection rate of 1 in 17,600. The incidence of neuroblastoma in Japan is 1in 7,300 so that this suggests an unacceptably high false negative rate if, as is suspected, in situ neuroblastoma is also detected. This has been confirmed by subsequent follow-up. Subsequently, Matsumoto et al (1985) in Tokyo applied the quantitative technique of high performance liquid chromatography (HPLC) to urine samples and in 12,500 children screened found 3 cases of neuroblastoma, with 2 false positive results (HPLC results can also be affected by dietary phenolic acids).

A recent report from Sapporo City, Japan (Nishi et al, 1987) reported a dramatic improvement in survival from less than 20% during the pre-screening period to 84% during the screening era. However it is well known that the comparison of survival rate for screened and unscreened populations can be misleading because of 'leadtime' bias and this is further complicated by the possible inclusion in the screened group of cases of in situ neuroblastoma which differ from those diagnosed clinically. Although not reported in their publications, the incidence of neuroblastoma in birth cohorts in Sapporo City has increased suggesting that 'in situ' cases are being detected which would almost certainly have regressed spontaneously. In the pre-screening era from 1974 to 1980 the incidence of neuroblastoma presenting clinically before the age of 5 years was 1in 7300. Screening commenced in 1981 and for the 1982 birth cohort the incidence was 1in 4041 and for the 1983 cohort 1in 3515 (Figures derived from data supplied by Takeda, Sapporo City, Japan).

There are considerable methodological uncertainties surrounding the reports from Japan making it difficult to interpret whether screening really has been beneficial. These include :
    Each prefecture in Japan directs its own screening programme independently and both qualitative and quantitative methods of analysis are used. Overall compliance is poor and coverage is at best 65-75% (Takeda, personal communication). Cancer registration in Japan is very patchy and in some prefectures is less than 5% complete and death certification is unreliable.

In their screening programme they describe a change in the pattern of stage of disease with an apparent reduction in advanced disease from 71.4% to 40.9% and an improvement in case survival. A fall in the proportion of older cases from 68% of cases presenting over the age of two years prior to screening to 32% after screening was also reported. However, the apparent increase in overall incidence following screening, probably due to the detection of "in situ " neuroblastoma, makes justification of this claim difficult.

Because of the complication of "in situ" neuroblastoma and possible lead time bias, the only way of evaluating neuroblastoma screening is by using mortality statistics, and adequate data are not available from Japan at the present time.

2 PILOT STUDIES IN THE NORTHERN REGION OF THE UK
In 1985 a Steering Group was established to conduct pilot studies aimed at assessing the feasibility of establishing neuroblastoma screening in the Northern Region.

In one health centre in North Tyneside health visitors (public health nurses) were asked to collect liquid urine samples from all six month old babies registered with them over a six month period. Whilst samples were obtained from 97% of children, this was a reflection of the health visitors' commitment to the project, and the method was abandoned as being too demanding on their time. Over the next six months urine samples were collected by blotting filter papers on wet nappies. This was much less time consuming and was acceptable to health visitors and parents alike. The urine samples were then analysed for VMA, HVA and creatinine content.

From January 1st 1987 this pilot study was extended to cover all births in North Tyneside and from January 1st 1988 to cover all births in four of the sixteen districts in the Northern Region, North Tyneside, North Tees, South Tyneside and Gateshead. The research nature of the study was explained to the parents by the health visitor and a written explanation given to them in the form of a letter. Details of these feasibility studies have been published (Craft et al, 1989).

During this pilot phase of the study the analytical methods available for the detection of urinary HVA and VMA have been evaluated both in urine from normal six month old babies and in urine from children known to have neuroblastoma.

2.1 Findings of the Pilot Studies
i) The La Brosse spot test was found to be insensitive with unacceptable rates of false positive and false negative results, confirming the reports of the Japanese.

ii) Thin layer chromatography (TLC) was found to be relatively cheap but only semi-quantitative. It is well known to be liable to errors of subjective interpretation.

iii) Gas-Chromatography - Flame ionisation detection (GC-FID). Of 1,500 urine samples analysed by this method, 199 (13%) had to be repeated because of interfering peaks. This was considered to be an unacceptably high repeat rate. Details of the analysis and the results obtained have been published (Dale et al, 1988).

iv) High performance liquid chromatography (HPLC) is generally regarded as the method of choice for routine laboratory estimation of HVA and VMA. HPLC is now used as the primary screening method in Kyoto and Sapporo Cities in Japan. Although the unit cost of the equipment is less than the preferred method described below, the slow analysis rate increases capital expenditure without significant gains in running costs. The assay is not absolutely specific and all abnormal results would have to be confirmed by an alternative method.

v) Gas chromatography - Mass spectrometry (GC-MS). Mass spectrometry is the most specific method of detection presently available. There should be neither analytical false positive nor false negative results. A Hewlett Packard 5970 GC-MS (Pascal based system), purchased by the North of England Children's Cancer Research Fund, was installed in the Department of Clinical Biochemistry at Newcastle General Hospital in April 1987. A reference range for VMA and HVA measurements was established and has been published (Seviour et al, 1988). There is now a new UNIX based GC-MS system which is faster and can assay up to 12 samples per hour, and a DOS based system which although it is slightly slower can still perform about 10 assays per hour.

There is little difference in overall cost between the GC-MS and HPLC methodologies, as shown in Table 3. While there is additional time spent in sample preparation with GC-MS in comparison with HPLC, overall the staffing levels required would not be dissimilar since with HPLC more staff would be required to operate and maintain a greater number of machines. The GC-MS based system also requires fewer skilled technicians.

Table 3 Comparative costs of HPLC and GCMS analysis

	HPLC	GC-MS
A Samples per machine per 250 day year	15,000	37,500
B Capital cost of instrument	£19,500	£40,000
C Running costs per instrument per year	£ 5,380	£ 6,300
D Sample preparation and analysis (per 1,000)	£ 240	£ 545
E* Cost per sample	£ 0.86	£ 0.93

$$*E=[B + (5xC) + (5xDxA/1000)]/(5xA)$$

Of the 2,470 babies born in North Tyneside in 1987, the first year of the study, cross checking with the birth register has shown that 95% were screened for neuroblastoma.

Refusals by parents were negligible. Up to December 1989, 22,100 babies have been screened.

During the initial phase of the pilot study reference ranges for VMA and HVA per mg creatinine for spot urine samples were established. These are shown in Table 4.

Table 4 Reference ranges for VMA and HVA in spot urine samples

	VMA*	HVA*
mean	11.4	17.0
SD	4.6	7.3
mean + 2SD	20.7	31.6
mean + 3SD	25.2	39.0

*mM/ mg Creatinine

All samples over mean + 2SD for either HVA or VMA were repeated and those higher than 3 SD above the mean were considered positive.   Using these criteria 7 clearly positive urine samples were identified. Of these two babies were diagnosed as having neuroblastoma. A third baby suffered from congenital muscular dystrophy and we believe that abnormally low excretion of creatinine resulted in spuriously high HVA and VMA/creatinine ratios. One baby had a chromosome abnormality and severe chronic respiratory disease probably resulting in high circulating levels of catecholamines. In the remaining three children, no specific reason for the high results was found and they are being followed up with regular liquid urine specimens. Urine HVA and VMA from all of these has returned to normal.

Two children who were screened and found to have normal results have subsequently developed neuroblastoma. Both had Stage IV disease on diagnosis. One child was only four and a half months old at screening. The criteria used for repeating samples and classifying them as 'positive' are under review in view of our experience to date.

Experience during the pilot phase of this investigation has lead to the conclusion that screening for neuroblastoma in six month old babies by analysis of urine collected on filter papers by health visitors is a readily workable system acceptable to parents, health visitors and biochemists.   Analysis by GC-MS provides a rapid and highly accurate method of assessment suitable for mass screening at a cost comparable to less sophisticated techniques. The specificity of the methodology is high with only 5 false positive cases requiring clinical evaluation and therefore giving a specificity of over 99.9%. Congenital muscular dystrophy is extremely rare and unlikely to cause major problems in a larger study.

An international meeting was held in Newcastle upon Tyne in 1988 to review the 'state of the art' of neuroblastoma screening. There was a consensus of opinion that although the preliminary reports from Japan were encouraging, they did not represent a prima facie case for the universal introduction of screening. It was recommended that well designed studies should be initiated on a sound epidemiological and statistical basis and that any such studies should collect common data (Draper, 1988). This feeling was reaffirmed at the International Society of Paediatric Oncology meeting in Prague in October 1989.

2.2 The Proposed Study

The study population size required to show a significant fall in mortality if neuroblastoma screening were effective has been calculated using information from two data sets. The first is the Northern Region Children's Malignant Disease Registry which provides accurate age specific incidence data for neuroblastoma in the Northern Region since 1968 (Craft et al, 1987). The relatively small number of cases in this register, however makes it inappropriate for survival calculations. The ENSG has provided information on 855 cases of neuroblastoma registered since 1982. This gives the best possible survival data but, as it is not population based, incidence and mortality rates cannot be calculated. A combination of these two data sets has allowed estimation of current age specific mortality rates from neuroblastoma. The overall incidence of neuroblastoma in the Northern Region is 1 in 10,580 births. This is similar to the rates found in the Manchester Children's Tumour Registry and in most of the rest of Europe (Parkin et al, 1988).

The following assumptions, which are based on the best available data from Japan, are made for estimating the effect of neuroblastoma screening on mortality:
1   Screening will detect 85% of those who would normally have presented from the age of 13-72 months.
2   Survival in this age group will be increased to 95% from its current level of 38%.
3   Screening will detect cases which would have presented between the ages of 6 and 12 months, but will not affect the survival of this group.
4   Screening is unlikely to detect the 5% of children who present after the age of 72 months.

The patients whose survival could be affected by screening are therefore only those who would normally have presented between the ages of 13 and 72 months ie. 5.95 per 100,000 births; 63% of all cases of neuroblastoma.

It is anticipated that the overall rate of neuroblastoma detected will be increased by 5 per 100,000, these being "in situ" cases which would otherwise have regressed spontaneously. While these cases will, at least initially, be indistinguishable from 'true' neuroblastoma, it is anticipated that their survival will remain unchanged and that detection of these cases will therefore make no contribution to reduction in mortality from neuroblastoma.

The end point of the evaluation is a comparison of the population death rate from neuroblastoma between screened and unscreened populations. It is essential that there is a comparison group since as is shown in Figure 1, overall mortality from neuroblastoma in Great Britain has tended to fall over the last 20 years.

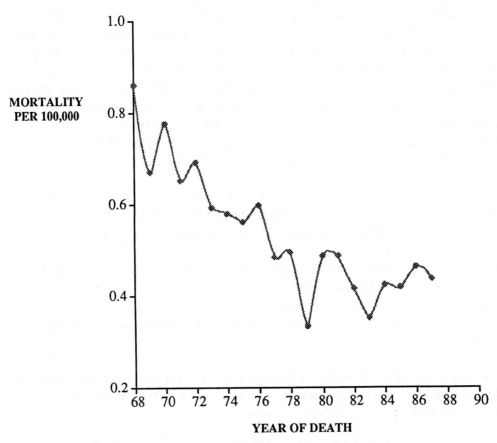

Figure 1 Overall mortality from neuroblastoma in Great Britain

On the basis of the above assumptions a screened population of about 500,000 with a similar sized control group would be necessary to be reasonably certain of detecting a significant fall in mortality. However the incidence rate of late-stage disease may be used as an intermediate indicator of the efficacy of screening. Careful observation of the distribution of stage of disease could give guidelines for future planning before the ultimate result of the study is known.

3 OVERALL STUDY DESIGN

A study is proposed of five administrative health regions in England (Northern, Mersey, North West, South West and Yorkshire Regions) plus Scotland. All cases of neuroblastoma diagnosed in children resident in the study regions at the age of 6 months over a six year period will be included in the study. The first year will be a control, unscreened period for all regions. One of the six regions will then commence screening and an additional region will then be included at four month intervals. Each region will be screened for one year followed by one year not screened, and a further screened year. Possible temporal and spatial differences in incidence and survival following treatment of neuroblastoma will therefore be taken into account in the study design. Each region will provide two 1-year birth cohorts to the screened population and four 1-year birth cohorts to the control population. Using 1986 birth figures (OPCS) this will provide a screened population of 561,600 and a control population of 1,123,200.

The design of the proposed study is shown in Figure 2. This proposal obviates the need for randomisation. The possibility of randomisation was discussed at great length both within the project team and with health visitors familiar with the screening process. The project team was concerned about the additional administrative procedures which randomisation would require and the probable reduction in coverage rate which would imply the need for a larger target population to ensure a statistically reliable result. Randomisation at the level of the child would lead to an enormous and unacceptable workload for each health visitor. Health visitors were also extremely concerned that, if randomisation at the level of the child were implemented, their role with families could be jeopardised if they were put in the difficult position of not screening a baby when there was pressure from the family to do so. Randomisation at a higher level - the health clinic or health district would bring with it a level of cross boundary contamination between control and screened populations both in space and time that could greatly undermine the controlled nature of the study. Even in the four districts screened at the present time there have been many mothers who have crossed district boundaries specifically to ensure that their babies are screened. Hence, after careful consideration, randomisation is felt to be impractical and would be excessively expensive as a result of the much greater demand on health visitor time and on the administrative structure of the project.

Cases detected, whether by screening or otherwise will receive similar treatment in each of the study regions. In order to identify any child who was not detected by screening and who subsequently develops neuroblastoma (a false negative) in one of the birth cohorts, a search will be made of the regional cancer registries and of the national registry held by the Childhood Cancer Research Group in Oxford. For the period of the study the place of residence at 6 months of age will be determined for each child developing neuroblastoma anywhere in the United Kingdom. All paediatric oncology centres in Great Britain will be given notification forms to be sent to the project administrator in Newcastle when a new case of neuroblastoma is diagnosed. This case will be checked immediately to ascertain whether or not it is in the study. It will be necessary, ultimately, to follow each birth cohort

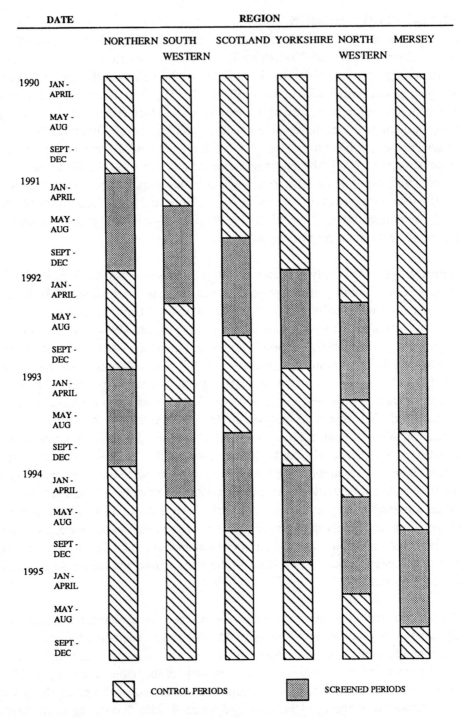

Figure 2 Plan for screening Scotland and five regions in England for neuroblastoma

for a period of 15 years, but as 95% of neuroblastoma will normally present by 72 months of age, a reasonably secure answer should be possible 66 months after the last child has been screened.

3.1 Sample Collection

Filter paper urine samples will be collected by health visitors from all babies at about six months of age in each region during screening periods. If no satisfactory result is obtained from this filter paper a second such sample will be requested. Failure to obtain an adequate result from this will lead to a request for a liquid urine specimen.

3.2 Biochemical Analysis

Analysis of VMA and HVA will be carried out on each sample using the GC-MS methodologies developed at Newcastle. Creatinine will be assayed by a standard colorimetric method using a plate reader. Any sample identified as abnormal, ie higher than 2 SD above the mean for either VMA or HVA, will have a repeat assay on the same specimen of urine and if this remains abnormal a second filter paper and then a liquid urine will be collected. If this is higher than 3 SD above the mean for either HVA or VMA, the baby will be referred to the regional paediatric oncology centre for investigation and treatment where appropriate.

3.3 Monitoring

Monitoring of the target population coverage rate will be undertaken by obtaining monthly birth counts in each region for each cohort screened. Any reduction in the proportion of babies screened in any district will be detected early and remedial action taken by the regional project health-visitor coordinator. It is not possible to cross check individual children with birth registers as it has been found to be difficult and time consuming in practice, not least because of inaccuracies in the birth registers.

3.4 The Study Population

The study population comprises all those children in the six study regions who reach the age of 6 months during the six year period 1st January 1990 to 31st December 1995. Any of these children who are diagnosed with neuroblastoma in Great Britain within the years of the study will be ascertained either by direct notification by the consultant in charge or by checking through the Childhood Cancer Research Group in Oxford. The number of children in the study will be approximated to that number of children born in the appropriate birth cohorts. While this is acknowledged to introduce a small error, the number of children moving out of a Region between birth and the age of 6 months will not be very different from those moving in.

3.5 Treatment of Children with Neuroblastoma

Children from the study birth cohorts presenting with neuroblastoma in any of the regions will be managed according to a protocol to be agreed by all the paediatric oncology units, so eliminating possible regional differences in treatment regimens and corresponding case survival. All regional centres are members of the ENSG which is designing standard treatment protocols.

3.6 Investigation of Diagnosed Cases of Neuroblastoma

This study will provide the opportunity to learn more about the biology of neuroblastoma. Investigation of the child and tumour will be standardised both for the screened and non-screened populations. It will include careful staging according to the TNM, Evans and the new International (Hilton Head) system and where possible appropriate biological samples will be collected for serum ferritin, NSE, nMyc amplification, tumour chromosomes and ploidy. All cases of neuroblastoma in any of the study populations will be notified to the study coordinator who will ensure collection of all relevant data on that child.

3.7 Statistical Analysis

Using the method of Armitage and Berry, 1987 for comparing binomial distributions with individual randomisation, a screened population of 561,000 would give a 75% probability (at the 5% significance level) of detecting a fall in mortality due to neuroblastoma from 3.27 to 0.96 per 100,000 in the 7-72 month age group. Analysis of the mortality data will be carried out using GLIM, 1978. It will be possible, using the the design of the study, to take into account any geographical differences and time trends in mortality. These estimates assume a minimum follow up of 66 months from screening.

3.8   Ethical Considerations

Ethical approval for a screening study has been obtained from all 16 districts in the Northern Region and will be sought for the remainder of the study area. The major ethical issue relates to the probable identification of patients with "in situ" neuroblastoma who would never have presented clinically. It is likely that these will be early stage disease and will require only an operation to remove the primary tumour. The 'cost' of identifying many cases early and thereby improving their chance of survival is that up to 5 in 100,000 babies may require an unnecessary operation.

This problem has been discussed at length in meetings of the research team and paediatric oncologists from the study regions and has been considered by all of the ethical committees in the Northern Region all of which accepted that the study proposal is reasonable. It was felt that parents should be given frank information about the screening process, ie. "screening may detect a tumour which could develop into a cancerous growth", and that on identification of a child with a tumour the course of action taken, including the information given to parents, would be that decided to be appropriate by the consultant concerned.

All parents of babies offered screening will have the research nature of the procedure explained to them. In the pilot studies in the Northern region an initial explanation by the health visitors followed by a written explanation has proved acceptable to both parents and health visitors. Paediatric oncologists in each region will produce an explanatory letter about the screening project to be given to parents. This will be translated into the primary languages spoken in each community and if appropriate audiotaped versions will be produced.

4   COST BENEFIT ANALYSIS

The second arm of the evaluation of neuroblastoma screening is a detailed assessment of the costs and possible benefits of the process and outcome of screening. Any reduction in mortality from neuroblastoma resulting from the screening procedure must be gained at reasonable financial cost. The figure of £450,000 per life saved was derived in 1987/8 and does not take into account the increasingly aggressive treatment with associated high drug and nursing costs which is now being given to children with this disease. A detailed analysis of the resources necessary to treat children with neuroblastoma is required to allow accurate calculation of the true costs of the treatment.

It is anticipated that screening will greatly reduce the number of children who experience late stage neuroblastoma and who are consequently exposed to costly and intensive therapy regimens. Most will have early stage disease and require little other than surgery. In addition to the cost of the testing procedure, screening for neuroblastoma will undoubtedly increase the number of normal children who undergo clinical investigation for possible malignant disease and the complication of in situ neuroblastoma implies that a proportion of children will undergo surgery for a tumour which would otherwise have remained asymptomatic and would not have been treated. The economic costs of these procedures must all be calculated in order that an estimate of the true financial costs of neuroblastoma screening can be estimated.

There are also, potentially, less tangible costs and benefits associated with the screening programme. Detection of false positive results will obviously involve families in a series of events which may well be very stressful to them, while there will be a great benefit for those families whose child undergoes only a surgical procedure as a result of early detection of disease in comparison with that for overt late stage malignant disease. The human benefit associated with saving a live is clear but its financial benefit is less so. How much it is worth spending to save one life has not been clearly defined for the Health Care Sector but in road transport terms a road improvement is worthwhile if it is predicted to be able to save one life for under £500,000 (Ramsey, personal communication). Taking into account the costs associated with screening outlined in this proposal along with approximate treatment costs, and should the assumptions made about the effect of screening be correct, then the cost of each additional life saved as a result of screening during the study will be in the region of £70,000. However the eventual costs of screening as a service will be considerably less than this.

4.1 Economic Costs

The proposed method of urine collection involves the health visitor. During the period of the study an evaluation of the amount of time they spend on this exercise will be assessed and this will be included in the final cost/benefit analysis. The pilot studies have shown that the additional workload is minimal and can be readily absorbed into the health visitors' routine work.

The cost of hospital investigation and treatment will be assessed using available budgetary information which, because of resource management, is being rapidly developed and refined. Over the study period detailed information will be collected on all investigative and treatment procedures undergone by all children with neuroblastoma diagnosed clinically in each of the screened regions. Similar information will be gathered for all children who are investigated following a positive urine test.

Detailed Health Service budgetary information will be collected from those centres where it is available and the number of days in hospital will be recorded for all patients in both screened and unscreened populations. Account will be taken not only of the investigative procedures undergone but also of the intensity of nursing and social support that is provided in specialist oncology units.

The additional cost of the screening programme will also be assessed. It is recognised that for a research project these will be higher than they would be for a routine service. In a research programme equipment has to be "written off" during the course of the study whereas it is likely to have a useful life of up to ten years and research coordinators would not be necessary if it were to become a service.

The analytical technique of Gas chromatography, mass spectrometry being used in the study may be replaced by a less expensive and less labour intensive process in a routine screening programme and this will be taken into account in the costing of the screening process. It is proposed that developmental work will proceed in parallel with this study to identify the best method should neuroblastoma screening become routine. For example, it is likely that immuno- or other binding assays which might present significant cost advantages will become available in the UK over the next few years (Mellow et al, in press). An immunoassay based kit is already available in Japan (Yokomori et al, 1989), but this is considered to be unsuitable for use in this evaluative study, GC-MS remains the Gold Standard.

4.2   Human Costs : Quality of Life

As with any screening programme there will be a proportion of cases in which repeat tests will need to be carried out and repeat specimens requested. Postal questionnaires will be used assess the degree of stress in parents resulting from the screening programme in regard to requests for repeat specimens.

Interviews will be conducted with the families of false positive cases, true positives and children who present clinically using validated questionnaires in addition to specific questionnaires to be designed for this study. These will address the issues of stress, anxiety, financial costs to families and of great importance, quality of life in the survivors and their families. Each family will be interviewed three times; at the time of investigation and then one and two years later. The families of all cases of neuroblastoma and all children who are investigated as a consequence of a high urine result will be interviewed in their homes by the project health visitors.

REFERENCES

Armitage P, Berry G. Statistical Methods in Medical Research. Oxford, UK: Blackwell Scientific Publications, 1987.

Beckwith JB, Perrin EV. In situ neuroblastoma: A contribution to the natural history of neural crest tumours. American Journal of Pathology 1963; 43:1089-1104.

Carlsen NLT. Why age has independent prognostic significance in neuroblastomas. Evidence for intra-uterine development and implications for the treatment of the disease. Anticancer Res 1988; 8:255-262.

Craft AW, Amineddine HA, Scott JES et al. The Northern Region Children's Malignant Disease Registry, 1986-1982. Incidence and survival. Br J Cancer 1987; 56:853-858.

Craft AW, Dale G, McGill A., et al. Biochemical screening for neuroblastoma in infants: A feasibility study. Medical and Pediatric Oncology 1989; 17:373-378

Dale G, McGill AC, Seviour JA et al. Urinary excretion of HMMA and HVA in infants. Ann Clin Biochem 1988; 25:233-236.

Draper GJ. Screening for neuroblastoma. Br Med J 1988; 297: 152-153

Draper GJ, Birch J et al. Childhood cancer in Britain. Incidence, survival and mortality. OPCS HMSO, London, 1982.

Evans AE, D'Angio GH et al. Prognostic factors in neuroblastoma. Cancer 1987; 59:1853-1859.

GLIM (Generalised linear interactive models) London, Royal Statistical Society, 1978.

Matsumoto M, Anazawa A, Zuzuki K et al. Urine mass screening for neuroblastoma by high performance liquid chromatography. Paediatric Research 1985; 19:625.

Mellow GW, Gallagher G, Landon J. Production and characterisation of antibodies to VMA. J Imm Methods - In Press.

Nishi M, Myake H, Takeda T, Shimada M, et al. Effects of mass screening of neuroblastoma in Sapporo City. Cancer 1987; 60:433-435.

Parkin DM, Stiller CA, Draper GJ et al. International incidence of childhood cancer. Lyon, France: IARC Scientific Publications No 87, 1988.

Sawada T, Nakata T, Takasugi N et al. Mass screening for neuroblastoma in infants in Japan. Lancet 1984; ii:271-273.

Seviour J, McGill AC, Dale G et al Method of measurement of urinary HVA and VMA by gas chromatography mass spectrometry. J Chromatography 1988; 432:273-277.

Shafford EA, Rogers DW, Pritchard J. Advanced neuroblastoma: Improved response rate using a multiagent regime (OPEC). J Clin Oncology 1984; 1:742-747.

Tuchman M, Ramnaraine HL et al. Three years experience with random urinary HVA and VMA levels in the diagnosis of neuroblastoma. Pediatrics 1987; 79:203-205.

Yokomori K, Hori T, Tsuchida Y et al. A new urinary mass screening system for neuroblastoma in infancy by use of monoclonal antibodies against VMA and HVA. J Pediatric Surgery 1989; 24:391-394.

36 Summary of Discussion on Screening for Neuroblastoma

Although the findings from Japan have been interpreted as indicating that the screening programme has been effective, it was pointed out that two different peaks of neuroblastoma incidence suggests that those cases detectable at 6 months may be prenatal in origin, while the later peak after 1 year may represent later onset and poorer prognosis disease, not so readily influenced by screening. It is not clear that screening at 6 months may suffice to bring forward the time of diagnosis for all in the later age peak, especially those normally diagnosed at the average of 4 years. It would therefore be appropriate to investigate screening at 1 year in comparison to screening at 6 months and no screening. There is also some concern on the appropriate management of children with positive tests in whom a tumour is not found on investigation. In such circumstances it would be appropriate to repeat tests after an interval, and possibly only perform a blind laparotomy if there was a rising titre in the test.

Additional studies have recently been proposed. In addition to the UK study a controlled study was started recently in North America with screening in the Canadian province of Quebec, with other regions in North America as control areas. In children with a long life expectancy a one time screen may be applicable for a rare disease, whereas a rare disease would not justify repeated screening in adults.

Section 8 Screening for Stomach Cancer

State of the Art on Screening for Stomach Cancer

There are data from Japan which suggest that stomach cancer screening can reduce mortality.

Screening programmes could continue in those regions with high stomach cancer incidence where they are already underway, but stomach cancer screening cannot be recommended in other countries as public health policy.

Recommendation for Research

Where screening has not already been implemented as public health policy (ie outside Japan), the opportunity should be taken to investigate the effectiveness of barium x-ray screening in high risk populations by means of a randomised controlled trial.

37 Evaluation of Mass Screening Programme for Stomach Cancer in Japan

S. HISAMICHI [1], A. FUKAO [1], N. SUGAWARA [2], M. NISHIKOURI [3],
S. KOMATSU [1], I. TSUJI [1], Y. TSUBONO [1] and A. TAKANO [4].

[1] Department of Public Health, Tohoku University School of Medicine, Sendai, Japan
[2] Cancer Detection Centre, Miyagi Cancer Society
[3] Department of Health and Environment, Miyagi Prefectural Office
[4] Miyagi prefectural Cancer Registry

1 INTRODUCTION

Worldwide stomach cancer is a relatively common cancer, and in many countries in the Western Pacific Region, Central and South America, and Northern Europe, there is a need to develop a stomach cancer control programme similar to that in Japan where there is a high mortality rate. Recently, mortality from stomach cancer in Japan has been decreasing. However, in 1988 the first ranking among all cancer deaths was still cancer of the stomach in both sexes, comprising 24.6% of deaths in males and 21.6% in females. Therefore, stomach cancer still constitutes a target of prime importance in cancer control in Japan.

The main purpose of mass screening for stomach cancer is early detection at the preclinical stage and prompt treatment with reduction of mortality from cancer at this site in the target population. In Japan, gastric mass screening by the barium x-ray method has been conducted nationwide since 1960. The Health and Medical Services Law for the Aged came into effect in 1983 and the Japanese government set up a public policy to try to screen 30% of people over the age of 40 each year. Since then, municipalities have had the responsibility for conducting the gastric screening programme. This article concerns the results and evaluation of gastric mass screening in Japan.

2 RESULTS OF GASTRIC MASS SCREENING

According to the report from the Japanese Society of Gastroenterological Mass Survey (Hisamichi, 1982), the number of examinees in Japan has been increasing year by year since 1968, and in 1987 the total number examined was 5,157,778. The number of cases of stomach cancer detected by the mass survey was 6,661 (0.13%). Among these cancer cases, surgical operations were performed in 97.2%. The proportion of cases of early stage gastric cancer was 52.1% of the detected cases and 60.7% of resected cases.

In the following discussion on evaluation of gastric mass screening, we will mainly use data from Miyagi Prefecture. Miyagi Prefecture is located in the north-eastern part of Honshu Island, the mainland of Japan. The 1985 census showed a population of 2,167,900. In this prefecture, the first mass screening for gastric cancer by mobile x-ray was started in 1960. During the 29-year period from 1960 to 1988 a total of 2,858,966 persons underwent the examination, and 5,350 cases of gastric cancer were detected (0.19%).

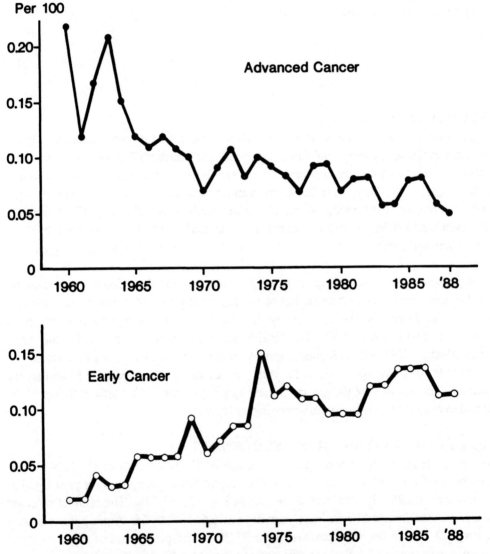

Figure 1 Trends in rate of detection of advanced and early cancer of the stomach (Miyagi Prefecture, Japan).

In 1988, the total number of persons examined in this prefecture was 187,316 and the coverage rate per year was 21.3% among the target population at risk who were recommended or invited to attend the annual gastric screening by the Japanese government, persons over 40 years of age. Figure 1 shows the trends in detection rate of advanced cancer and early cancer of the stomach. The detection rate of early stage cancer has been increasing year by year since 1970, and in recent years was approximately 0.12%. In contrast, the detection rate of advanced cancer has decreased from 0.2% to 0.05%.

3 EVALUATION OF THE EFFECTIVENESS OF GASTRIC MASS SCREENING

There have been many studies to evaluate the effectiveness of gastric mass screening in Japan (Table 1).

Table 1 Studies to evaluate the effectiveness of gastric mass screening (Japan)

Research design	Studies carried out	Result
1. Randomized controlled trial		
a. Individual randomisation	None	-
b. Group randomization	On-going	?
2. Time trend analysis (incidence and mortality)	Done	effective
3. Retrospective cohort study	Done	effective
4. Correlation of screening rate and change in mortality	Done	effective
5. Case-control study	Done	effective

The findings from these studies (Hisamichi, 1989; Hisamichi, 1984; Hisamichi,1988; Oshima 1979; Oshima, 1986; Annual Report, 1980, 1981, 1982, 1984; Annual Report, 1985; Annual Report 1986, 1987, 1988) suggest that the widespread application of gastric mass screening as a public health service in Japan has contributed towards reducing the mortality from stomach cancer. However, none of the studies carried out in Japan were randomized controlled trials; other so-called second-best methods, such as time trend analysis, retrospective cohort study, correlation of screening rate and change of mortality, and case-control study have been used instead. Therefore, the possibility of several kinds of potential biases cannot be ruled out.

In this paper, in order to update the previous presentation by Dr. Oshima, Osaka, Japan (Oshima, 1988), we show the result of the time trend analysis between incidence and mortality from 1960-1985, and provide an interim report of a randomized controlled trial (group randomization) which has been initiated in Miyagi Prefecture. In this prefecture, population-based cancer registration was started in 1952 by the late Dr. M. Segi, Professor, Tohoku University School of Medicine, and has been continued. The reliability of cancer registration is considered high with 9.5% of cases recorded as Death Certificate Only, an incidence to death ratio of 1.78, and histological identification of 81.7% of reported cases in 1984-86. Therefore, we have data on both incidence and mortality from cancer over a long time period.

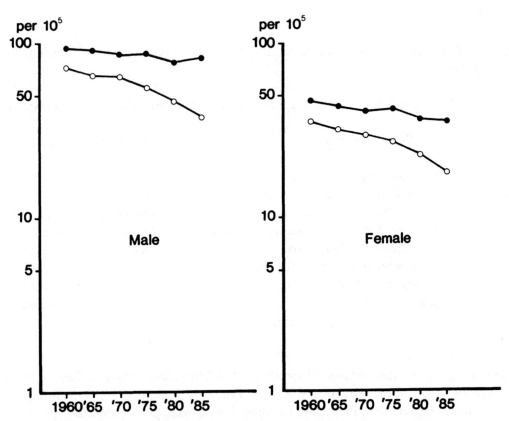

Figure 2 Trends of age-adjusted incidence and mortality rates of stomach cancer (Miyagi Prefecture, Japan).

3.1 Time Trend Analysis
Figure 2 shows the age-adjusted trends of incidence and mortality from stomach cancer in Miyagi Prefecture from 1960 to 1985. Incidence in both males and females shows a decreasing trend, and this trend has slowed down in recent years. On the other hand, until around 1970 the mortality rate decreased in parallel with the decreased incidence; however, since 1975 the decreasing trend has become more prominent and a definite separation of the two curves can be seen. The reasons for the reduction in the incidence rate are believed to be the Westernization of the Japanese diet and other changes in life style and environment.

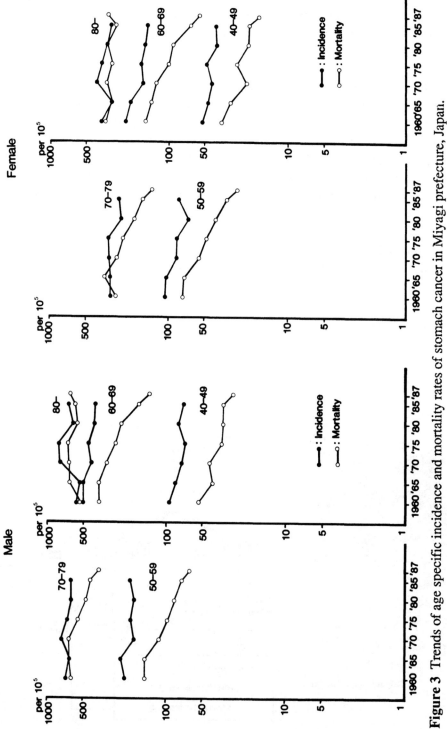

Figure 3 Trends of age specific incidence and mortality rates of stomach cancer in Miyagi prefecture, Japan.

However, the separation of the mortality rate cannot be explained by the reduction in incidence alone. We consider that this separation between the two decreasing trends is due to improved techniques for early detection and widespread application of the mass screening programme, as well as the progress in related therapy.

Figure 3 shows the same data analysed by age specific groups in males and females. The separation between the trends of incidence and mortality is demonstrated especially in the age group 50 to 79 in both sexes, the main target age population for gastric mass screening. Therefore, we consider this separation of the two curves in these age groups to be attributable to the effect of the widespread screening programme for 25 years in Miyagi Prefecture. However, the time trend analysis is also influenced by medical technology, the medical care system, and the reliability of data collection methods during the periods in question.

3.2 Randomized Controlled Trial

In Japan, it is very difficult to conduct a randomized controlled trial (RCT), because many municipalities all over Japan have been voluntarily conducting gastric mass screening for a long time. We started a specially designed RCT for evaluating the gastric mass screening programme in Miyagi prefecture in 1985.

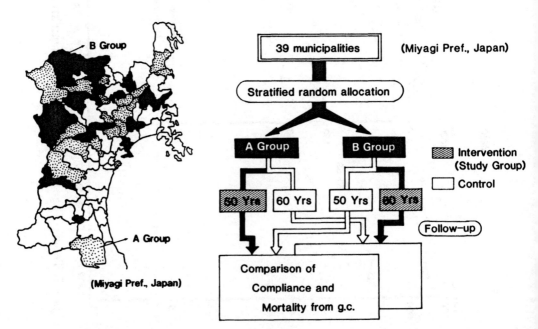

Figure 4 Randomized controlled trial; Group randomization, 1985-

Allocation to the trial is by group randomization, and not individual randomization. Furthermore, this trial is not in previously unscreened populations, because in Japan the special law on cancer screening programmes mentioned above has been implemented since 1983 and there is no longer the possibility to conduct a study using individual-based randomization.

We asked 63 municipalities in this prefecture to participate in the trial, and 39 municipalities agreed to join the trial. They were allocated to two groups (A and B group) by a method of stratified random sampling. In the municipalities allocated to the A group, 50-year-old people in 1985 were encouraged to attend gastric screening by means of a direct postal invitation specially written by the head of local government. Screening for people of other age groups was conducted in the usual way without an intensive screening campaign. On the other hand, in the municipalities allocated to the B group, 60-year-old people in 1985 were likewise encouraged to attend a gastric mass screening, and screening for people of other age groups was conducted in the usual way. From these methods, the study group of the trial consisted of an intensive screening campaign group (50 year-olds in the A group and 60 year-olds in the B group), and the control group consisted of a non-intensive screening campaign group (50 year-olds in the B group and 60 year-olds in the A group) (Fig.4).

The objectives of this trial are as follows:
(a) to compare the coverage rate (the rate of compliance) between the study group and the control group,
(b) to clarify behavior change associated with attending a screening as part of the intensive screening campaign, and
(c) to provide data on comparison of the mortality rates from stomach cancer in the two groups.

As this trial is on-going, we present the design of the trial and an interim report of the results, especially on the coverage rate (the rate of compliance).

Figure 5 shows the coverage rate of gastric mass screening of subjects who were 50 and 60 years old in 1985 and the trend until 1988. Intervention in the study group for this trial was done only once for people age 50-59 and 60-69. After that, screening continued in the usual way of the screening campaign that the government would conduct and similarly for the control group. Incidentally, in Japan there is the belief in a "critical age (the age of knots)"; for example, when a person reaches the age of 40, 50, or 60 years old, he or she is thought to have reached a turning point in terms of his/her work and health. Using this belief, the mayor's office conducted the intensive screening campaign. For example, one catch phrase in a direct mail was, "You are now at an important age point in your life. Please have a cancer check-up!"

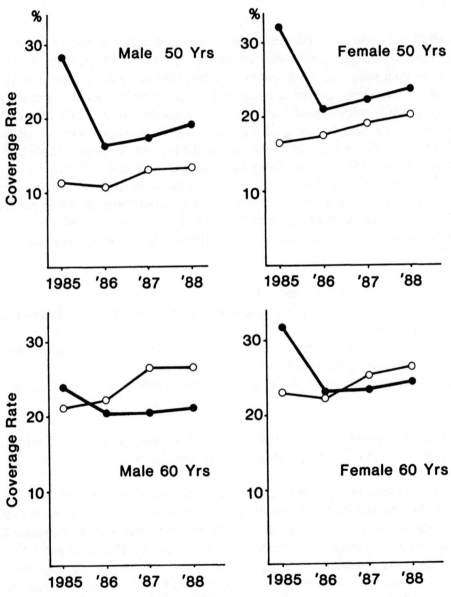

Figure 5 Coverage rate (compliance) and its trend

The results of the RCT conducted since 1985 with 5,723 subjects in the study group and 6,087 subjects in the control group are shown in Figure 5. In addition to this, we conducted a RCT in a similar way with another group of people who had just turned 50 and 60 years old in 1986. Both the men and women in the 50 year-old group showed a high compliance rate of gastric mass screening for their first year, showing a clear difference from the control group. However the trend thereafter showed a sharp decline for the second year and, after maintaining a difference of coverage rate of 4 or 5%, is slowly rising. On the other hand, among the 60 year-olds, although there was some difference at the time of initial screening, the trend even showed a decrease from the next year. A similar trend was seen in the women as well. There was a distinct difference between the 50 and 60 year-olds in terms of their compliance with gastric mass screening, but the reason for this was not immediately known and will be the subject of further investigation.

3.3 Case-Control Study

Fukao et.al. (Fukao, 1987) conducted a case-control study to evaluate the effectiveness of gastric mass screening and the optimal interval of screening. The methodology of this study is as follows. The cases consisted of all patients with advanced cancer detected by gastric mass screening during the period from 1979 to 1983 in Miyagi Prefecture; there were 241 male and 126 female cases. For each case, one control of the same sex who was age matched (within 3 years) with the case was selected randomly from the examinees of the same precinct who were not diagnosed with advanced stomach cancer. There were 367 controls. From the files of gastric mass screening of the Cancer Detection Centre, Miyagi Cancer Society, it was determined whether the cases and controls had ever had screening tests before the date of diagnosis of advanced stomach cancer.

Table 2 shows the results of the case-control study evaluating the relative protective effect of mass screening for stomach cancer. Relative protection was first used in a Toronto Case-Control Study on optimal frequency of screening for cervical cancer by Clarke et al (1979, 1986); relative protection was calculated by comparing examinees who had one or more negative results with those who had never been screened.

Table 2 Optimal interval for screening for stomach cancer (Fukao et al, 1987)

Time since last negative result (years)	No. of cases of advanced cancer	No. of controls	Relative protection	95% Confidence interval
Never screened	156	89	1.00	
1	132	220	2.92	2.09-4.08
2	40	31	1.36	0.80-2.32
3	23	18	1.37	0.70-2.67
4	16	9	0.99	0.42-2.32
Total	367	367		

A significant protective effect of screening in examinees who were screened a year before with a negative result was shown as a relative protection of 2.92 (95% confidence interval: 2.09-4.08). This means that people who were screened every year had approximately 3 times the chance of not getting advanced cancer in comparison with those who had never been screened or not screened for more than 5 years. The relative protection is highest in the group receiving screening every year. The trend of positive relative protection continued until the last negative screen was performed three years before diagnosis. This trend, although not statistically significant, seems like a dose-response relationship. From the result, Dr. Fukao and his co-investigators consider that screening intervals for gastric cancer should not be greater than 3 years.

4 COST-EFFECTIVENESS/BENEFIT ANALYSIS

We conducted a cost-effectiveness analysis of gastric mass screening. Table 3 shows the sensitivity, specificity and positive predictive value of gastric mass screening. These figures are average and actual data given from the gastric mass screening in Miyagi Prefecture.

Table 3 Sensitivity and specificity of gastric mass screening

	Cancer	No cancer	Total
Test positive	170	9,830	10,000
Test negative	30	89,970	90,000
Total	200	99,800	100,000

Sensitivity = 85%, Specificity = 90%
Rate of positive test = 10%
Positive predictive value = 1.7%

Figure 6 is the decision tree of gastric mass screening. The numerical values in the figure were calculated from data on people of average age 55 years with stomach cancer detected by screening, with estimated life expectancy of 20 years. We conducted this decision analysis on the assumption of a target population for screening of 100,000 people. The numbers for cured cancers in Figure 6 were calculated from our experience; for example, the 5-year relative survival rate among the 554 patients with stomach cancer detected by mass screening was approximately 70%, while that among the 3,375 patients with stomach cancer presenting at the out-patient clinic with symptoms was approximately 25%. In Figures 6 and 7 we used the numbers of lives saved of cancer patients to derive the numbers of cured cancers.

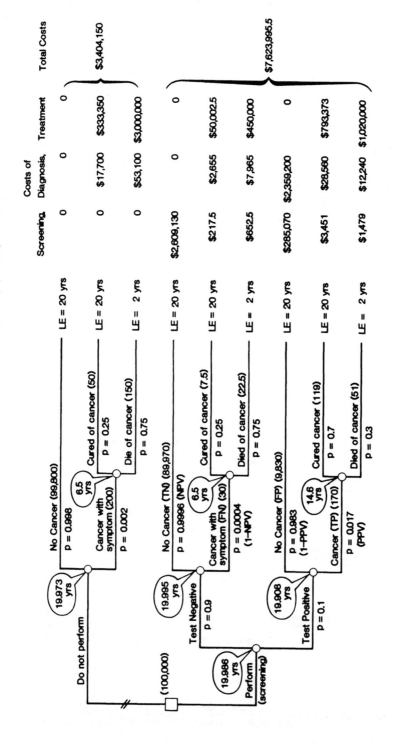
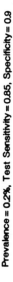

Figure 6 Decision tree of Gastric Mass Screening (Original tree). Based on 100,000 persons, 55 years old, of both sexes Miyagi Prefecture, Japan.

The total costs include the costs of screening, diagnosis and treatment, i.e. cost of screening = $29, diagnosis (B) (includes fibrescopic examination and biopsy) = $240, diagnosis (A) (includes fibrescopic examination, direct x-ray and biopsy) = $354, treatment of early stomach cancer = $6,667, treatment of advanced stomach cancer = $20,000. As this original decision tree is very complicated, a reduced decision tree is shown in Figure 7. In Figure 7, we use the number of lives saved of cancer patients as a value of the effectiveness instead of life expectancy in figure 6.

The marginal cost-effectiveness of mass screening for stomach cancer is equal to the cost with (B) minus the cost with (A), divided by the number of lives saved by (B) minus the number of lives saved by (A) (Figure 7). If 100,000 people at age 55 are the target population for the cost-effectiveness analysis of gastric mass screening, the numbers of lives saved by conducting the screening in addition to those saved without screening was 76.5 (126.5-50). The marginal cost-effectiveness becomes approximately $55,000 (US) per life saved. However, it depends on the economic situation, the cost value applied to human life and the levels of medical technologies used in the usual way, etc., which differ considerably from country to country, whether the mass screening programme is regarded as expensive or not.

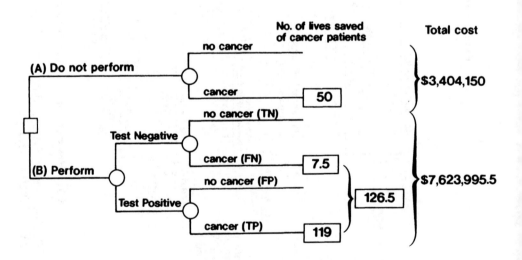

$$\text{Marginal cost - effectiveness} = \frac{\text{Costs with (B)} - \text{Costs with (A)}}{\text{No. of lives saved (B)} - \text{No. of lives saved (A)}}$$

Figure 7 Reduced decision tree of gastric mass screening

In today's Japan, the monetary value of the life of a 55 year-old male is estimated approximately at $200,000-300,000 (US). Therefore, from the stand-point of cost-benefit analysis, it is appropriate that mass screening for gastric cancer should be conducted in Japan.

5 CONCLUSION

From the time trend analysis and the case-control study described here and many other studies undertaken to evaluate the effectiveness of gastric mass screening, the widespread programme of gastric mass screening in Japan is considered to be effective in reducing the mortality rate from stomach cancer in the target age population at risk, especially from 50 to 79 years old.

As the RCT very carefully designed by us in Miyagi Prefecture, Japan is now on-going, we described in this paper an interim report of the RCT; i.e. the rate of compliance and its trend compared between the study group and the control group. It is necessary to wait for at least two or three years before the final results of this trial will be available. Stomach cancer is still one of the very common cancers in the world. The importance of comprehensive cancer control, using both primary prevention and secondary prevention should be emphasized. Furthermore, it is important that the decreasing trend of mortality from stomach cancer, observed to be separating from the decreasing trend of incidence, is speeded up.

Acknowledgement

This work was supported partly by a grant from the Ministry of Health and Welfare for the Comprehensive 10-year Strategy for Cancer Control, Japan. The authors are grateful to Mrs. Y. Okuno, a committee member of Miyagi Prefectural Cancer Registry, Miyagi Cancer Society, and Miss Y. Nakata, a member of the staff of the Department of Public Health, Tohoku University School of Medicine, for their technical assistance and help with data collection, etc.

REFERENCES

Annual Report 1980, 1981, 1982, 1984 of Research Committee of Studies on Evaluation of Mass Screening for Stomach Cancer, Hisamichi S, Ed. (Chairman of the Committee), Department of Public Health, Tohoku University School of Medicine, Sendai, 1981, 1982, 1983, 1985. (in Japanese)

Annual Report 1985 of Research Committee of Studies on Evaluation of Mass Screening for Stomach Cancer, Tamura K, Ed. (Chairman of the Committee), Cancer Detection Centre of Hokkaido Cancer Society, Sapporo, 1986. (in Japanese)

Annual Report 1986, 1987, 1988 of Research Committee of Studies on Quantitative Analysis on Effect of Mass Screening for Stomach Cancer, Ed. by Tamura K. (Chairman of the Committee), Cancer Detection Centre of Hokkaido Cancer Society, Sapporo, 1989. (in Japanese)

Clarke EA, Anderson TW. Does screening by 'Pap' smears help prevent cervical cancer? A case-contol study. Lancet 1979; ii:1-4.

Clarke EA, Hilditch S, Anderson TW. Optimal frequency of screening for cervical cancer: a Toronto case-control study. In Screening for Cancer of the Uterine Cervix. (M Hakama, AB Miller, NE Day, eds.) IARC Scientific Publications: Lyon, International Agency for Research on Cancer, 1986, No. 76, pp.125-131.

Fukao A, Hisamichi S, Sugawara N. A case-control study on evaluating the effect of mass screening on decreasing advanced stomach cancer. (in Japanese) J Jpn Soc Gastroenterol Mass Survey 1987; 75:112-116.

Hisamichi S. Screening for gastric cancer. World J Surg 1989; 13:31-37.

Hisamichi S, Iwasaki M, Arisue T, et al. Nationwide statistics of mass screening for digestive organs in 1987. (in Japanese) J Jpn Soc Gastroenterol Mass Survey 1982; 85:180-201.

Hisamichi S, Sugawara N. Mass Screening for gastric cancer by x-ray examination. Jpn J Clin Oncol 1984; 14:211-223.

Hisamichi S, Sugawara N, Fukao A. Effectiveness of gastric mass screening in Japan. Cancer Detec Prev 1988; 11:323-329.

Oshima A. Screening for stomach cancer: the Japanese program. In Screening for Gastrointestinal Cancer. (J Chamberlain, AB Miller, eds.) Hans Huber: Toronto, 1988, pp.65-70.

Oshima A, Fujimoto I. Evaluation of mass screening program for cancer. In Second Symposium on Epidemiology and Cancer Registries in the Pacific Basin. (JC Bailar, ed.) Bethesda, NCI Monograph 53 NIH, 1979, pp.181-186.

Oshima A, Hirata N, Ubukata T, et al. Evaluation of a mass screening programfor stomach cancer with a case-control study design. Int J Cancer 1986; 38:829-833.

38 Summary of Discussion on Screening for Stomach Cancer

Stomach cancer is one of the most common cancers in the Western Pacific, Central and South America and Eastern Europe and the possibility that screening can reduce mortality requires careful consideration.

Studies to evaluate the effectiveness of the Japanese screening programme have used several designs including time trend analyses, case control studies and a trial with group randomization of a special invitation letter to encourage participation currently in progress. Completed studies have suggested a benefit, but several possible biases cannot be ruled out. Reduction in incidence raises the question as to whether a major part of the effect is due to dietary change or change in other etiological exposure as screening for stomach cancer can be expected to reduce mortality but not incidence. Indeed, a general compliance of 40% with screening would not normally be expected to have a major effect on mortality trends. However, recently completed time trend analyses show a drop in mortality which cannot be explained by decreased incidence. Lesser falls in incidence than mortality could be explained by the effect of screening in detecting earlier disease or lesions which would not have surfaced otherwise without having an important effect on the disease that results in death. Correlation studies do show that the degree of reduction in mortality is related to the extent of screening. In order for the mortality trends to be accounted by bias, the dietary changes and screening should be correlated. This is not totally unrealistic, because both appear first in the well to do areas. It was pointed out that although the recent case-control study obtained a relative protection of 65%, no attention was paid to the possibility that the underlying risk was different in the two groups. One difficulty that has arisen in the Japanese program is deciding at what age screening should be stopped. It is recognised that the prognosis of the disease is poorer at older ages. One proposal is to stop at 74, but it may be more realistic to stop at 69, recognising that the effect of screening in the 60s if effective will help to reduce mortality at least in the early 70s.

In Venezuela a programme of screening people over the age of 40 using the barium x-ray has been in progress in a high risk area of the country for the last 9 years. This programme involves two mobile screening units, suspicious findings resulted in referral to a centre for diagnosis. A case control study has recently been initiated with deaths from the disease as the cases and population controls. It was suggested that another approach to evaluate such a programme would have been to randomise districts to be screened or not from the beginning.

Although screening for stomach cancer is public policy in Japan, it is unlikely to become public policy elsewhere unless the Japanese findings can be replicated. The priority that countries are likely to give to evaluation of screening for stomach cancer will depend on the priority given to control of stomach cancer in the relevant population, and the resources available.

State of the Art on Screening for Nasopharyngeal Cancer

While the existing screening tests show some promise, no study has been done to examine the impact of screening on mortality. Therefore, screening for nasopharyngeal cancer cannot currently be recommended as public health policy.

Recommendations for Research
Standardize available tests with respect to definitions of positives and negatives.
Estimate sensitivity and specificity of the tests under screening conditions.
Evaluate therapy for cancers suspected on the basis of abnormal serology.
A randomized controlled trial should be conducted in unscreened high risk areas using mortality from the disease as the endpoint.

39 Screening for Nasopharyngeal Carcinoma

A. J. SASCO

Unit of Analytical Epidemiology, International Agency for Research on Cancer
Lyon, France

1 INTRODUCTION

Nasopharyngeal carcinoma (NPC) is a rare cancer in most populations of the world. The vast majority of reported incidence rates are below 1 case per 100,000 person-years (Muir et al., 1987) among males and even lower among females. The male to female ratio in most parts of the world is of the order of 2. The highest reported rate (age-standardized to the world population) occurs in Hong Kong with a figure of 30 per 100,000 person-years for males and 12.9 for females. Other populations with rates higher than 10 in men are the Chinese in the Bay Area of the USA (14.8 in men; 8.0 in women), the Chinese in Singapore (18.1 in men; 7.9 in women), the Chinese in Hawaii (11.2 in men; 4.9 in women) and in New Zealand, the population of the Pacific Polynesian Islands (14.1 in men; 1.5 in women).

Other incidence rates, not reported in Cancer Incidence in Five Continents, indicate that the Chinese in the south-eastern part of the People's Republic of China (Guangxi autonomous region, Guang Dong province and, to a lesser extent, Fujian and Hunan) have rates in the order of 20 (17 per 100,000 in Wuzhou, Guangxi for example (Zeng et al., 1982)). Chinese migrating to other parts of the world also have high rates such as those found in Taiwan (Chen et al., 1988), Singapore (Lee et al., 1988) as well as in the USA (Muir et al., 1987). High rates are also reported for Eskimo populations in Alaska (Lanier et al., 1980), Canada (Schaefer and Hildes, 1986) and Greenland (Nielsen et al., 1977). Finally, intermediate rates, estimated at 10 to 15/100,000, but with a high proportion of young cases, are found in northern Africa (Ellouz et al., 1978) and some other parts of Africa (Hidayatalla et al., 1983). The rest of the world's population has low rates of the disease (Muir et al., 1987). In northern Africa, the incidence curve differs from that seen in China, with a noticeable proportion of cases occurring in late adolescence and young adulthood (Ellouz et al., 1978). Among Chinese migrants, the risk decreases mainly with the second and third generation.

Three factors are thought to play an important role in the etiology of NPC: a virus, the Epstein-Barr virus (EBV), diet and genetics. Presence of EBV DNA in the malignant cells has been constantly demonstrated in undifferentiated NPC tumours in various parts of the world (Henlé and Henlé, 1985). Such a close link between a virus and a cancer is a remarkable etiologic feature of NPC and is used for screening, early diagnosis and surveillance of NPC cases. Genetics also play a role in the etiology of NPC, as demonstrated by the studies of HLA profile (Chan et al., 1983, 1985) and as supported by the notion of an increased risk among relatives of NPC cases (Lanier et al., 1986; Ireland et al., 1988).

The main environmental risk factor for NPC is diet, either loosely defined as traditional diet or more specifically studied in some Chinese populations. The consumption of Cantonese salted fish has been linked to NPC occurrence, in particular when heavily consumed at a young age, and as a weaning food (Ho, 1971, 1972; Geser et al., 1978; Armstrong et al., 1983; Yu et al., 1986, 1988, 1989; Yan et al., 1989). This repeatedly found association is supported by experimental data (Fong and Walsh, 1971; Huang et al., 1978; Yu et al.,1989). A recent study also found an increased risk for salted fish and for other traditional food in a low-risk region of China (Ning et al., 1990). Further environmental risk factors include occupational exposures to dust and fumes (Armstrong et al., 1983) and possibly to formaldehyde (Roush et al., 1987) although this latter association is still controversial (Purchase and Paddle, 1989); use of nasal oil (Lin et al., 1973; Shanmugaratnam et al., 1978) and finally exposure to smoke, either domestic exposure to various smokes and fumes (Djojopranoto and Soesilowati, 1967; Armstrong et al., 1978) or exposure to environmental tobacco smoke as a child (Yu et al., 1988). A positive role of active smoking has been found in three studies (Hu and Huang, 1972; Lin et al., 1973; Mabuchi et al., 1985) while in another study the inclusion of lung cancer cases among the controls (Geser et al., 1978) leading to an underestimation of the risk does not rule out an etiologic role for smoking. Two other studies did not find any association (Henderson et al., 1976; Shanmugaratnam et al., 1978).

2 NPC AS A CANDIDATE DISEASE FOR SCREENING

In order to qualify for being considered for a screening programme, a disease needs to fulfill several criteria (Cole and Morrison, 1980). One has to demonstrate that:
- the disease has serious consequences;
- early treatment is more effective than treatment started at a later date
  corresponding to the time of diagnosis based on clinical symptoms;
- the prevalence of the detectable pre-clinical phase (DPCP) is high enough
  among the people screened.

The first point is easy enough to fulfill. NPC is responsible for considerable morbidity, represents a heavy financial and social burden for some specific population groups (mainly south-eastern Chinese, Eskimos, Alaskan, Canadian and Greenland natives and, to a lesser extent, northern African populations) and is a major cause of cancer mortality at a relatively young age for these ethnic groups. The third point is also not difficult to fulfill for these same peoples. In contrast, the degree to which the second point can be satisfied is less clear. Radiotherapy is the treatment of choice. Five year survival rates as high as 84% are reported for stage I tumours (Ho, 1978), whereas advanced tumours are associated with a much poorer survival rate. Therefore, theoretically NPC seems a good candidate for screening, but the proof of the efficacy of screening needs to be established. In particular, the advantages of earlier treatment have to be quantified.

3 SCREENING FOR NPC: AVAILABLE METHODS

Given the constant association of EBV with NPC, serological markers of EBV immunity have been proposed and accepted as diagnostic aids in head and neck cancers, as well as for the surveillance of the evolution of NPC (Coates et al., 1978; Naegele et al., 1982; Cevinini et al., 1986; Gurtsevitch et al., 1986; Hadar et al, 1986; Bogger-Goren et al., 1987; Coyle et al., 1987; Faggioni et al., 1987; Ammatuna et al., 1988; Levine et al., 1988; de Vathaire et al., 1988). Several tests have also been proposed for screening (Table 1).

Table 1 Proposed NPC screening methods

I. EBV serological determinations:

Determination of presence and titers of:
  • Immunoglobulin A/Viral Capsid Antigen (IgA/VCA)
  • Immunoglobulin A/Early Antigen (IgA/EA)
  • Immunoglobulin A/Membrane Antigen (IgA/MA)
  • EBV specific DNase activity

by the following methods:
  • Immunoenzymatic test (IE)
  • Immunofluorescence (IF)
  • Immunoautoradiography (IR)
  • Enzyme-linked immunoabsorbence (ELISA)
  • Use of preabsorbed sera (staphylococcus aureus or antihuman IgG)
    for IgA/EA and IgA/MA

II. Determinations in exfoliated cells:
  • Simple cytology
  • Use of anticomplement immunoenzymatic method (ACIE)
    for identification of Epstein-Barr Nuclear Antigen (EBNA) in cells
  • Binding with 125 I monoclonal selective antibodies

EBV serological markers were used for screening for NPC for the first time in 1978-80 in Zangwu, a rural county of the Guangxi autonomous region of the People's Republic of China by Zeng and his collaborators. Since these initial surveys, other population studies have been conducted in Guangxi and Guang Dong, as well as some surveys restricted to high risk individuals in other Chinese groups. Populations, methods used and results will be discussed below. To our knowledge, no populations other than the Chinese have yet been the object of mass screening. Most of the evidence has been collected by one team of investigators and the tests used for screening have changed over time. Those studies which are available on the prevalence screen are summarised in Table 2.

Table 2 Main results of published population screening surveys - prevalence screen

Reference	Screen population	Number screened	Method used & test	Positivity (%)	NPC detected
Zeng et al., 1979, 1980	Zangwu (rural)	148,029 (aged 30+)	IE IgA/VCA	3,533 (2.4)	55
Zeng, 1985	Moloas (rural)	15,324	IE IgA/VCA	151 (1.0)	7
Zeng et al., 1982	Wuzhou City	12,932 (aged 40-59)	IE IgA/VCA	680 (5.3)	13
		680 IgA/VCA positive	IE IgA/EA	30 (4.5)	9
		507 IgA/VCA negative	IE IgA/EA	0 (0)	
Chen et al., 1989	Taiwan govt employees high risk population	22,596 9,869	EBV specific DNase activity	1,250 (5.5) 1,176 (11.9)	14

The first study published concerned a population survey conducted in the Zangwu rural county of the Guangxi autonomous region (Zeng et al., 1979). Of a population of 450,000 individuals, all persons aged 30 and above were asked to be screened and 148,029 persons were bled (proportion of refusers or unavailable not given). An immunoenzymatic test was used for the detection of immunoglobulin A to the Viral Capsid Antigen (IgA/VCA); 3,533 were found to be positive, representing 2.4% of all those screened (Zeng et al., 1980). Among the 3,533 individuals having IgA/VCA antibodies, 460 or 13.0% of the positives had a titer greater or equal to 1/80 or 0.3% of those screened. These 460 individuals were submitted to a clinical examination; 55 NPC were found on clinical grounds and verified histologically, representing 11.9% of the screened positives or 0.37 prevalent case per 1,000 screened. The stage distribution indicates a clear shift towards earlier stages than commonly found in this rural population (1 in situ; 12 stage I; 19 stage II; 17 stage III; 6 stage IV). No measures of sensitivity, specificity or any other characteristics of the test were presented.

An additional serological survey was carried out among a minority group in another rural county of the Guangxi region (Zeng, 1985). In Laucheng county, 15,324 Molaos were screened for IgA/VCA; 151 were found to be positive (1.0% of those screened) and among these 7 cancers were diagnosed (5.9% of the screened positive or 0.46 prevalent case per 1,000 screened).

Another population serological survey was carried out in the urban population of Wuzhou City, situated in the centre of Zangwu county. The results of the initial survey were presented for 12,932 persons screened in the 40 to 59 year age-group (Zeng et al., 1982). Once again, the rate of compliance is not stated. IgA/VCA was detected by an immunoenzymatic method as for the rural population. Of the 12,932 persons screened, 680 were found positive or 5.3% of those screened, which is considerably higher than the positivity rate reported for the rural population (Zeng et al., 1979), with 204 (30%) having titers greater than 1/40 or 1.6% of those screened. The positivity rate of IgA/VCA increased with age as did the geometric mean titer. The frequency of IgA/VCA was similar for males and females. All 680 positive individuals were examined (independently of the Ig/VCA titer) and 13 NPC were detected, representing 2.0% of people with any level of IgA/VCA antibodies or 1 prevalent case per 1,000 screened. Of the 13 cases, 9 were in stage I and 4 in stage II.

In addition to having a clinical examination, all 680 IgA/VCA positive individuals had a determination of their immunoglobulin A to the Early Antigen levels (IgA/EA) by an immunoenzymatic method (Zeng et al., 1982). This test was also done on 507 IgA/VCA negative individuals. No IgA/EA positive subjects were found among the IgA/VCA negative individuals, whereas 30 of the IgA/VCA positive persons were also IgA/EA positive (or 4.5% of IgA/VCA positive). These include 9 NPC cases out of 13 (or 30.0% of IgA/EA positive).

Because the immunoenzymatic test for the detection of IgA/EA among NPC patients fails to be positive for about 30 to 50% of NPC cases, a more sensitive test was elaborated (Zeng et al., 1983a) using an immunoautoradiographic method. The positivity for IgA/EA was increased, as well as the geometric mean titer in NPC cases and in subjects with nasopharyngeal chronic inflammation, but also in persons with other tumours. No positive results were described among normal subjects. Therefore, it was recommended that a two-step procedure for serological mass surveys be carried out, first by using an immunoenzymatic test or immunofluorescence test for the detection of IgA/VCA and then among positive subjects by proceeding to the detection of IgA/EA antibody by immunoautoradiography.

It has also been proposed that an anticomplement immunoenzymatic (ACIE) method be used to detect EBV nuclear antigen (EBNA) in exfoliated carcinoma cells of IgA/VCA positive individuals without any clinical signs (Zeng et al., 1984). This method was applied to 64 IgA/VCA positive individuals and 4 cases of NPC were found, all in stage I. It was concluded that ACIE could be proposed for following up IgA/VCA positive individuals.

The most recently reported mass survey comes from Taiwan (Chen et al., 1989) where, over a three-year period, 22,596 sera from government employees and 9,869 sera from a high-risk NPC region were screened for the presence of antibody to EBV specific DNase. All subjects were males, between the ages of 20 and 70, the majority being between 35 and 60 years of age. Positive individuals were asked to come to a special Ear, Nose and Throat clinic, but over the study period only 54% of those positive were examined. Among these, 14 NPC cases were found, 10 of them already known. The follow-up revealed one additional case. There were therefore only five new cases found (3 stage II and 2 stage III). Estimates from a previous study on NPC patients and controls indicated specificity of 94.7% and sensitivity of 90.3% (Chen et al., 1987).

Finally, one study from Singapore (Chan, 1989) reports figures for sensitivity and specificity of IgA/VCA and Ig/EA detection but without specification of the methods used either for the test itself or for the determination of these values. For IgA/VCA, the sensitivity is estimated at 95% and the specificity at 97% which, with an estimate of the prevalence of the DPCP set equal to the NPC incidence rate, leads to a predictive value positive of 0.6%. For IgA/EA, corresponding figures are 90% sensitivity, 99% specificity and 2% predictive value positive. A double step procedure is therefore proposed with a first screen for IgA/VCA to be followed among positive individuals by an IgA/EA determination. The predictive value positive would then increase to 36%. Such a procedure is considered by the author to be labour intensive and somewhat subjective. The recommendation is only to screen family members of NPC patients, where HLA haplotype could also be determined. No population screening is proposed. Relatives of NPC patients are also screened in Hong Kong.

Only some of the reports on the studies described above provided follow-up information on individuals found to be positive on testing but not found initially to have NPC (Table 3). Over a three-year period, follow-up of 3,478 individuals found positive in Zangwu revealed 32 additional cases (10 stage I; 9 stage II; 11 stage III; 2 stage IV) (Zeng et al., 1983b). The methods of follow-up of positive subjects were not specified and no follow-up was carried out for negative individuals.

Table 3 Main results of published population screening surveys - follow-up of positive individuals

Reference	Screen population	Number screened positive	Method used & test	Duration of follow-up and results
Zeng et al., 1983b	Zangwu (rural)	3478	IE IgA/VCA	1 to 3 years 32 NPC
Zeng et al., 1985	Wuzhou City (20,726 screened)	1136	IE IgA/VCA	4 years 17 NPC
Zeng et al., 1986	Wuzhou City	1138	IE IgA/VCA	1 year 4 NPC

Follow-up of the individuals found positive in the 1980 survey conducted in Wuzhou was continued for up to four years and results reported (Zeng et al., 1985). While the paper on the initial survey done in Wuzhou only concerned 12,932 subjects aged 40-59, with 680 IgA/VCA positive, the follow-up was carried out on 1,136 IgA/VCA positive found among 20,726 screened individuals. Among these 5.5% positive, 18 cases of NPC were found at the initial screening (10 stage I; 6 stage II; 2 stage III) including 14 with an IgA/VCA titer equal to or greater than 1/40. Over a period not precisely defined but probably shorter than four years for some of these individuals, subsequent annual clinical and histological examinations revealed 17 additional NPC cases (5 stage I; 11 stage II and 1 stage III). The only stage III tumour occurred in a patient who had refused biopsy. This permits the estimation of an incidence rate among IgA/VCA positive individuals which is 7.5 times higher than among the total Wuzhou population. It is claimed that not a single case of NPC occurred among 19,590 IgA/VCA negative individuals which would mean that there were no false negative subjects, but no formal follow-up of these negative subjects was set up. The article does not present any figures for sensitivity or specificity, but it can be estimated that specificity is of the order of 95%. Follow-up was then extended for one more year which revealed four new NPC cases. In this latter study (Zeng et al., 1986), among the 20,726 subjects screened, 1,138 (instead of 1,136 as previously reported (Zeng et al., 1985)) were described as IgA/VCA positive. A subset of 494 individuals were subjected to annual retesting of IgA/VCA; 63.4% were stable, 10.9% lost their positivity, 11.7% increased their titers by four dilutions or more and 10.7% had decreasing levels. Eighty-eight percent of NPC patients were diagnosed among the subjects with stable or increasing IgA/VCA titers. Follow-up was also carried out among 259 IgA/VCA negative subjects.

Over a four-year period, 93.1% remained negative, 5.4% became positive (14 subjects including 12 with low titers) and 1.5% fluctuated from negative to positive to negative again.

Comparison of enzyme-linked immunoabsorbent assay (ELISA) versus immunoenzymatic test was presented for detection of IgA/EA positive individuals. ELISA was more sensitive than the immunoenzymatic method, but also slightly less specific. Another method to improve the sensitivity of the test for the detection of IgA/EA is to use staphylococcus aureus or antihuman immunoglobulin G (IgG) preabsorbed sera. Finally, it is also possible to detect immunoglobulin A against the Membrane Antigen (IgA/MA) or IgG/MA and to increase the sensitivity of the test detecting IgA/MA by the use of staphylococcus aureus preabsorbed sera. A more detailed description of the test for IgA/MA was later presented (Pi et al., 1987). Preabsorption by removing competing IgG increases the sensitivity of the test, making it similar to the detection of IgA/EA while being more specific, but it is still not as sensitive as IgA/VCA.

4 EVALUATION OF THE SCREENING TESTS

Estimates of sensitivity and specificity of various virological tests were presented based on serological evaluation of NPC diagnosed cases and normal controls and, for some of these tests, a group of NPC suspected cases or some other pathological group were also included (Zeng et al., 1983; Zhu et al., 1986; Zeng et al., 1986; Pi et al., 1987; Chen et al., 1987). No valid estimates have yet been presented based on populations of apparently asymptomatic individuals. In particular, no strict follow-up of all negative individuals has ever been set up to pick up false negative cases. Also, it is worth remembering that so far, available data on population surveys only describe the results from a prevalence screen with no subsequent re-screening on any substantial number of individuals. In addition, all published population surveys have been conducted by one team of investigators in one region of China. No precise data on the cost of various tests have yet been reported.

5 FOLLOW-UP AND EVALUATION OF POSITIVE SUBJECTS

Subjects found positive on a first level screening test, such as IgA/VCA are then submitted to a second test, usually the determination of IgA/EA. They are also the object of a detailed clinical investigation including a nasopharyngoscopy and biopsy of either suspicious lesions or randomly done in apparently normal mucosa of individuals with an indicative serological profile.

To date, a shift in stage distribution has been documented in Wuzhou (Zeng et al., 1982, 1985) and in rural Zangwu (Zeng et al., 1980), either among the cases found at first screening or during the follow-up of positive individuals. This information has been used as evidence that there will be an effect on the mortality rate, but it should be strongly emphasized that such an effect has not yet been demonstrated in any published study, no study yet having looked at NPC mortality rates among screened versus unscreened populations. In fact, unpublished evidence from at least one Chinese cancer registry shows that over the years, and even before the introduction of large scale serological screening, there has been some stage shift towards earlier stages at diagnosis but no decrease in NPC mortality rates.

6 SUMMARY AND CONCLUSIONS

At the present time, no strong evidence exists in favour of screening for NPC, but it has to be recognised that the use of serological tests looks promising because it brings about a considerable shift in the stage distribution at diagnosis. It would therefore seem imperative that a proper large scale randomised trial of screening for NPC in a high risk population be set up and conducted in the near future. Its aim should be to assess the impact of screening on mortality from NPC in a screened as compared to an unscreened group. Given the nature of the test being used and the fluctuation of antibody status and titers, it will be important to repeat the screening test at regular intervals, both among positive and negative subjects. The problem is compounded by the fact that serological testing identifies high-risk individuals who are more likely to develop NPC in the (near) future, but cannot by itself identify subjects with or without cancer at the time of the initial serological examination. The issue of defining properly the criteria for serological and clinical follow-up of positive as well as negative individuals is crucial. The frequency and serious nature of NPC in certain population groups justifies such a study and it should be carried out before the large scale introduction of an as yet unproven method of screening. It is urgent to study the mortality rates of screened and unscreened populations adequately and not rely merely on assumed survival rates based on a modified stage distribution.

REFERENCES

Ammatuna P, de Thé G, Speciale R et al. Serological and immunohistological assessment of Epstein-Barr virus infection in Sicilian patients with suspected nasopharyngeal carcinoma. Microbiologica 1988; 11:89-94.

Armstrong RW, Kannan Kutty M, Armstrong MJ. Self-specific environments associated with nasopharyngeal carcinoma in Selangor, Malaysia. Soc Sci Med 1978; 12D:149-156.

Armstrong W, Armstrong MJ, Yu MC et al. Salted fish and inhalants as risk factors for nasopharyngeal carcinoma in Malaysian Chinese. Cancer Res 1983; 43:2967-2970.

Bogger-Goren S, Gotlieb-Stematsky T, Rachima M et al. Nasopharyngeal carcinoma in Israel: epidemiology and Epstein-Barr virus related serology. Eur J Cancer Clin Oncol 1987; 23:1277-1281.

Cevenini R, Donati M, Caliceti U et al. Evaluation of antibodies to Epstein-Barr virus in Italian patients with nasopharyngeal carcinoma. J Inf 1986; 12:127-131.

Chan SH. Screening for NPC. Ann Acad Med Singapore 1989; 18:80-82.

Chan SH, Chew CT, Prasad U et al. HLA and nasopharyngeal carcinoma in Malays. Br J Cancer 1985; 51:389-392.

Chan SH, Day NE, Kunaratman N et al. HLA and nasopharyngeal carcinoma in Chinese. A further study. Int J Cancer 1983; 32:171-176.

Chen GJ, Chen JY, Hsu MM et al. Epidemiological characteristics and early detection of nasopharyngeal carcinoma in Taiwan. In: Wolf GT, Carey TE (eds). Head and Neck Oncology Research. Amsterdam-Berkeley: Kugler Publications, 1988, pp 505-513.

Chen JY, Chen CJ, Liu MY et al. Antibodies to Epstein-Barr virus-specific DNase in patients with nasopharyngeal carcinoma and control groups. J Med Virol 1987; 23:11-22.

Chen JY, Chen CJ, Liu MY et al. Antibody to Epstein-Barr virus-specific DNase as a marker for field survey of patients with nasopharyngeal carcinoma in Taiwan. J Med Virol 1989; 27:269-273.

Coates HL, Pearson GR, Neel HB et al. An immunologic basis for detection of occult primary malignancies of the head and neck. Cancer 1978; 41:912-918.

Cole P, Morrison AS. Basic issues in population screening for cancer. JNCI 1980; 64: 1263-1272.

Coyle PV, Wyatt D, Connolly JH et al. Antibodies to Epstein-Barr virus in patients with nasopharyngeal carcinoma in northern Ireland. IJMS 1987; 156:182-184.

Djojopranoto M, Soesilowati. Nasopharyngeal cancer in East Java (Indonesia). In: Muir CS, Shanmugaratnam KS (eds). Cancer of the nasopharynx (UICC Monograph Series Vol. 1). Copenhagen: Munksgaard, 1967, pp 43-46.

Ellouz R, Cammoun M, Ben Attia R et al. Nasopharyngeal carcinoma in children and adolescents in Tunisia: clinical aspects and paraneoplastic syndrome. In: de Thé G, Ito Y (eds). Nasopharyngeal carcinoma: Etiology and control. IARC Sci Pub No. 20, International Agency for Research on Cancer, Lyon, 1978, pp 115-130.

Faggioni A, Corradini C, Venanzoni M et al. Nasopharyngeal carcinoma: the diagnostic value of the antibody-dependent, cellular cytotoxicity test and EBV serology. J Experim Pathol 1987; 3:471-477.

Fong YY, Walsh FO. Carcinogenic nitrosamines in Cantonese salt-dried fish. Lancet 1971; ii:1032.

Geser A, Charnay N, Day NE et al. Environmental factors in the etiology of nasopharyngeal carcinoma: report on a case-control study in Hong Kong. In: de Thé G, Ito Y (eds). Nasopharyngeal carcinoma: etiology and control. IARC Sci Pub No. 20, International Agency for Research on Cancer, Lyon, 1978, pp 213-229.

Gurtsevitch V, Ruiz R, Stepina V et al. Epstein-Barr viral serology in nasopharyngeal carcinoma patients in the USSR and Cuba and its value for differential diagnosis of disease. Int J Cancer 1986; 37:375-381.

Hadar T, Rahima M, Kahan E et al. Significance of specific Epstein-Barr virus IgA and elevated IgG antibodies to Viral Capsid Antigen in nasopharyngeal carcinoma patients. J Med Virol 1986; 20:329-339.

Henderson BE, Louie E, Soohoo Jing J et al. Risk factors associated with nasopharyngeal carcinoma. New Eng J Med 1976; 295:1101-1106.

Henlé W, Henlé G. Epstein-Barr virus and human malignancies. Adv Viral Oncol 1985; 5:201-238.

Hidayatalla A, Malik MOA, El Hadi AE et al. Studies on nasopharyngeal carcinoma in the Sudan. I. Epidemiology and Aetiology. Eur J Cancer Clin Oncol 1983; 19:705-710.

Ho JHC. Genetic and environmental factors in nasopharyngeal carcinoma. In: Nakahara W, Nishioka K, Hirayama T et al (eds). Recent advances in human tumor virology and immunology. University of Tokyo Press, Tokyo, 1971, pp 275-295.

Ho JHC. Nasopharyngeal carcinoma (NPC). Adv Cancer Res 1972; 15:57-92.

Ho JHC. Stage classification of nasopharyngeal carcinoma: a review. In: de Thé G, Ito Y (eds). Nasopharyngeal carcinoma: etiology and control. IARC Sci Pub No. 20, International Agency for Research on Cancer, Lyon, 1978, pp 99-113.

Hu MS, Huang HL. Retrospective study on the etiological factors of nasopharyngeal carcinoma. New Med (Canton) 1972; 12:10.

Huang DP, Ho JHC, Saw D et al. Carcinoma of the nasal and paranasal regions in rats fed Cantonese salted marine fish. In: de Thé G, Ito Y (eds). Nasopharyngeal carcinoma: etiology and control. IARC Sci Pub No. 20, International Agency for Research on Cancer, Lyon, 1978, pp 315-328.

Ireland B, Lanier A, Knutson L et al. Increased risk of cancer in siblings of Alaskan native patients with nasopharyngeal carcinoma. Int J Epidemiol 1988; 17:509-511.

Lanier A, Bender T, Talbot M et al. Nasopharyngeal carcinoma in Alaskan Eskimos, Indians and Aleuts: a review of cases and study of Epstein-Barr virus, HLA and environmental risk factors. Cancer 1980; 46:2100-2106.

Lanier A, Clift S, Ireland B et al. Cancer risks and EBV antibody patterns in NPC families. In: Proceedings of the Second Symposium on EBV and associated malignant diseases. October 1986, St Petersburg FL, 1986, pp 85-89.

Lee HP, Day NE, Shanmugaratnam K (eds). Trends in cancer incidence in Singapore, 1968-1982. IARC Sci Pub No. 91, International Agency for Research on Cancer, Lyon, 1988.

Levine PH, Connelly RR, Milman G et al. Epstein-Barr virus serology in the control of nasopharyngeal carcinoma. Cancer Detect Prev 1988; 12:357-362.

Lin TM, Chen KP, Lin CC et al. Retrospective study on nasopharyngeal carcinoma. JNCI 1973; 51:1403-1408.

Mabuchi K, Bross DS, Kessler II. Cigarette smoking and nasopharyngeal carcinoma. Cancer 1985; 55:2874-2876.

Muir C, Waterhouse J, Mack T et al (eds). Cancer Incidence in Five Continents, Volume V. IARC Sci Pub No. 88, International Agency for Research on Cancer, Lyon, 1987.

Naegele RF, Champion J, Murphy S et al. Nasopharyngeal carcinoma in American children: Epstein-Barr virus-specific antibody titers and prognosis. Int J Cancer 1982; 29: 209-212.

Nielsen NH, Mikkelsen F, Hansen JPH. Nasopharyngeal carcinoma in Greenland: the incidence in an Arctic Eskimo population. Acta Pathol Microbiol Scand, Sect A, 1977; 85: 850-858.

Ning JP, Yu MC, Wang QS et al. Salted fish and other risk factors for nasopharyngeal carcinoma in Tianjin, a low risk region of China. JNCI 1990; 82:291-296.

Pi GH, Zeng Y, Wolf H. Detection of IgA antibody to EBV membrane antigen using Staphylococcus aureus preabsorbed sera is closely associated with nasopharyngeal carcinoma. J Virol Meth 1987; 15:33-39.

Purchase IFH, Paddle GM. Does formaldehyde cause nasopharyngeal cancer in man? Cancer Letters 1989; 46:79-85.

Roush GC, Walrath J, Stayner LT et al. Nasopharyngeal cancer, sinonasal cancer and occupations related to formaldehyde: a case-control study. JNCI 1987; 79:1221-1224.

Schaefer O, Hildes JA. Canada (Eskimos): Inuit Cancer Register 1950-1980. In: Parkin DM (ed). Cancer Occurrence in Developing Countries. IARC Sci Pub No. 75, International Agency for Research on Cancer, Lyon, 1986, pp 159-163.

Shanmutgaratnam K, Tye CY, Goh EH et al. Etiological factors in nasopharyngeal carcinoma: a hospital-based retrospective, case-control, questionnaire study. In: de Th G, Ito Y (eds). Nasopharyngeal carcinoma: etiology and control. IARC Sci Pub No. 20, International Agency for Research on Cancer, Lyon, 1978, pp 199-212.

de Vathaire F, Sancho-Garnier H, de Thé H et al. Prognostic value of EBV markers in the clinical management of nasopharyngeal carcinoma (NPC): a multicenter follow-up study. Int J Cancer 1988; 42:176-181.

Yan L, Xi Z, Drettner B. Epidemiological studies of nasopharyngeal cancer in the Guanzhou area, China. Preliminary report. Acta Otolaryngol (Stockh) 1989; 107: 424-427.

Yu MC, Ho JHC, Lai SH et al. Cantonese-style salted fish as a cause of nasopharyngeal carcinoma: report of a case-control study in Hong Kong. Cancer Res 1986; 46:956-961.

Yu MC, Mo CC, Chong WX et al. Preserved foods and nasopharyngeal carcinoma: a case-control study in Guangxi, China. Cancer Res 1988; 48:1954-1959.

Yu MC, Huang TB, Henderson BE. Diet and nasopharyngeal carcinoma: a case-control study. Int J Cancer 1989; 43:1077-1082.

Yu MC, Nichols PW, Zou XN et al. Induction of malignant nasal cavity tumours in Wistar rats fed Chinese salted fish. Br J Cancer 1989; 60:198-201.

Zeng Y. Seroepidemiological studies on nasopharyngeal carcinoma in China. Adv Cancer Res 1985; 43:121-138.

Zeng Y, Gong CH, Jan MG et al. Detection of Epstein-Barr virus IgA/EA antibody for diagnosis of nasopharyngeal carcinoma by immunoautoradiography. Int J Cancer 1983a; 31:599-601.

Zeng Y, Liu YX, Liu CR et al. Application of immunoenzymatic method and immunoautoradiographic method for the mass survey of nasopharyngeal carcinoma. Chinese J Oncol 1979; 1:2-7.

Zeng Y, Liu YX, Liu CR et al. Application of an immunoenzymatic method and immunoautoradiographic method for a mass survey of nasopharyngeal carcinoma. Intervirology 1980; 13:162-168.

Zeng Y, Pi GH, Deng H et al. Epstein-Barr virus seroepidemiology in China. AIDS Res 1986; 2:S7-S15.

Zeng Y, Shen SJ, Deng H et al. Early nasopharyngeal carcinoma among IgA/VCA antibody-positive individuals detected by anticomplement immunoenzymatic method. Chin Med J 1984; 97:155-157.

Zeng Y, Zhang LG, Li HY et al. Serological mass survey for early detection of nasopharyngeal carcinoma in Wuzhou City, China. Int J Cancer 1982; 29:131-141.

Zeng Y, Zhang LG, Wu YC et al. Prospective studies on nasopharyngeal carcinoma in Epstein-Barr virus IgA/VCA antibody-positive persons in Wuzhou City, China. Int J Cancer 1985; 36:545-547.

Zeng Y, Zhong JM, Li LY et al. Follow-up of studies on Epstein-Barr virus IgA/VCA antibody-positive persons in Zangwu County, China. Intervirology 1983b; 20:190-194.

Zhu XX, Zeng Y, Wolf H. Detection of IgG and IgA antibodies to Epstein-Barr virus membrane antigen in sera from patients with nasopharyngeal carcinoma and from normal individuals. Int J Cancer 1986; 37:689-691.

40 Summary of Discussion on Screening for Nasopharyngeal Cancer

Populations at high risk for nasopharyngeal cancer include those in South Eastern China, Taiwan, Chinese migrants to Singapore and the USA, natives of Alaska, Canada and Greenland, with intermediate risk in Thailand, Vietnam, the Philippines and certain North African groups. The disease seems a good candidate for screening in high risk populations because it is a very serious health problem in countries with a high prevalence. However, it is not known that treatment of "early" disease is effective, nor has the optimal test been identified. Tests based on Epstein Barr virus (EBV) serology are available, and several different methods are used to perform the tests.

Population screening programmes have been initiated in the Guang Xi and Guang Dong areas of the People's Republic of China. Data are not available for complete evaluation, however, as exemplified by information from China in which prevalence screens were performed with no repeat screens. There are no data on selection of screenees, compliance or active follow-up of negatives, so no valid estimation of sensitivity and specificity is possible. A stage shift to stage I and II disease from 30% to 70% has been reported, but no mortality data.

Section 10 Methodological Issues

41 Surrogate Measures in the Design of Breast Screening Trials

N.E. DAY

Medical Research Council Biostatistics Unit, Cambridge, England

1 INTRODUCTION

The natural history of most cancers is markedly heterogeneous. The relationship between detectability and curability is complex, and the effect of earlier detection on prognosis is unpredictable. Randomised trials with mortality from the relevant cancer as the endpoint are therefore of fundamental importance in the evaluation of mass screening for cancer. Their purpose is to establish in an unbiased quantitative manner the reduction in specific cancer mortality that can be achieved. Breast screening of women under 50 years of age and a combination of radiological cytological screening for lung cancer in high risk groups are both examples where randomised trials have failed to demonstrate any appreciable reduction in mortality, notwithstanding clear indication that cancers were being diagnosed earlier. In both these cases, in the absence of results on mortality from randomised trials, use of surrogate endpoints might have lead to erroneously optimistic conclusions on efficacy. Once the value of a particular screening modality has been established, however, there are clearly going to be a range of further questions concerning the optimum application of the screening modality. Modifications of the screening technique, choice of the appropriate interval between screening tests, extension to a broader age group, are all areas where fine tuning of the screening programme may lead to a substantial improvement in benefit, or in the cost benefit ratio. Randomised trials with cancer mortality as the endpoint are large, lengthy and very costly operations, and it would not be appropriate to adopt them as the means to answer all the questions that arise. The rest of this paper refers specifically to breast cancer, since it is the only malignancy for which randomised trials have unequivocally demonstrated benefit and for which the aim of screening is to detect invasive cancer earlier. For cervical cancer, where the benefit of screening has also been established, screening aims to detect pre-invasive lesions and the use of invasive cancer incidence rather than mortality is already accepted as a valid, early outcome measure.

Examination of the results of the randomised trials on which the value of a screening modality is based should indicate the relationship between earlier detection and better prognosis, i.e. should identify the tumour characteristics which are changed by earlier detection, changes which effect the overall improvement in survival and reduction in mortality. This process should enable one to define predictors of the change in mortality brought about by earlier diagnosis, based on the characteristics and time of diagnosis of the cancers that arise during a screening programme. A distinction needs to be made between predictors which can be used in a qualitative manner to monitor the progress of a programme, and predictors which one attempts to use in a more formal, quantitative way to estimate future mortality.

The former are basically early evaluation (or quality assurance) measures, the purpose of which is to ensure that ongoing or newly instituted public health programmes are following the same course as the randomised trials which demonstrated benefit (Day et al, 1989). No precise prediction of the effect on mortality is attempted, nor could quantitative comparisons be made between programmes of the expected future mortality. For breast screening, suggested measures of this type have been prevalence at the initial screening round, proportion (or rate) of small cancers (e.g. less than 15mm), detected at the first and later screen and the proportionate rate of interval cancers in each successive 12 months period after a negative screening test.

The latter have been termed surrogate measures, their use requires quantitative justification, and their purpose is to replace mortality as the major endpoint in a trial or programme.

2 SURROGATE MEASURES – DEFINITION AND VALIDITY

The definition of surrogate endpoint used here follows that proposed by Prentice (1989). Suppose measures $(Z_1, Z_2, ...) = Z$ are made on each diagnosed cancer (e.g. size, grade, etc.), and a trial of different screening modalities is undertaken with arms $X_1, X_2, ...$ etc. (e.g. different frequencies of screening). Then the condition that Z is an adequate surrogate measure of mortality, in this trial, is that the survival distribution, $\lambda(t;Z, X)$ given the value of this surrogate is independent of the arm of the trial, i.e.:

$$\lambda(t;Z, X) = \lambda(t;Z). \tag{1}$$

The survival in each arm of the trial can be predicted in unbiased manner if one knows the value of the surrogate variables, Z, for each cancer diagnosed in the trial..

The probability of death before time T for a case with covariate Z is given by:

$$1 - \exp\left(-\int_o^T \lambda(u;Z)\right) du$$

Thus, if on arm X_i of the trial one has observed R_i cases with surrogate variables $Z_{i1}, Z_{i2}, ... Z_{in}$, then the expected number of deaths E(Di) before time T is given by:

$$E(Di) = \sum_{j=1}^{Ri} \left(1 - \exp\left(-\int_o^T \lambda(u;Zij)\, du\right)\right) \tag{2}$$

If the number of individuals on arm X_i of the trial is N_i, taken to be orders of magnitude larger than R_i, then the expected cumulative mortality rate to time T is:

$$E(D_i) / N_i$$

and the ratios of this value between the different arms of the trial gives the appropriate estimates of the breast cancer mortality rate ratios.

3 SURROGATE MEASURES -- POWER AND EFFICIENCY

Expression (1) is the condition for a set of covariates to be valid surrogates of mortality. The value of a set of surrogates lies not just in their validity, but also in their efficiency. For this purpose, it is of interest to compare the variance of the estimate generated by the use of surrogate variables to the variance of the estimate one would have based on breast cancer deaths:

Writing
$$P(Z_{ij}) = 1 - \exp(-\int_o^T \lambda(u;Z_{ij}))da$$

we have
$$Var(E(D_i)) = \sum_{j=1}^{R_i} Var(P(Z_{ij})) \tag{3}$$

if one ignores uncertainty in the specification of the function $\lambda(u;Z)$. To ensure that the inference is made conditional on the total number of individuals in each arm, rather than on the number of cancer cases, it is important that expression (3) is computed, treating R_i as a (Poisson) random variable. If inferences are made conditional on the R_i, then one would be considering the distribution of the surrogate variables, rather than the absolute incidence of different values of the surrogates.

Assuming an underlying Poisson distribution the variance of the actual number of deaths as given by
$$Var(D_i) = E(D_i).$$

The estimate of interest when there are two arms to the trial is the relative hazard of cancer mortality, estimated when using surrogates
by $\quad N_2 E(D_1) / N_1 E(D_2)$
and by $\quad N_2 D_1 / N_1 D_2$
when cancer deaths are used as the endpoint. With equal numbers on each arm, the asymptotic variances of the logarithm of the two estimates are then given by:

$$\frac{\sum\limits_{j=1}^{R_1} \mathrm{Var}\,(P_T(Z_{1j}))}{(E(D_1))^2} \quad + \quad \frac{\sum\limits_{j=1}^{R_1} \mathrm{Var}\,(P_T Z_{2j}))}{(E(D_2))^2}$$

for surrogate endpoints, and

$$\frac{1}{E(D_1)} \quad + \quad \frac{1}{E(D_2)}$$

for mortality taken as an endpoint.

An important special case occurs when Z is discrete, taking values $Z_1, \dots Z_n$. With a two-armed trial with equal allocation, one would have the following schema:

Arm 1   Arm 2

N individuals in each arm
Observed proportions in each trial arm with covariate =

$Z_1 \dots\dots\dots\dots\dots Z_n$		$Z_1 \dots\dots\dots\dots\dots Z_n$	
q_{11}	q_{1n}	q_{21}	q_{2n}

We suppose both Σq_{1i} and Σq_{2i} to be small, so that the great majority of individuals in the trial do not present as cases.

Putting P_i as the proportion of cases with covariate $= Z_i$ dying before time T, irrespective of the study arm and assumed known from previous studies, then the predicted number of deaths t_i on arm 1 is given by

$$t_i = N \sum_j P_j\, q_{ij}$$

The total number of cases R_i on arm i is of course given by

$$R_i = N \sum_j q_i$$

The parameter of relevance is the logarithm of the ratio of the number of deaths on each arm, with variance given by:

$$\frac{\overline{\sum_1 Pi^2 q_{1i}}}{N(\sum Pi \, q_{1i})^2} + \frac{\overline{\sum Pi^2 q_{2i}}}{N(\sum Pi \, q_{2i})^2} \tag{4}$$

(dropping terms in q_i^2, $i>1$) which can be written as:

$$\frac{1}{t_1}\left(1 - \frac{N\sum q_{1i}Pi\,(1-Pi)}{t_1}\right) + \frac{1}{t_2}\left(1 - \frac{N\sum q_{2i}Pi\,(1-Pi)}{t_2}\right)$$

From this last expression, one can see that the variance of the log odds ratio estimate based on a surrogate variable is never greater than the variance based on mortality, given by:

$$\frac{1}{t_1} + \frac{1}{t_2}$$

The largest value of the variance occurs when all the Pi are either 1 or 0, in which case knowledge of the surrogate removes all uncertainty on the mortality outcome, i.e. the surrogate is precisely equivalent to mortality. This situation might be thought intuitively to be the most powerful for the use of a surrogate; it is in fact the least powerful.

The minimum value of this variance is given by

$$\frac{1}{R_1} + \frac{1}{R_2}$$

i.e. is related to the number of cases rather than the number of deaths. If one is considering breast screening trials, with mortality at ten years, the difference between the number of cases and number of deaths could be over 5 fold. An example of a trial with different breast screening frequencies is given in a later section, where a three-fold increase in efficiency is obtained using surrogate endpoints. It is evident that a major shortening of the trial will also result.

It is interesting to note that the power of a surrogate is maximised when uncertainty in the mortality outcome, given the surrogate, is greatest rather than least. The power is at a minimum when the surrogate is equivalent to mortality, i.e. when uncertainty is least. The reason for this apparent paradox is that use of the surrogate involves taking expectations over the mortality uncertainty, the expectation being based on prior knowledge. The more this prior knowledge is used, the greater the power achieved. The cost one pays is the dependence on prior information, which may be incorrect.

One final point that requires elaboration is that in most trials, the cancers would not all be diagnosed at the same time. In order to calculate mortality at a fixed time T after the start of the trial, the survival time from diagnosis for each individual cancer will have to vary. The expressions given above then have to be generalised to allow individual survival time T_i. This generalisation is straightforward, and follows the lines developed by Flanders and Longini (1990). The example given in the next section illustrates the approach.

4 AN EXAMPLE - THE FREQUENCY OF BREAST SCREENING

Considerable doubt exists as to the relative benefits of different screening intervals for women aged over 50. Extensive data are available from randomised trials establishing that screening is of benefit in this age group, but much of the data refers to a screening interval between 30 and 36 months (Rutqvist et al, 1990). In the United Kingdom, breast screening has been adopted nationally for women aged 50 to 64 years, with an interval of 3 years. It is apparent from earlier data (Tabar et al, 1987) that the incidence of interval cancers will increase markedly in the second, and especially, the third year after screening (see Table 1a). The reduction in the proportion of cancers that would surface clinically as interval cancers would be reduced if the inter-screening interval were reduced.

Table 1   Interval cancers in the years following a negative
          mammographic test

a) Proportionate incidence

1	2	3
13%	29%	47%

b) Expected proportion of interval cancers if screening frequency is

1 year	2 years	3 years
13%	21%	30%

Table 1b indicates the degree of such reductions once a steady screening state is reached, i.e. after the prevalence screen if high sensitivity is achieved. The difference between yearly and 3 yearly screening is not large. Reducing the proportion of interval cancers however is not the only benefit to be expected from more frequent screening. One also expects the cancers found at screening to be less advanced if the time since the last screening test is shorter. Table 2 compares when one might expect cancers to be diagnosed with yearly, as opposed to 3 yearly screening. An increased lead time of 1 or 2 years can be expected for a considerable proportion of screen detected cancers. The question to be addressed is the extent to which prognosis is improved by this increase in lead time. A randomised trial to estimate the change in breast cancer mortality could be based on breast cancer mortality as the endpoint. Alternatively, one could examine the use of surrogate measures. The results of the WE trial will be used to compare the two approaches. We consider the former first.

Table 2 Cross-tabulation of expected time of occurrence and diagnostic category of breast cancer diagnosed among women screened yearly and screened three yearly - indicating how time of diagnosis is changed (assuming a population from which 100 cases per year can be expected in the absence of screening)

Yearly Screening

		Year 1		Year 2		Year 3		Total
		Interval	Screen detected	Interval	Screen detected	Interval	Screen detected	
	Year 1 Interval Cancers	13	–	–	–	–	–	13
3 Yearly Screen- ing	Year 2 Interval Cancers	–	16	13	–	–	–	29
	Year 3 Interval Cancers	–	18	–	16	13	–	47
Screen detected cancers at end of Year 3			53[1]		71[2]		87	211
TOTAL		13	87	13	87	13	87	300

[1] Increase in lead time of 2 years [2] Increase in lead time of 1 year

5 FREQUENCY TRIAL WITH MORTALITY AS AN ENDPOINT

The results of the Swedish WE trial indicated that for women in the age group 50 to 69 who accepted screening, a reduction of 40% was seen in breast cancer mortality, compared to the unscreened control group. Other trials have shown similar differences (Day, 1991). This reduction was associated with an average inter screening interval of 33 months. If a trial were to be launched comparing an interval of approximately 33 months with a shorter interval, then one would clearly expect fewer breast cancer deaths on the trial arm with the shorter screening interval for a given number of woman years of observation. Thus, for a similar relative reduction in risk, to obtain equal power to the WE study will require a large study. Specifically, if a further 40% reduction (i.e. from 60% to 36% of mortality) in breast cancer mortality is obtained with yearly screening, compared to screening on average

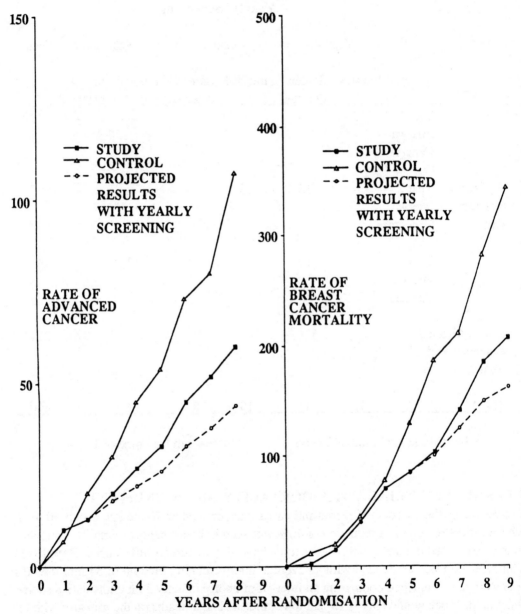

Figure 1 Observed results in the Swedish Breast Screening Trial and
projected results with yearly screening

every 33 months, then the variance of the logarithm of the risk ratio is larger, compared to the original trial, by a factor of:

$$(.36^{-1} + .60^{-1}) / (1 + .60^{-1})$$
$$= 1.67$$

for trials of the same size. To obtain equal power, a 67% increase in trial size would be needed.

In terms of the study length, one can assume that in the WE study, most of the initial effect on breast cancer mortality would arise from the prevalence screen. The effect of later screening tests will therefore be slower to appear. Figure 1 indicates the results one might envisage.

6 FREQUENCY TRIAL WITH SURROGATE ENDPOINTS
Crude differences in survival in the Swedish WE trial are shown in Figure 2, with large differences between screen detected and clinically detected cancers (Tabar et al, 1991). The difference in survival between interval cancers and cancers detected at incidence screens disappears after adjusting for tumour size, malignancy grade and nodal status (see Table 3).

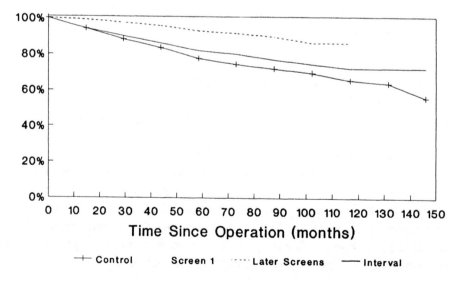

Breast cancer cases only

Figure 2 Cumulative survival by detection method; WE Trial, age 70-74

Table 3   Relative hazards of screen detected, interval and control group cancers, before and after adjustment for prognostic factors

Breast cancer category	Unadjusted relative hazard	Adjusted* relative hazard
Control group	1.0	1.0
Prevalence screen detected	0.29	0.57
Incidence screen detected	0.27	0.73
Interval cancers	0.76	0.74

* Adjusted for tumour size, nodal status and malignancy grade

Each of these three variables has an independent effect on survival. The most appropriate design for a trial of screening frequency is to consider as eligible only those women who have had a prevalence screen, since this forms the group for whom the benefit of additional screening tests can be assessed. The cancers that are diagnosed from immediately after one screening test to immediately after a later screening test form a group of cancers from which length bias has been removed provided the initial screening test is of good sensitivity. Results on interval cancers from the WE study (Tabar et al, 1987) demonstrate that sensitivity close to or better than 90% was achieved. The design of a trial of different screening frequencies based on surrogate endpoints would have:

6.1   Endpoints
The three prognostic variables (size, nodal status and malignancy grade) potentially available on all cancers diagnosed in the trial are valid surrogate endpoints, provided one includes only those cancers arising at incidence screen or between screening tests.

6.2   Comparison Groups and Duration of Trial
With two screening frequencies (intervals of r_1, and r_2 years between screen), the duration of the trial, at a minimum, should be R years, where R is the lowest common multiple of r_1 and r_2. Arm one has R/r_1, screening tests, arm two has R/r_2 tests. Included in the trial are all cancers diagnosed from immediately after the prevalence screen until immediately after the test that takes place R years after the prevalence screen. Because length bias is absent from both sets of cancers, equal numbers are expected on each arm.

As an example, consider a trial comparing screening every 3 years with screening every year. The trial lasts three years, with three annual tests on one arm and one test at the end

Table 4   Size distribution of cancers from the Swedish WE trial in the control group and the combined interval and incidence screen cancers in the study group, together with a hypothetical size distribution or yearly screening – invasive cancers only

| Size distribution (mms) | Observed in the WE study | | Hypothesised from yearly screening interval and incidence cancer | Approximate 10 year breast cancer mortality from the WE study |
	Controls	Interval and incidence screens		
	%	%	%	%
< 10	7	25	35	5
10 - 14	16	25	35	10
15 - 19	20	15	20	20
20 - 29	30	15	5	40
30 - 49	20	15	5	60
50+	7	5	–	60
Total	100	100	100	
Average 10 year mortality	35.5%	22.7%	14.3%	

of three years on the other arm. For illustrative papers, the following power considerations were calculated using tumour size alone as the surrogate variable. Table 4 gives the distribution of size from the WE trial of cancers in the control (unscreened) arm and of the combined interval and incidence screen cancers. Also given are the approximate 10 year breast cancer mortality rates for each size of tumour. The expected average ten years mortality i the two groups is shown, with a difference of 36%, close to the reduction observed (the difference between this value and the observed reduction in breast cancer mortality of 40% is due to the worse malignancy grade in the assessed control group. The difference is slight).

The last column of Table 4 gives a hypothetical size distribution for the cancers diagnosed among women screened every year. The predicted 10 year breast cancer mortality in this group is approximately 36% lower than in the 3 yearly screening group, i.e. the same difference between no screening and 3 yearly screening. With different screening frequencies, some allowance should be made for different lead time distributions. Their effect, however, is small and for the sake of simplicity they have been ignored in this paper.

The variance (large sample) of the logarithm of the predicted mortality rate ratio is given by expression (4), and equals 3.84, if one ignores the factor N. The corresponding variance, again ignoring N, of the rate ratio based on breast cancer mortality is 11.41, almost three fold greater.

If screening more frequently does not change the size distribution of diagnosed cancers (an improbable hypotheses but corresponding to the null), then the ratio of the two variances (i.e. estimate based on actual mortality to estimate based on predicted mortality), in 2.25.

Thus in the region of the null and plausible alternative hypotheses, the design using surrogate variables is two to three times more powerful and efficient than the design using breast cancer mortality. It will also produce a result (equivalent to 10 year mortality) within 3 years of the last date of entry into the trial. A trial based on observed 10 year mortality for all diagnosed cases would have to continue for 13 years after the last date of entry into the trial. In many respects, this is the difference in terms of size and duration between a feasible study and one not worth undertaking.

7   CONCLUSION

The use of surrogate measures clearly needs to be approached with care. There are, however, a substantial number of modifications which might be made to an ongoing public health screening programme to improve its performance, and it is not practicable to consider trials with mortality as endpoint being undertaken for each. One approach is through the development of models which can be used to guess at the cost effectiveness of different choices (Habbema 1991). The problem is that the assumption fed into such models to replace the uncertainty in the available data are usually crude and unverifiable. The example of cancer of the cervix is salutary in this respect. Cervical screening had been an area which attracted extensively the attention of model developers. In the two critical areas of the age to target screening and screening frequencies, it is difficult to identify a single contribution derived from models which has had a significant effect on policy. The crucial contributions came from observational studies (IARC, 1986), exploiting the extensive experience built up over 25 years in population based screening programmes. For breast screening, it will be some years before equivalent data are likely to be available. Furthermore, since smaller effects are seen with breast screening, the problems of bias arising from uncontrolled observational studies are more acute. The use of surrogate measures then has three advantages. First, it makes full use of the information available from past studies. Second, it concentrates attention on the specific variables for which information is lacking and third, it leads to the design of feasible trials.

REFERENCES

Day NE, Williams DRR and Khaw K-T. Breast cancer screening programmes: the development of a monitoring and evaluation system. Brit J Cancer 1989; 59:954-958.

Day NE. Screening for breast cancer. Brit Med Bulletin 1991. In press.

Flanders WD and Longini IM. Estimating benefits of screening from observational cohort studies. Stats Med 1990; 8:959-981.

Habbema D. This volume 1991.

IARC Working Group. The duration of protection given by a negative cervical cytological test. Br Med J 1986; 293:659-664.

Prentice RG. Surrogate endpoints in clinical trials: definitions and operational criteria. Stats Med 1990; 8:431-441.

Rutqvist LE, Miller AB, Andersson I, Hakama M, Hakulinen T, Sigfússon BF, Tabar L. Reduced breast cancer mortality with mammography screening - an assessment of currently available data. Int J Cancer Supplement 1990; 5:76-84.

Tabar L, Fagerberg G, Day NE and Holmberg L. What is the optimum interval between mammographic screening examinations? An analysis based on the latest results of the Swedish two county breast cancer screening trial. Brit J Cancer 1987; 55:547-551.

Tabar L, Fagerberg G, Duffy SW and Day NE. This volume. 1991.

42 Recent Developments in Cancer Screening Modeling

S. G. BAKER, R. J. CONNOR and P. C. PROROK

Biometry Branch, Division of Cancer Prevention and Control, National Cancer Institute, Bethesda, MD, USA

1 INTRODUCTION

A wide variety of models has been developed over the past several decades for the purpose of examining information related to cancer screening. These have ranged from being largely conceptual with relatively little mathematical content, to more complex analytic formulations, to very comprehensive, computer intensive models. This paper focuses on four recently developed analytic models which, taken together, offer the possibility of more informative and reliable inferences from both experimental and observational screening studies. Two of the models deal with approaches to drawing conclusions about screening effectiveness in the absence of a controlled study. Another looks in detail at staging information to gain greater insight into the mechanism by which screening generates an effect. The fourth model is a preliminary approach to obtaining a more efficient and accurate assessment of screening benefit in a trial by adjusting for both a lag period before which the benefit begins to appear, and a dilution effect created by continued acquisition of data after screening ceases.

2 THE WALTER-STITT MODEL

This model (Walter and Stitt, 1987) extends an earlier modeling effort (Day and Walter, 1984; Walter and Day, 1983), and is aimed at evaluating the survival experience of cancer cases detected by screening. The objective is to estimate the magnitude of survival benefit for screen detected cases while allowing for lead time, length, and selection biases. If this can be accomplished using data only from a screened group of individuals, then the approach would have the potential for evaluation of screening benefit in community settings or other non-experimental environments.

The main features of the underlying model (Day and Walter, 1984) are as follows. Individuals in a healthy state may develop asymptomatic or preclinical disease. After some time the disease progresses to the point at which the screening method can potentially detect disease. The time interval during which the disease remains preclinical but detectable by the screen is termed the detectable preclinical phase (DPCP). If the person is not screened, the disease may advance to become symptomatic, at which time it is diagnosed in the usual way without screening. If screening detects a cancer during its DPCP, the date of diagnosis is advanced by the lead time interval.

Under the assumptions of the model, one can derive expressions for the anticipated incidence rates of clinical disease among groups of people with particular screening histories, and for the anticipated prevalence of preclinical disease found at the various screens. These incidence and prevalence functions depend on the incidence rate of clinical disease expected in the population in the absence of screening, the distribution of the DPCP duration, and the screen sensitivity, which is assumed constant. One can estimate relevant parameters by fitting observed incidence and prevalence data using standard statistical methods.

To extend these results to permit an analysis of the survival experience of screen-detected cancers, the total survival time for such cases is the sum of two components: (i) the lead time, and (ii) the survival time after the point of clinical diagnosis until death. Let t denote the lead time, and x the 'extra' survival after the expected time of clinical detection. The total survival time from diagnosis by screening is $z = x + t$. The objective of the analysis is to estimate the distribution of x for screen-detected cases. It is claimed that one can then compare this distribution to the survival in various other groups of cases not detected by screening, to examine whether improvement has occurred.

The survival of screen-detected cases is characterized by a hazard function $h(y,t,z)$ that in general depends on the DPCP duration (y), the lead time time (t), and the total survival time since diagnosis by screening (z). From this, the marginal distribution of x is

$$\int_0^\infty \int_0^y h(y,t,x + t) \exp\left[- \int_0^{x+t} h(y,t,u)du \right] g(t|y)f(y)dtdy.$$

If observable, this distribution could be compared to the survival experience of cases not diagnosed by screening. For a given patient, however, only z is observable, while x, y and t are unknown. Therefore, parameter estimation must use the empirical survival time since diagnosis of the screen-detected cases. One can then infer those parameters specifically related to the post-lead time component of survival.

One particularly simple hazard function used for analysis was

$$h(y,t,z) = \begin{cases} 0, & \text{for } z \leq t \\ \theta, & \text{for } z > t \end{cases}.$$

This function assumes there is no additional hazard associated with early detection by screening, and that the hazard is constant (at θ) after the time of usual clinical diagnosis in the absence of screening. Under this model, x follows an exponential distribution with parameter θ. To estimate θ, the marginal distribution of z is derived by integrating out the distribution of t. If the parameters characterizing the distribution of t are estimated exogenously, $\hat{\theta}$ is computed by maximizing the distribution of z over θ.

The suggested analysis is to determine an adjusted survival curve of x for the screen-detected cases, and compare it with the empirical survival observed in other case groups. Possible comparison groups mentioned are the interval cases that arise among persons previously screened, or cases among persons offered screening but who refuse. In a randomized trial, one can also make a comparison with the survival in the control group not offered screening. If randomized controls are unavailable, one might perform an external comparison using survival data from an unscreened part of the general population. This suggested approach, however, leads to a major concern about the model, since the other case groups mentioned would be expected to be different from the screen-detected cases even in the absence of screening because of length bias. The comparison one would ideally like to make is with the survival distribution of the screen-detected cases in the absence of screening.

The method was applied to the survival experience of the 132 cases of breast cancer detected by screening during the HIP study (Shapiro, Venet, Strax, et al, 1988). A previous analysis of the HIP data (Walter and Day, 1983) had shown that an exponential distribution for the DPCP duration gave a good fit to the incidence and prevalence figures for the screened women; the estimated value of the exponential parameter λ was 0.585, corresponding to a mean DPCP duration of $1/0.585 = 1.71$ years. Using maximum likelihood, the parameter estimate for the present model was $\hat{\theta} = 0.03664$, which led to the following comparable estimates for the observed and predicted cumulative survival:

Years since diagnosis

	1	2	3	4	5	6	7	8	9	10
Observed	0.977	0.939	0.939	0.924	0.878	0.840	0.832	0.799	0.791	0.740
Predicted	0.991	0.971	0.944	0.915	0.885	0.854	0.824	0.795	0.767	0.739

Using the estimated value of $\theta = 0.03664$, the survival of the screen-detected cases was compared to that of other case groups. Table 1 gives the adjusted cumulative survival distribution of x, the 'extra' survival component of the screen-detected cases, as well as the empirical survival data for the interval cases, and the refusers. The screen-detected cases have a survival benefit relative to the other groups, which have rather similar survival curves.

From this, the authors concluded that careful use of an appropriate model may yield reasonable estimates of the survival benefit conferred on screen-detected cancer cases. Randomization, if employed, is invaluable in validating many assumptions of the model, which in turn lends greater credibility to the model results. This model may also be used with non-randomized data, as illustrated, but requires much greater care in interpretation of results. The HIP example produced reasonably satisfactory estimates of benefit in the survival experience of screen-detected breast cancer. However, in other data sets, this might be more problematic.

Table 1 Estimated post-lead time cumulative survival of screen-detected cases, and empirical cumulative survival for other case groups from the Walter-Stitt model.

		Case group	
Years since diagnosis	Screen-detected post-lead-time survival	Interval cases	Refusers
1	0.964	0.936	0.875
2	0.929	0.849	0.757
3	0.896	0.767	0.731
4	0.864	0.720	0.697
5	0.833	0.690	0.671
6	0.803	0.636	0.644
7	0.774	0.611	0.609
8	0.746	0.587	0.591
9	0.719	0.560	0.581
10	0.693	0.536	0.548
Number of cases	132	173	120

3 PERIODIC SCREENING EVALUATION

In common with the Walter-Stitt approach, an important motivation for this model stems from the recognition that it is sometimes necessary to evaluate screening without a randomized control group. Every method for such an analysis requires certain assumptions or has certain limitations. The choice of method depends on the purpose of the study and knowledge about the screen and disease. Some methods have been developed to estimate preclinical duration and sensitivity of the screen, but not mortality (Day and Walter, 1984; Baker, 1990; Goldberg and Wittes, 1978; Louis, Albert, and Heghinian, 1978; Brookmeyer, Day and Moss, 1986). Other methods require strong parametric assumptions (Walter and Stitt, 1987; Flehinger and Kimmel, 1987). Still other methods require an assumption that the age-specific incidence rates estimated from a nonrandomized control group are unbiased (Morrison, Brisson, and Khalid, 1988).

Periodic Screening Evaluation (PSE) refers to a new method for analyzing screening data (Baker and Chu, 1990). It uses a different set of assumptions and limitations which, in some cases, may be preferable to those of other methods. Unlike other methods, PSE estimates cancer mortality rates without making strong parametric assumptions and without using a nonrandomized control group to estimate age-specific incidence. Instead, PSE employs two other approaches. First, to estimate the age-specific probability of cancer incidence in the absence of screening, PSE uses older screened persons as controls for younger screened persons. This approach is the principal innovation of PSE. Second, to estimate case-fatality rates, i.e., rates of cancer mortality following diagnosis, in the absence of screening, PSE uses a nonrandomized control group. This use of a non-randomized control group is likely to introduce less bias than the use of a nonrandomized control group to estimate age-specific incidence rates. Although PSE bypasses some limitations of other methods, it introduces other limitations. In particular PSE assumes that, given age at screening, year of birth is not a predictor of cancer incidence and that a nonrandomized control group yields an unbiased estimate of case fatality rates in the absence of screening. Other limitations are that PSE applies only to persons who would accept a screening offer, requires data from persons offered at least two screens, and needs a large sample size. Nevertheless, the limitations of PSE seem preferable for many applications to the limitations associated with other methods.

PSE requires that data be generated in the following way. At least two screens are offered to persons who are asymptomatic and have not had a prior screen. The interval between successive screens is the same for all persons. The age distribution of persons offered screening should be approximately uniform. A person can either accept or refuse the offer of screening. All accepters and, ideally, all refusers are followed for the duration of screening unless they are censored. Accepters and, ideally, refusers diagnosed with cancer are followed after screening stops.

In the PSE framework, a diagnosis of cancer can arise in one of two ways: either an asymptomatic person is screened, the screen is positive, a biopsy is taken, and the biopsy is positive; or a person visits a physician because he has symptoms which possibly indicate the presence of cancer, and the physician diagnoses cancer. PSE makes the following assumptions:

3.1 Assumption 1
For a given person, the youngest age when a screen, if given, would result in a diagnosis is equal to or less than the youngest age when, in the absence of screening, symptoms would arise and result in a diagnosis. This assumption is similar to the progressive disease assumption used in other models (e.g. Albert, Gertman and Louis, 1978; Louis, Albert and Heghinian, 1978; Zelen and Feinleib, 1969; Prorok, 1976; Shwartz, 1978; Blumenson, 1976).

3.2 Assumption 2
For a given person, if a screen does not result in a diagnosis, a screen at a younger age would not have resulted in a diagnosis. Given Assumption 1, this is equivalent to the assumption of a progressive test; i.e., if a screening test is positive at a given age, it will be positive at an older age.

3.3 Assumption 3
If a person's age is known, knowledge of his year of birth adds no information for predicting cancer diagnosis. In other words, there is no birth-cohort effect.

3.4 Assumption 4
Case-fatality rates depend on time since diagnosis.

3.5 Assumption 5
Due to length bias sampling (Zelen and Feinleib, 1969; Morrison, 1985; Prorok, 1984), case-fatality rates depend on whether the diagnosis occurred in the absence of screening, on the first screen, in an interval between screens, or on a screen subsequent to the first.

3.6 Assumption 6
For all screened individuals with cancer, there exists a group of individuals with cancer which provides an unbiased estimate of the case-fatality rate in the absence of screening; e.g., those with cancer among individuals refusing screening might be such a group.

Note that these assumptions do not mention quantities described in many other models such as the rate of tumor growth, the duration of early stage cancer, and the sensitivity of the screen. This does not mean that there are hidden assumptions about these quantities. It simply means that PSE bypasses these quantities.

The key idea of PSE is that older screened individuals provide information about younger screened individuals. Two aspects are crucial to this idea: the requirement that individuals are screened more than once and the assumption of no birth cohort effect. To see why, suppose a group of asymptomatic individuals age 40 (denoted by G40) and a group of asymptomatic individuals age 41 (denoted by G41) are given a screen immediately, and another one year later. Consider a subgroup of G41 who are negative on the first screen, i.e, the screen does not lead to diagnosis at age 41, and are symptomatically detected within a year. Also consider a subgroup of G40 who are negative on the second screen (at age 41, and hence on the first screen at age 40) and are symptomatically detected within a year. In each subgroup, individuals have a negative screen at age 41 and are symptomatically detected within a year. The estimated probability of having a negative screen at age 41 and being symptomatically detected within a year, given asymptomatic at age 41, is the fraction of individuals in G41 who have a negative screen at age 41 and are symptomatically detected within a year. Similarly, the estimated probability of having a negative screen at age 41 and being symptomatically detected within a year, given asymptomatic at age 40, is the fraction of individuals in G40 who have a negative screen at age 41 and are symptomatically detected within in year. Under the no birth cohort assumption, the event of having a negative screen at age 41 and being symptomatically detected within a year is the same in the two groups. Therefore, one minus the ratio of these two estimated probabilities is an estimate of the probability of symptomatic detection between ages 40 and 41, given asymptomatic at age 40. This is a probability which is usually observed in a control group of individuals who are not screened; in PSE, it is estimated using only information from the individuals who were screened. Because PSE's estimate of the probability of symptomatic detection involves a ratio of rare events, it is not surprising that the sample size must be large to achieve adequate precision. Precision can also be improved by additional screens, which serve to increase the number of events common to different age cohorts. Because there are usually multiple common events, estimation is often complicated; it is most easily accomplished by likelihood-based methods and use of the EM algorithm (Dempster, Laird and Rubin, 1979).

Using the aforementioned data and assumptions, PSE estimates the age-specific mortality rate from cancer given asymptomatic status at a certain age, and under various ages when periodic screening might begin (Baker and Chu, 1990; Baker, 1989). As a check of PSE, its estimates were compared with those obtained when the mortality rate in a randomized control group was known. Data from women offered screening as part of the HIP study (Shapiro, Venet, Strax, et al, 1988) were used. Among these women, 9,982 refused screening and the remaining 20,133 accepted the screening invitation. Four consecutive screens were offered an average 1.1 years apart, and this interval was used in the analysis. Refusers were selected as a nonrandomized control group. In support of Assumption 6, survival curves based on estimated case-fatality hazards among refusers and controls over 14 time intervals were very similar.

For purposes of validation, the number of deaths from cancer for 9 intervals after entry, which equals almost 10 years, was examined. To avoid extrapolations after age 63, the validation was confined to women ages 40 to 54 at the start of the study. Applying PSE, the number of deaths from cancer among screened women had they not been screened was estimated using only data from these screened women. To estimate the number of deaths from cancer in the controls, the aforementioned estimate was added to the observed number of deaths from cancer in the refusers, and the total was adjusted by the age distribution at entry in the control group. The estimated cumulative number of deaths from cancer in the control group was then compared with the observed cumulative number (Figure 1). The agreement was good. Thus, for at least one site and one screening modality, PSE performed well, although the sample size was insufficient for a definitive test. Whether PSE will perform well for other sites or modalities remains to be determined.

4 STAGE-SHIFT MODEL

The stage-shift cancer screening model (Connor, Chu and Smart, 1989) allows an exploratory analysis of a completed cancer screening randomized controlled trial (RCT). Specifically, in the model screen-detected cancers can be shifted either from one stage to the next lower stage, or within a given stage to an earlier time of diagnosis. Associated with these shifts, the model provides measures of benefit at each stage with regard to cancer deaths. Using the model, the extent of these shifts, between and within stages, can be estimated, and the mortality benefits associated with these shifts can be examined stage-by-stage. Thus the model can provide valuable insight into the interrelationships between the screening, the stage shifts, and the mortality benefits at each stage.

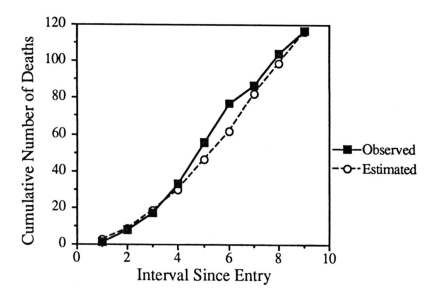

Figure 1   Cumulative breast cancer deaths for women in HIP randomized control group ages 40 to 54 at entry. Estimated deaths are based on PSE applied only to data from women offered screening. Intervals are in lengths of 1.1 years.

The model, in its basic format, requires that the screening RCT have two equal-sized groups, an intervention group offered screening and a control group not offered screening, with individuals randomly assigned to each group. It also requires that active screening is ended but follow-up is continued. Additionally, it is assumed that at some point in time the numbers of cancers in the two groups become equivalent and form comparable cancer groups. That is, it is assumed that the cancers found in the intervention group would have had the same natural history distribution as those found in the control group had there been no screening. The numerical equivalency essentially precludes screening detecting "latent cancer" (i.e., "cancer" that does not progress beyond the preclinical stage), and the random assignment of individuals to the two groups is expected to yield equivalent natural history distributions. Clearly, the comparability assumption must be investigated (e.g., the histologic distribution of the cancers in the two groups should not differ) before the model is used to examine the results of a RCT. To fit the model, data from the RCT should include for each cancer: randomized group, stage at diagnosis, and survival or mortality history from entry to the end of follow-up. For each cancer in the intervention group the mode of detection (i.e., whether it was screen-detected or not) is required.

The assumptions that underlie the model are quite simple. They are:
1. Screen detected cancers are shifted from their usual (in the absence of screening) stage at diagnosis to either one stage lower, say from stage k to stage k-1, or to an earlier time in the usual stage; shifts of greater than one stage are not permitted.
2. Cancers not screen-detected are found at their usual stage and time.

3. Screen-detected cancers are not more likely to die than they would have been had there been no screening.

From the RCT assumptions and the model assumptions, the following stage shift relationships are derived:

$$T_k = \underline{D_k} - \sum_{k+1}^{K} \underline{C_j} + \sum_{k+1}^{K} \underline{S_j}$$

and

$$T_{k,k-1} = \sum_{k}^{K} \underline{C_j} - \sum_{k}^{K} \underline{S_j},$$

where T_k is the number of cancers internally shifted at stage k,
          $T_{k,k-1}$ is the number of cancers shifted from stage k to stage k-1,
          $\underline{D_k}$ is the number of cancers screen-detected at stage k,
          $\underline{C_k}$ is the number of stage k cancers in the control group,
          $\underline{S_k}$ is the number of intervention group cancers at stage k,

and K is the highest (worst) stage of the cancer. The underlined variables are observed in the RCT. The other variables are not observable. Values for these other variables are obtained by substituting the observed quantities in the model relationships.

The model defines external (internal) stage-shift death reduction benefits at stage k as the difference between the deaths that would have occurred among the cancers shifted to stage k-1 (to an earlier time in stage k) in the absence of screening and the deaths that did occur among the cancers so shifted. The total death reduction at stage k is the combination of the external and internal deaths prevented at stage k. It is given by

$$TSDB_k = \underline{DC_k} - \underline{DND_k} - DT_k - DT_{k,k-1}$$

where $\underline{DC_k}$ is the number of cancer deaths among the stage k control group cancers,
          $\underline{DND_k}$ is the number of cancer deaths among the not detected stage k intervention group cancers,
          DT_k is the number of cancer deaths among the internally shifted stage k cancers, and
          $DT_{k,k-1}$ is the number of cancer deaths among the cancers externally shifted from stage k to stage k-1.

DT_k and $DT_{k,k-1}$ cannot, in general, be uniquely fitted by the model; only a range of possible values is obtainable. Hence, the death reduction benefits are given by a range of values.

In addition to death reduction benefits associated with the stage shifts, the model allows the prognosis, with respect to cancer death, of the detected cancers to be estimated. The ratio of the proportion of cancer deaths among the usual stage k cancers that are screen-detected to the proportion of cancer deaths among the usual stage k cancers is the measure of the death prognosis of the detected cancers. It is given by

$$\text{Prog}_k = \left((DC_k - DND_k) \, / \, (C_k - ND_k) \right) / (DC_k/C_k)$$

where ND_k is the number of stage k cancers in the intervention group that are not screen-detected. A value less than one indicates that the detected cancers would, in the absence of screening, have a better than average prognosis for stage k cancers.

Table 2   Results of fitting the stage-shift model:
Breast cancers shifted

		Shifts	
Stage[1]	Internal $\left(\tilde{T}_k\right)$[2]	External $\left(\tilde{T}_{k,k-1}\right)$	Total $\left(\tilde{T}_k + \tilde{T}_{k,k-1}\right)$
4	1	4	5
3	1	23	24
2	3	28	31
1	72	--	72
All	77	55	132

[1] Stage is stage at which cancer would have been diagnosed if there had been no screening.

[2] The tilde is used to denote the fitted value for an unobservable variable.

Table 3   Results of fitting the stage-shift model:
Breast cancer deaths prevented

		Shifts	
Stage	Internal $\left(IS\tilde{D}B_k\right)$	External $\left(ES\tilde{D}B_k\right)$	Total[1] $\left(TS\tilde{D}B_k\right)$
4	0	0-1	0-1
3	0-1	3-7	3-7
2	0-3	6-28	6-30
1	9-30	---	9-30
All[2]	9-34	9-34	43

[1] The total deaths prevented is not a simple sum of the internal and external deaths prevented in a stage, due to the interdependence of variables.

[2] The deaths prevented are not simple sums of the deaths prevented in individual stages due to interdependence.

Data from the HIP breast cancer screening trial (Shapiro, Venet, Strax, et al, 1988) were used with this model. It was assumed that the cancers found through year six of the study formed comparable case groups, and these were used to fit the model. There was essentially complete follow-up of these cases through year 18 from entry. The fitted values for stage shifts, deaths prevented, and prognosis are given in Tables 2, 3, and 4.

Table 4   Results of fitting the stage-shift model: Proportion of breast cancer deaths for shifted and control group cancers and measure of prognosis

Stage	$\dfrac{(DC_k-DND_k)}{(C_k-ND_k)}$	$\dfrac{DC_k}{C_k}$	$\widetilde{\text{Prog}}_k$
4	5/5 (1.000)	22/22 (1.000)	1.000
3	19/24 (0.792)	38/43 (0.884)	0.896
2	30/31 (0.968)	84/125 (0.672)	1.440
1	30/72 (0.417)	52/181 (0.287)	1.451

The results from fitting the stage-shift model assuming the six-year case groups are comparable suggest:

1. Screening advanced the time of diagnosis of the usual stage 3, 2, and 1 cancers; the former two were predominantly detected a stage lower than usual and the last at an earlier time in stage 1.
2. Screening detected the usual stage 2 and 1 cancers which had a poorer than usual death prognosis for their stage. If this is not entirely due to selection bias, it would be inconsistent with length biased sampling.
3. Screening prevented the majority of breast cancer deaths by earlier than usual detection and treatment of poorer prognosis stage 2 and 1 cancers.

5   PEAK   ANALYSIS

A standard model for the analysis of survival data arising from a randomized trial is proportional hazards (Cox, 1972). The advantage of a proportional hazards model is that the effect of an intervention on survival is summarized by a single quantity, and estimation of this quantity does not depend on nuisance parameters. A drawback to using a proportional hazards model to analyze mortality data from a screening trial is that the proportional hazards assumption is not likely to be valid throughout the entire follow-up period. A plausible alternative is that proportional hazards is valid only over some time interval when the constant of proportionality is smallest, that is, when the effect of the intervention is greatest. The rationale for this alternative in a screening trial is that there is generally some lag before the screening reduces mortality, if this happens at all. Further, if follow-up continues after screening ceases, then at some time after the last screen, the reduction in mortality must diminish.

Peak analysis is the name given to a method which estimates the minimum mortality hazard ratio from data of the aforementioned form. The word "peak" refers to the assumption of a time period during which the ratio of the hazard of cancer mortality in the screened group to that in the control group is smallest, which means that the effect of screening has peaked.

Other approaches to this problem which focus on significance tests based on weighted rank statistics are under development (Zucker and Lakatos, 1990; Self, 1990).

In the peak analysis approach, time since start of the study is divided into discrete intervals: $i = 1, 2, ..., I$. Let h_{si} and h_{ci} denote the hazard for cancer mortality at time i in the screened and control groups, respectively. The model assumes that the ratio of the hazard in the screened group to the hazard in the control group is constant over some interval $[j,k]$, as given by:

$$h_{si} = \begin{cases} \phi_i \, h_{ci}, & \text{for } i = 1, 2, ..., j\text{-}1, \\ \phi_{jk} \, h_{ci}, & \text{for } i = j, j\text{+}1, ..., k, \\ \phi_i \, h_{ci}, & \text{for } i = k\text{+}1, k\text{+}2, ..., I. \end{cases} \tag{1}$$

Furthermore, the model assumes that the constant hazard ratio in $[j,k]$ is smaller than the hazard ratio for any other interval, i.e.,

$$\phi_{jk} < \phi_i \quad \text{for } i = 1, 2, ..., j\text{-}1, k\text{+}1, k\text{+}2, ..., I. \tag{2}$$

For the screened and control groups, respectively, let x_{si} and x_{ci} denote the number of cancer deaths in interval i, and n_{si} and n_{ci} denote the number of individuals at risk of cancer death at the start of interval i. Also let $y_{si} = n_{si} - x_{si}$ and $y_{ci} = n_{ci} - x_{ci}$. Adopting a binomial model for grouped survival data (Cox and Oakes, 1984), we have $x_{si} \sim$ Binomial (h_{si}, n_{si}) and $x_{ci} \sim$ Binomial (h_{ci}, n_{ci}).

Let $\theta_{jk} = \{\phi_{jk}; h_{cm}, m = j, ... , k; \phi_i \text{ and } h_{ci}, i \notin [j,k]\}$. The likelihood is given by

$$L(\theta_{jk}) = \prod_{i \notin [j,k]} [\phi_i h_{ci}]^{x_{si}} [1 - \phi_i h_{ci}]^{y_{si}} h_{ci}^{x_{ci}} (1 - h_{ci})^{y_{ci}}$$

$$\cdot \prod_{i \in [j,k]} [\phi_{jk} h_{ci}]^{x_{si}} [1 - \phi_{jk} h_{ci}]^{y_{si}} h_{ci}^{x_{ci}} (1 - h_{ci})^{y_{ci}}.$$

For a given (j,k), the maximum likelihood estimates are

$$\hat{\phi}_i = \frac{x_{si}}{x_{ci}} \frac{n_{ci}}{n_{si}} \qquad \text{for } i \notin [j,k], \text{ and}$$

$$\hat{h}_{ci} = \frac{x_{ci}}{n_{ci}} \qquad \text{for } i \notin [j,k],$$

while in general, $\hat{\phi}_{jk}$ and $\hat{h}_{ci}$ for $i \in [j,k]$ must be determined by an iterative procedure.

However, under some additional assumptions, approximate closed-form estimates can be obtained for these parameters. The first assumption is that the probability of surviving death from cancer in interval $i \in [j,k]$ can be approximated by an estimate under a model in which the hazard ratio varies among intervals; i.e.,

$$(1 - \hat{h}_{ci}) \doteq y_{ci} / n_{ci} \quad \text{and} \quad (1 - \hat{\phi}_{jk}\hat{h}_{ci}) \doteq y_{si} / n_{si}.$$

Since these probabilities are close to one, regardless of the model, misspecification errors are likely to be small. The second assumption is that the death rate from competing risks is likely to be the same in both groups, and the death rate from the cancer under study is relatively small, so that one can write $n_{si} \doteq n_s \psi_i$ and $n_{ci} \doteq n_c \psi_i$, where ψ_i denotes the probability of surviving competing risks to time i, and n_s and n_c denote the numbers of individuals in the screened and control groups, respectively, at the start of the study. The approximate closed-form estimates are then

$$\hat{\phi}_{jk} = n_c \sum_{i=j}^{k} x_{si} \Big/ \left(n_s \sum_{i=j}^{k} x_{ci} \right), \text{ and}$$

$$\hat{h}_{ci} = (x_{si} + x_{ci}) \Big/ (\hat{\phi}_{jk} n_{si} + n_{ci}), \quad i \in [j,k].$$

Because (j,k) is not known, the data must be used to estimate (j,k), as well as θ. The value of (j,k) selected is the one which gives the best fit to the data. For each combination of j and k $(k \geq j)$, $L(\theta_{jk})$ is maximized; this yields $\hat{\phi}_i$ for $i = 1, 2, ..., j-1, k+1, ... I$ and $\hat{\phi}_{jk}$. To adjust for equation (2), one might conclude that a particular model (j,k) is inadmissible if $\hat{\phi}_{jk} > \hat{\phi}_i$ for $i = 1, 2, ... j-1, k+1, k+2, ..., I$. However, this is not advisable because $\hat{\phi}_i$ may be a poor estimate of ϕ_i, particularly when the number of deaths is small. This may occur when i is less than some value, say g, because of, for example, small numbers of deaths in the early years of a study. A more robust strategy is to identify the interval, call it v, having the minimum hazard ratio (i.e., $\hat{\phi}_v < \hat{\phi}_i$ for $i \neq v$) and select only j and k which include v. Nevertheless, because the variability of $\hat{\phi}_i$ may still be large for $i < g$, it might be necessary to restrict the search for $\hat{\phi}_v$ to $v \geq g$.

When all intervals [j,k] under consideration are nested, one could use the maximum of the log-likelihood to compare goodness of fit. Otherwise, one could use the Akaike information criterion (AIC) to compare goodness of fit. This equals minus twice the maximum of the log-likelihood plus twice the number of independent parameters (Akaike, 1973). The AIC for this model, denoted by AIC(j,k), is given by:

$$\text{AIC}(j,k) = -2 L(\hat{\theta}_{jk}) + 2 \{(j-1) + (I-k) + 1 + I\}.$$

The AIC is computed for each (j,k) which includes the minimum hazard ratio. The interval [j,k] which minimizes AIC(j,k) is selected, and the constant of proportionality, ϕ_{jk}, is estimated. The standard error of $\hat{\phi}_{jk}$ is computed using the bootstrap approach (Efron, 1982), where replicated samples are generated according to the following distributions: $x_{si} \sim$ Poisson(x_{si}) and $x_{ci} \sim$ Poisson(x_{ci}). If a lower or upper bound is known for either j or k, the standard error will be reduced.

REFERENCES

Akaike H. Information theory and an extension of the maximum likelihood principle. In: Petrov BN, P. Czaki P. (eds). 2nd International Symposium on Information Theory. Budapest: Akademiai Kiado, 1973, pp.267-81.

Albert A, Gertman PM, Louis T. Screening for the early detection of cancer. I. The temporal natural history of a progressive disease state. Math Biosci 1978; 40:1-59.

Baker SG. Innovations in screening: evaluating periodic screening without using data from a control group. In: Engstrom P, Anderson P, Mortenson L (eds). Advances in cancer control: innovations and research. New York: Alan R. Liss, 1989, pp.15-21.

Baker SG. A simple EM algorithm for capture-recapture data with categorical covariates. Biometrics 1990. To appear.

Baker SG, Chu KC. Evaluating screening for the early detection and treatment of cancer without using a randomized control group. J Am Stat Assn 1990; 410:321-327.

Blumenson LE. When is screening effective in reducing the death rate? Math Biosci 1976; 30:273-303.

Brookmeyer R, Day NE, Moss S. Case-control studies for estimation of the natural history of preclinical disease from screening data. Stat Med 1986; 5:127-138.

Connor RJ, Chu KC, Smart CR. Stage-shift cancer screening model. J Clin Epidemiol 1989; 42:1083-1095.

Cox DR. Regression models and life tables (with discussion). J R Stat Soc B 1972; 34:187-220.

Cox DR, Qakes D. Analysis of survival data. London: Chapman and Hall, 1984, p.103.

Day NE, Walter SD. Simplified models of screening for chronic disease: estimation procedures from mass screening programs. Biometrics 1984; 40:1-14.

Dempster AP, Laird NM, Rubin DB. Maximum likelihood from incomplete data via the EM algorithm. J Royal Stat Soc 1979; 39:1-38.

Efron B. The jackknife, the bootstrap, and other resampling plans. Philadelphia: Society for Industrial and Applied Mathematics, 1982.

Flehinger BJ, Kimmel M. The natural history of lung cancer in a periodically screened population. Biometrics 1987; 43:44-53.

Goldberg JD, Wittes JT. The estimation of false negatives in medical screening. Biometrics 1978; 34:77-86.

Louis TA, Albert A, Heghinian S. Screening for the early detection of cancer. III. Estimation of disease natural history. Math Biosci 1978; 40:111-144.

Morrison AS. Screening in chronic disease. New York: Oxford University Press, 1985.

Morrison AS, Brisson J, Khalid N. Breast cancer incidence and mortality in the Breast Cancer Detection Demonstration Project. J Natl Cancer Inst 1988; 80:1540-1547.

Prorok PC. The theory of periodic screening I: lead time and proportion detected. Adv Applied Prob 1976; 8:127-143.

Prorok PC. Evaluation of screening programs for the early detection of cancer. In: Cornell RG (ed). Statistical methods for cancer studies. New York: Marcel Dekker, 1984, pp.267-328.

Self S. An adaptive weighted long-rank test with application to cancer prevention and screening trials. 1990. Submitted.

Shapiro S, Venet W, Strax P, et al. The Health Insurance Plan project and its sequelae, 1963-1986. Baltimore: The Johns Hopkins University Press, 1988.

Shwartz M. A mathematical model used to analyze breast cancer screening strategies. Oper Res 1978; 26:937-955.

Walter SD, Day NE. Estimation of the duration of a pre-clinical disease state using screening data. Am J Epidemiol 1983; 118:865-886.

Walter SD, Stitt LW. Evaluating the survival of cancer cases detected by screening. Stat Med 1987; 6:885-900.

Zelen M, Feinleib M. On the theory of screening for chronic diseases. Biometrika 1969; 56:601-614.

Zucker DM, Lakatos E. Weighted linear rank statistics for comparing survival curves when there is a time lag in the effectiveness of treatment. 1990. Submitted.

43 Case-Control Studies of Screening

S.M. MOSS

Cancer Screening Evaluation Unit, Institute of Cancer Research Section of Epidemiology, 15 Cotswold Road, Sutton, Surrey SM2 5NG, U.K.

1 INTRODUCTION

Randomised controlled trials of screening are often difficult to conduct, both for ethical and for logistic reasons. In recent years, case-control studies have been used on a number of occasions to evaluate screening programmes where there is no control population available. The design of such studies and the selection of both cases and controls has been discussed in some detail (Morrison, 1982; Weiss, 1983). Sasco et al (1986) differentiate between two types of study according to whether the screening test is designed to detect early-stage cancer or a pre-cancerous state.

Cases should be subjects with the stage of disease which screening aims to prevent e.g. deaths or advanced stage disease for a test to detect early stage cancer, or invasive disease for a test to detect a pre-cancerous state. Controls should be selected from the general population, and not early stage disease, since the latter are more likely to have experience of screening, or indeed to have been diagnosed by screening. Most studies have recorded screening history in cases and controls up the date of diagnosis of the case, and have then compared the risk of a screened person dying (or developing invasive disease) with that of an unscreened person.

The three main potential sources of bias in the evaluation of cancer screening are lead-time bias, length bias and selection bias. Lead-time bias arises due to the fact that the date of diagnosis is automatically advanced for those cases detected by screening. Length bias is the tendency of screening to detect cancers which spend longer in the asymptomsatic state. Both these biasses can be avoided in case-control studies, as in prospective studies, by the correct study design. However, selection bias - the tendency for the non-acceptors of screening to be at higher or lower risk of developing and/or dying from this disease than the general population, cannot easily be excluded.

This paper reviews the evidence from case-control studies of screening, discusses possible design problems, and attempts to assess to what extent the results may be biassed.

2 BREAST CANCER SCREENING

The first published case-control studies of breast cancer screening were from Nijmegen

(Verbeek et al, 1984) and Utrecht (Collette et al, 1984) in the Netherlands. Both included deaths from breast cancer as cases, with age-matched controls drawn from the general population. The Nijmegen study found a relative risk of 0.48 (95% Confidence Interval 0.23 - 1.00) in ever screened women compared with never screened, while the Utrecht study found a relative risk of 0.30 (95% CI 0.13 - 0.70). The studies are compared in Table 1.

Table 1   Case-control studies of breast cancer screening.

	Nijmegen (Verbeek et al)	Utrecht (Collete et al)	Florence (Palli et al)
Age-range	35+	50 -69	40-70
Intake to screening	1975-76	1975-77	1970-81
Cases died in:	1975-81	1975-81	1977-84
% cases screened	57%	20%	49%
% controls screened	70%	43%	65%
Attendance at round 1	74%	72%	60%
Relative risk (ever vs never screened)	0.48	0.30	0.53
[95% C.I.]	[0.23-1.00]	[0.13-0.70]	[0.29-0.95]

There are two possible explanations for the difference in the findings. The first is the more restricted age range in the Utrecht study; only women aged 50-64 were included in the screening programme, and this is the age-group in which randomized trials mainly show a benefit of screening. The second is the way the cases were selected. The Nijmegen study included only deaths in women with breast cancer diagnosed after they had been invited to screening, whereas the Utrecht study included all deaths in women with breast cancer diagnosed after the introduction of the screening programme (de Waard et al, 1984). Since it took approximately two years to invite the whole population, this has the effect of reducing the percentage screened in both cases and controls, since the screening history of a control is counted only up to the time of diagnosis of the case. This approach therefore necessarily includes some cases diagnosed before receiving an invitation to screening who could not benefit from the programme, although these should in theory be counterbalanced by the inclusion of controls who did not have the opportunity of screening by the time of diagnosis of the case.

At first sight, the study by Palli et al (1986) from Florence looks similar to the Nijmegen one, and gives a correspondingly similar relative risk. However, there is again a difference in study design; the initial invitations to screening in Florence took place over a period from 1970 to 1981, but deaths are only included in the study for the period 1977-84. Since one expects a difference in mortality to become evident only after screening has been in progress for several years, the exclusion of some cases dying shortly after their date of entry would tend to increase the estimated benefit of screening. It can be argued that this gives a truer indication of the long-term effect of screening, but it means the relative risk is not directly comparable with those from the other studies.

This study did attempt to adjust for potential confounding factors such as marital status and level of education; this adjustment made only small differences to the overall relative risk, with most difference seen in the 40-49 age group. A subsequent paper (Palli et al, 1989) updated these results with the inclusion of breast cancer deaths for 1986-7; the overall adjusted relative risk was 0.53. This paper looked at risk for time intervals of <30 months and 30+ months between the last screen and date of diagnosis. However, since cancers detected by screening are included in the '<30 months' category, it is perhaps surprising that there is still an apparent beneficial effect of a previous screen 30 or more months previously compared with never screened, and this may again be a result of selection bias.

A case-control study carried out within the UK Trial of Early Detection of Breast Cancer (UK TEDBC, 1990) attempted to demonstrate to what extent the results of previous studies might have been affected by selection bias. Whilst not a randomized trial, the UK Trial of Early Detection of Breast Cancer included four separate "comparison" populations, from which the same data on breast cancer incidence and mortality was collected as in the four "intervention" districts (UK TEDBC, 1981). The first results on mortality from this trial showed a reduction in breast cancer mortality in the two districts offering annual screening of 14% relative to the comparison districts; this reduction increased to 20% when the breast cancer mortality in the different districts in the 10-year period before the start of the trial was taken into account (UK TEDBC, 1988).

Two separate case-control analyses were carried out. The first compared the risk of breast cancer death in women in one of the screening districts with that in one of the comparison districts. The cases consisted of all breast cancer deaths in cases diagnosed after entry to the trial in the two districts, with the controls drawn from the two populations combined. The second study had a similar design but was conducted solely in one of the screening districts and compared the risk of breast cancer death in screened and unscreened women.

As in many screening programmes, the analysis of the UK TEDBC is complicated by a two-year intake period into the screening districts, whilst all the subjects in the comparison district entered on 1st January 1980. This problem was solved in the case-control study by measuring time from each subject's date of entry, rather than as calendar time.

Table 2 shows the results of the two analyses, and compares them with the results of the cohort mortality analysis (UK TEDBC, 1988). The difference between the relative risk associated with the population offered screening, compared with that not offered it, as estimated by the case-control analysis and that resulting from the cohort analysis is due to the failure of the former to take account of the variable length of follow-up. Thus the comparison of the age-standardized mortality rates with no adjustment for period in trial,

Table 2   Relative risk of death from breast cancer from case-control studies A (comparison vs screening district) and B (ever vs never screened within screening district) and from cohort analysis of the same two districts of the UK TEDBC

	Case-control studies		Cohort studies
	A	B	
Comparison population	1.0 1.0		1.0
Population offered screening	0.76		0.79
Never screened	1.13	1.0	1.0
Ever screened	0.63	0.51	0.41

yields the same relative risk as the case-control approach. This bias could have been adjusted for by censoring all the data at the time of shortest follow-up, but this would have meant discarding data from the period when screening would be expected to have greatest effect. This problem would not arise in a study of a single population offered screening, unless there is reason to suppose that those with an early date of entry are more or less likely to accept screening.

It is clear from the results of this study that a comparison of screened and never screened women within the population offered screening gives a biassed estimate of the overall benefit of screening to the population. The equality of breast cancer incidence in non-attenders for screening with that in a control population has been used elsewhere as evidence against the existence of selection bias (Verbeek et al, 1984); likewise other studies have used risk factors associated with increased incidence to adjust for possible bias (Palli et al, 1986). An attempt in this study to adjust for factors influencing incidence between the two districts was unsuccessful due to the incompleteness of the data collected. However, since the incidence rate in the non-attenders in the screening district was similar to that in the comparison population as a whole, it appears that in this instance the bias results from the cases in women not attending for screening being those with a poor prognosis relative to those in a comparison population.

The increased scope for selection bias to occur as compliance decreases to 50% can be illustrated as follows. Suppose, with no effect of screening, 100 deaths occur in 100,000 women. If compliance were 80%, then to achieve an apparent relative risk of 0.25 in the acceptors would need 50 deaths in each group - a rate of 2.5 per 1000 in the non-acceptors. However, if compliance were only 50%, the same relative risk would be achieved with 20 deaths in the screened group and 80 in the non- screened - a rate of only 1.6 per 1000 in the non-acceptors.

This should lead to some caution in the interpretation of the results from the Nottingham case-control study of the effect of education in breast self-examination (Locker et al, 1989) The attendance at education sessions on BSE was 49% as a result of two rounds of invitations. The study shows an overall relative risk of 0.70 in women attending for education. However there is no difference between the survival of the whole case series and that of a series of historical controls. Further, just under half of the study populations formed one of the BSE districts in the UK Trial of Early Detection of Breast Cancer. The first results on mortality from this study showed a risk of breast cancer mortality in two BSE centres (Nottingham & Huddersfield) of 1.10 relative to the comparison centres, with no significant difference between the two BSE centres (Nottingham having the higher risk of the two) (UK TEDBC, 1988). As these results would suggest, the breast cancer mortality rate in the non-attenders in both districts was higher than in the comparison districts, indicating that selection bias had occurred.

It is of interest to note that the cohort analysis comparison of screened vs not screened gives a lower estimate of relative risk than the case-control analysis. The explanation for this is that women first attending for screening some time after entry contribute person-years both in the screened and not-screened groups; although their 'screening' person-years will be after the date of diagnosis for a number of the cases; this will tend to decrease the rate in the screened and increase that in the not-screened.

3 CERVICAL SCREENING

The case-control approach has been frequently used in the evaluation of cervical screening (Clarke et al, 1979; van der Graaf et al, 1988; Celentano et al, 1988; Aristazabel et al, 1984; La Vecchia et al, 1984; Raymond et al, 1984; Olesen, 1988), since screening has generally been introduced on a population-wide basis, and no randomized controlled trial has ever been conducted.

One problem with case-control studies of cervical screening, as discovered by Morrison (1982), is the handling of cases of invasive disease detected by screening. The exclusion of such cases would result in a deficit of screen-detected cases and hence overestimate the benefit of screening; their inclusion, however, may lead to an underestimate of benefit, since the effect of lead-time may lead to a surplus of such cases. The latter will be less of a problem where a screening programme has been in existence for some time.

A related problem is the difficulty in differentiating between 'symptomatic' and 'screening' smears. If smears taken because of symptoms are included, this will again lead to an underestimate of the benefit of screening since cases are more likely to have had such smears. Most studies have tried to identify and exclude smears taken because of symptoms; most have also addressed this problem by excluding, in both cases and controls, smears taken within 6 or 12 months of the date of diagnosis of the case, as suggested by Sasco et al (1986). However, none of the above studies appears to have matched screen-detected cases with controls screened at the same time, and this will bias the results in favour of screening, since for example a case of invasive disease diagnosed at a first screen will count as never screened, whereas a control screened only once a year previously will count as 'ever screened'.

Table 3 Case-control studies of cervical screening

	Toronto (Clarke)	Netherlands (van der Graaf)	Maryland (Celentano)	Cali (Aristazabel)	Milan (La Vecchia)	Geneva (Raymond)	Denmark (Olesen)
Screening introduced		1976		Late 1960's		1962-	1968
Cases diagnosed in:	1973-6	1979-85 (Aged <70)	1982-84	1977-81 + cases diagnosed 1971-76 under treatment/obsvn.	1981-3	1970-6	1983
Matching of controls	Age, neighbourhood, type of dwelling	Age, district	Age, race, neighbourhood	Age, neighbourhood	Age	Age, nationality, civil status	Age, area
% cases screened	32%	47%		4%	31%	18%	45%
% controls screened	56%	68%		31%	64%	38%	67%
Definition of screening history	'Screening' smears 12-72 months before diagnosis	'Preventive' smears 12+ months before diagnosis	Screened within 3 years	'Screening' smears 12-72 months before diagnosis	'Screening' smears	Negative smears 0-120 months before diagnosis	6+ months before diagnosis
Relative risk (ever vs never screened)	0.37	0.32	0.29	0.10	0.26	0.31	0.25

The first case-control study of cervical screening was published by Clarke and Anderson (1979), and the majority of subsequent studies have used a very similar design. Table 3 compares the study design and major findings of the various studies. (The study by La Vecchia et al (1984) also studied the effect of screening for cases of CIN. However, as has been pointed out (Parkin & Moss, 1984) this is not an appropriate analysis, and this part of the study is not included here). The relative risks for ever vs never screened range from 0.37- 0.25, with the exception of the study by Aristazabel et al (1984), which found a relative risk of 0.10 using neighbourhood controls, or even lower if clinic controls were used. It can be seen from Table 3 that the percentage of both cases and controls ever-screened is low compared with the other studies, and this is particularly true of the cases. This may be a reflection of the problem described above with the exclusion of smears taken within a year of diagnosis, if a substantial proportion of women had only one smear.

A distinction should be drawn between studies evaluating the benefit of screening, and studies looking at the benefit of a previous negative smear. The latter approach has been used to study the relative benefits of a previous smear at different times in the past (Macgregor et al, 1985; Geirsson et al, 1986), and hence to draw conclusions on the optimal frequency of screening (IARC Working Group, 1986).

The study by Raymond et al (Raymond et al, 1984) in fact only included previous negative smears in the screening history, and it is perhaps surprising that this did not result in a greater relative risk in the 'never screened'; however, this may be due to the relatively early time period (1970-6) during which the cases were collected.

The possible effect of selection bias on the results of the various studies is difficult to ascertain. It is generally believed that women at highest risk of developing cervical cancer are those least likely to attend for screening, and if this is the case then this would lead to the case-control approach over-estimating the benefit of screening, except in as much as the bias is due to age, or other factors which are controlled for. However, there are little hard data to support this supposition or to use to quantify the effect.

A number of the studies have attempted to adjust for confounding factors in the analysis, and in general this made little difference to the relative risk. Indeed in one study, the relative risk in the never screened increased after adjustment for age at first intercourse (van der Graaf et al, 1988). However, the factors determining attendance for rescreening are complex, and the existence of a bias cannot be discounted. The various difficulties described may account for the fact that mortality from cervical cancer and incidence of invasive disease have not fallen to the extent that might be predicted from the relative risks found and the percentage of the population screened (Macgregor et al, 1986).

Case-control studies looking at time intervals from a negative smear have largely taken selection bias into account to some extent by including only women with at least one Pap smear. However, the possibility that level of risk is associated with number of smears or time between smears cannot be ignored, and should be borne in mind when considering inferences on the natural history of the disease drawn from such data (Brookmeyer, et al, 1986)

4 SCREENING FOR OTHER SITES

A case-control study has showed no benefit of screening by biennial chest X-rays in preventing death from lung cancer (Ebeling & Nischan, 1987). In this study smoking did not appear to be correlated with participation in screening, and overall participation was high (75-80%).

A case-control study has also been conducted of screening for stomach cancer in Japan (Oshima et al, 1986). A notable feature of the results of this study is the different relative risks observed in males (0.59) and females (0.38), with only the latter being significantly different from unity. The authors have also attempted to discount symptomatic screens by excluding those within 12 months of diagnosis; this should bias the results in favour of screening, since some screen-detected cases will appear unscreened; however whilst the relative risk for males decreases that for females increases with this procedure. Little is known about the association of risk factors with participation in screening for stomach cancer.

5 SUMMARY

As screening for cancer of various sites becomes more widespread, the use of case-control studies in their evaluation is likely to increase. The various problems discussed above suggest the approach should be used with some caution, and the design of the study, and in particular the calculation of screening history, should be clearly stated in any publication.

It would appear dangerous to try to quantify the benefit of offering screening to a population from the results of such studies comparing acceptors and non-acceptors of screening. The approach may be more valuable in considering the effects of different screening intervals, but even then considerable care is needed to avoid bias in the results.

REFERENCES

Aristazabel N, Cuello C, Correa P et al. The impact on vaginal cytology on cervical cancer risk in Cali, Colombia. Int J Cancer, 1984; 34: 5-9.

Brookmeyer R, Day NE and Moss SM. Case-control studies for estimation of the natural history of preclinical disease from screening data. Stat. Med, 1986; 5: 127-138.

Clarke EA and Anderson TW. Does screening by "Pap" smears help prevent cervical cancer? A case-control study. Lancet,1979; ii: 1-4.

Celentano D, Klassen A, Weisman C et al. Cervical cancer screening practices among older women: results from the Maryland cervical cancer case-control study. J Clin

Epidemiol, 1988; 41: 531-541.

Collette HJA, Day NE, Rombach JJ et al. Evaluation of screening for breast cancer in a non-randomised study (the DOM Project) by means of a case-control study. Lancet, 1984; i: 1224-1225.

de Waard F, Collette HJA, Rombach JJ et al. The DOM project for the early detection of breast cancer, Utrecht, The Netherlands. J Chron Dis,1984; 37: 1-44.

Ebeling K and Nischan P. Screening for lung cancer: results from a case-control study. Int J Cancer, 1987; 40: 141-144.

Geirsson G, Kristiansdottir R, Sigurdsson K. et al. Cervical cancer screening in Iceland: a case-control study. In: Screening for Cancer (eds. Hakama M, Miller AB and Day NE). IARC Scientific Publications No. 76, Lyon, International Agency for Research on Cancer, 1986 pp 37-41.

IARC Working Group on Evaluation of Cervical Cancer Screening Programmes. Screening for squamous cervical cancer: duration of low risk after negative results of cervical cytology and its implication for screening policies. BMJ, 1986; 293: 659-664.

La Vecchia C, Decarli A, Gentile A et al. "Pap" smear and the risk of cervical neoplasia: quantitative estimates from a case-control study. Lancet, 1984; ii: 770-782.

Locker AP, Caseldine J, Mitchell AK et al. Results from a seven-year programme of breast self-examination in 89,010 women. Br J Cancer, 1986; 60: 401-405.

Macgregor JE, Moss SM, Parkin DM, et al. Case-control study of cervical cancer screening in North-East Scotland. BMJ, 1985; 290: 1543-1546.

Macgregor JE, Moss SM, Parkin DM et al. Cervical cancer screening in North-East Scotland. In: Screening for Cancer (eds. Hakama M, Miller AB and Day NE). IARC Scientific Publication, No. 76, Lyon, International Agency for Research on Cancer, 1986; pp 25-36.

Morrison AS. Case definition in case-control studies of the efficacy of screening. Am J Epidemiol, 1982; 115: 6-8.

Olesen F. A case-control study of cervical cytology before diagnosis of cervical cancer in Denmark. Int J Epidemiol, 1988; 17: 501-508.

Oshima A, Hirata N, Ubukata T et al. Evaluation of a mass screening program for stomach cancer with a case-control study design. Int J Cancer, 1986; 38: 829-833.

Palli D, Rosselli del Turco M, Buiatti E et al. A case-control study of the efficacy of a non-randomised breast cancer screening program in Florence (Italy). Int J Cancer, 1986; 38: 501-504.

Palli D, Rosselli del Turco M, Buiatti E et al. Time interval since last test in a breast cancer screening programme: a case-control study in Italy. J Epid and Comm Health, 1989; 43: 241-248.

Parkin DM and Moss SM. Papanicolaou smears and risk of cervical neoplasia. Lancet, 1984; ii: 1099.

Raymond L, Obradovic M and Riotton G. A case control study to estimate the detection of cancer of the cervix uteri by cytology. Rev. Epidem et Sante, 1984; 32: 10-15.

Sasco AJ, Day NE and Walter SD. Case-control studies for the evaluation of screening. J Chron Dis, 1986; 39: 399-405.

UK Trial of Early Detection of Breast Cancer Group. Trial of Early Detection of Breast Cancer: description of method. Br J Cancer, 1981; 44: 618-627.

UK Trial of Early Detection of Breast Cancer Group. First results of mortality reduction in the UK Trial of Early Detection of Breast Cancer. Lancet, 1988; ii: 411-4

UK Trial of Early Detection of Breast Cancer Group. A case-control evaluation of the effect of breast cancer screening in the UK Trial of Early Detection of Breast Cancer In preparation, 1990.

van der Graaf Y, Zielhuis G, Peer P et al. The effectiveness of cervical screening: a population-based case-control study.   J Clin Epidemiol, 1988; 41: 21-26.

Verbeek ALM, Hendricks JHCL, Holland R et al. Reduction in breast cancer mortality through mass screening with modern mammography. (First results of the Nijmegen Project 1975-81). Lancet, 1984; i: 1222-1224.

Weiss NS. Control definition in case-control studies of the efficacy of screening and diagnostic testing. Am J Epidemiol, 1983; 118:457-460.

44 Summary of Discussion on New Approaches to the Evaluation of Screening

It was emphasised that it was only appropriate to use intermediate outcomes to assess the effectiveness of screening when previous data provided evidence on the determinants of the ultimate outcome, reduction in mortality or incidence, as appropriate to the screening process. This was only so for breast cancer, and perhaps specifically in the Swedish two-county trial, where the effect of screening is completely explained by three prognostic factors, tumour size, nodal status and tumour grade. For a situation where this had not been demonstrated to be so it was still necessary to use the ultimate outcome measure, mortality, in evaluation of effectiveness. In relation to screening for lung cancer, for example, application of the approach would have been deceptive. The reason is that although lung cancer screening resulted in the diagnosis of "early" cancers, these were largely "benign", a form of over-diagnosis, with no reduction in the amount of advanced disease. The advantage of the approach when used when the process leading to reduction in mortality is known and understood, is the improvement in power over mortality as the endpoint as well as more rapid determination of outcome. In addition providing the determinants of effect are precisely known, it can provide quantitative estimates of the degree of effect.

It is important to avoid confusing process and outcome measures under circumstances when the effect of screening on reduction in mortality or incidence was not precisely known, such as in screening for breast cancer in women under the age of 50. Such measures, appropriate as intermediate outcome measures in women over the age of 50 were necessary but not sufficient as surrogates for the definitive mortality outcome in the younger age group. However, the results of large randomized trials should be used to help understand the process, which was a continuum over time resulting eventually in the definitive outcome. Further, difficulties could arise over situations where the overall effect was influenced by non-responders. Clearly, extrapolation under these circumstances would be less secure, unless the proportion of non-responders and their incidence and mortality was duplicated in the new situation. Further, although this approach may enable one to act on the assumption that mortality reduction would follow in a circumstance where it was appropriate to expect mortality reduction to follow, it was still necessary to validate the model assumptions eventually by confirming that mortality reduction of the order anticipated did indeed follow. Such a validation of the approach will be facilitated if investigators with data from randomized trials attempted to validate the approach on their own data.

Although validation is the ideal to aim for, it was pointed out that there could be a practical problem as it might have been considered unethical to have waited for the mortality reduction before acting, while if your investigation had been planned to capitalise on the power advantage the new approach provided, there might never be sufficient power to detect an eventual mortality difference. Thus you would have to fall back on the overriding requirement to monitor screening policies put in place in the population to verify that eventually the anticipated benefits did in fact occur, if it was decided to use the trial with intermediate outcome events to guide decisions on introduction of screening in the population. It was also noted that the approach depended on ensuring that some of the measures used had minimal error, such as the grading of breast cancer malignancy by one pathologist, which could not be duplicated when applied to the evaluation of a programme with many pathologists involved. Thus for complete evaluation, it will be necessary to search for new markers of outcome that could be measured precisely and could replace more subjectively measured parameters. There is also a potential problem with simpler measures such as the size of the tumour, which in the UICC TNM classification depends on the size of just the invasive component, as used in the Swedish WE trial, while in routine practice in North America, and therefore in the Canadian NBSS, precise measurement of size of such components was often not available. Indeed some macroscopic measures of size that were recorded were often misleading, as they included fibrosis associated in some instances with a large intraductal component. Thus, even for this measure in trials, the recorded size measure may not be comparable.

Caution was advised over drawing inferences from the first screen, as the extent to which prevalence was a multiple of the expected annual incidence was dependent on the degree of over-diagnosis in that setting. Further, although for breast cancer screening using mammography a prevalence to expected annual incidence ratio of 3 can be anticipated, there may not be as high a prevalence: expected incidence ratio for cancers other than breast cancer. Only when it was possible to compare the interval cancers after the first screen as a fraction of the expected incidence would it be possible to conclude that the screen had adequate sensitivity.

When more than one screening test is used detecting different segments of detectable cancer (as for mammography and physical examination for breast cancer, or possibly multiple tumour markers for ovarian cancer) sensitivity is improved but at a cost of reduced specificity, or with a different cut off between positive and negative, specificity can be improved at a cost of reduced sensitivity. If increased sensitivity is the aim, it needs to be shown if the increased sensitivity affects proportionate incidence. If not, the increased sensitivity was obtained only at a cost of over-diagnosis. [Note that some over-diagnosis could still have occurred even if proportionate incidence was reduced to a degree. It is not clear that there is a direct relationship between classical measures of sensitivity and proportionate incidence, except under circumstances where the lead time distribution is accurately computed.]

Concerning the use of models, there was a danger that if too many parameters were assumed, you could infer a spurious effect, and that these would then be published, whereas less conservative approaches, with no effect inferred, would not be published. There was also concern over the Peak Analysis Model, in that its use might enable investigators to select an approach to analysis which maximized the effect, after looking at the data. Therefore the use of such an approach, to be valid, should have been specified in advance in the protocol of the study, based on previous research. However, if an effect had been demonstrated using more conventional approaches, the model might be used for estimation, rather than significance testing.

It is clear that models already developed or under consideration may enhance our understanding of the natural history of screen detected lesions and the process of screening. However, they require validation with the best available data, which is preferably derived from randomized trials, before they could be extrapolated in ways that might guide policy decisions. It was noted that the models so far developed for evaluation of screening for breast cancer have largely been validated on data from the HIP study. It was important that they be validated on other data sets from other trials. As such data become available assumption-based models need to be modified to incorporate this extra information, in order to improve the extrapolations needed to make policy decisions.

Concerning the selection bias demonstrated in case control studies of screening for breast cancer, there was a possibility that it could be controlled for if data on risk factors for prognosis of breast cancer were available. There were, however, two difficulties with this. The first was that insufficient knowledge exists on the factors that determine prognosis, and second, data on these factors were not likely to be derivable in a case-control study, especially if the cases are deaths from the disease. There could be a temptation to attempt to control for differences in cancer treatment. However, to control for such differences might introduce bias, as treatment would be influenced by stage and this was influenced by screening. A further caution relates to risk factors for incidence. If such factors were unrelated to prognosis, to adjust for them might introduce bias. Some factors related to prognosis are behavioural. Compliance with invitations to attend screening is clearly related to attitude to health care in general. Such factors could also be related to outcome.

It was asked whether a comparison had been made between the effect estimated in case-control studies of screening for cancer of the cervix and cohort or time-trend studies from the same region. This was evaluated in Aberdeen, and it was noted that the reduction of disease in the population was not as great as that anticipated from the case control studies. However, in part, at least, this must be due to the dilution of effect by the non-responders in the population, and was not necessarily an indication of bias. For other cancers, caution is appropriate in using the case-control approach, as in any observational study. The design does, however, have application in considering questions such as frequency of rescreening. However, it is important that the findings of all case-control studies should be interpreted with care before they can be extrapolated in ways that could guide policy decisions.

It was suggested that for cancer of the cervix detection of stage 1a could be regarded as a benefit of screening, and that some of the problems of case-control studies could be avoided if they were not counted as cases, the degree of protection being based on the stage 1 b or worse cases. Another difficulty lessened by such an approach could be the fact that it is often difficult to identify in records those cases diagnosed by screening, compared to those cases who have a smear because of symptoms. There is also a possibility that the degree of protection could vary according to the quality of cytology in different laboratories. This was evaluated in one case-control study and the degree of relative protection was found to be greater for tests done in the central laboratory than for tests done in other laboratories.

In some countries data relevant to ongoing screening programmes are kept in a way which makes them inaccessible for evaluating the effectiveness of the programme. This problem is caused by attitudes towards data privacy and the confidentiality of medical information. The restrictions caused by this inhibit research on the provision of optimal cost-efficient health services. It is clear that this deterrent to health service evaluation is not in the best interests of public health. Overly restrictive rules on the confidentiality of medical and other records and their linkage, where they can be shown to be inhibitory to such research, should be reconsidered.

It was noted that a case-control study does not provide evidence of the potential effect of screening in the population, unless special approaches are made to ensure that the results can be extrapolated to the population. This should be possible if there is evidence on the compliers, and the background mortality in the compliers and non-compliers. Data on a non-invited but comparable group is not sufficient. In an analysis of the screening programme for cancer of the cervix in Finland it was found that the compliers and non-compliers had the same distribution of the known risk factors. However, in a cohort analysis the relative risk for compliers vs non-compliers was 1.7.

These considerations suggest that it would be appropriate as a research objective to attempt to develop methods that would facilitate the estimation of the effect in the total population from case-control studies.

Index

Lightning Source UK Ltd.
Milton Keynes UK
UKOW02f0425111013

218896UK00007B/191/P